ALLE ZEIT WACH 1842

Mental Health in the Elderly

A Review of the Present State of Research

Edited by
H. Häfner, G. Moschel, N. Sartorius

With 37 Figures and 31 Tables

Springer-Verlag
Berlin Heidelberg New York Tokyo

Dr. Dr. Heinz Häfner

Professor of Psychiatry, University of Heidelberg
Director, Central Institute of Mental Health
P.O. Box 5970
D-6800 Mannheim/FRG

Dr. Günther Moschel

Chairman, Department of Medical Sociology
Central Institute of Mental Health
P.O. Box 5970
D-6800 Mannheim/FRG

Dr. Norman Sartorius

Director, Division of Mental Health
World Health Organization
CH-1211 Geneva 27/Switzerland

ISBN 3-540-16182-1 Springer-Verlag Berlin Heidelberg New York Tokyo
ISBN 0-387-16182-1 Springer-Verlag New York Heidelberg Berlin Tokyo

Library of Congress Cataloging in Publication Data
Main entry under title: Mental health in the elderly.
1. Geriatric psychiatry. 2. Aged–Mental health services. I. Häfner, H. (Heinz), 1926–. II. Sartorius, N. III. Moschel, G., 1932–. [DNLM: 1. Health Services for the Aged. 2. Mental Disorders–in old age. 3. Mental disorders–psychology. 4. Mental Health–in old age. WT 150 M5492]
RC451.4.A5M446 1986 362.2′0880565 85-32330

Typesetting: With a system of the Springer Produktions-Gesellschaft
Dataconversion: Brühlsche Universitätsdruckerei, Giessen;
Offsetprinting: Ruksaldruck, Berlin; Bookbinding: Lüderitz & Bauer, Berlin
2125/3020-543210

List of Contributors

Alavi, Professor Dr. Abass,
Division of Nuclear Medicine, Hospital of the University of Pennsylvania, 3400 Spruce Street/G 1, Philadelphia, PA 19104, USA

Bergmann, Professor Dr. Klaus,
Consultant Psychiatrist, The Bethlem Royal Hospital and the Maudsley Hospital, Denmark Hill, London SE5 8AZ, GB

Bickel, Dr. Horst,
Sonderforschungsbereich 116 an der Universität Heidelberg, im Zentralinstitut für Seelische Gesundheit, N 5, D-6800 Mannheim 1, FRG

Carlsson, Professor Dr. Arvid,
Farmakologiska Institutionen, Göteborg Universitet, P.O.Box 33031, S-400 33 Göteborg, Sweden

Cooper, Professor Dr. Brian,
Epidemiologische Psychiatrie, Zentralinstitut für Seelische Gesundheit, J 5, P.O. Box 5970, D-6800 Mannheim 1, FRG

Davies, Professor Dr. A. Michael,
Director, The School of Public Health and Community Medicine, P.O.Box 1172, Jerusalem 91010, Israel

Diekstra, Professor Dr. René F. W.,
Rijksuniversiteit te Leiden – Faculteit der sociale Wetenschappen, Klinische Psychologie, Hoolgracht 15, 2312 KM Leiden, Netherlands

Evans, Professor Dr. John G.,
Dept. of Geriatric Medicine Radcliff Infirmary Woodstock Rd., Oxford OX2, 6HE, UK

Frackowiak, Dr. Richard S. J.,
MRC Cyclotron Unit, Hammersmith Hospital, Ducane Road, London W12 OHS, GB

Godber, Dr. Colin
Consultant Psychogeriatrician, Psychogeriatric Unit Moorgreen Hospital, Southampton and South West Hampshire Health Authority, Botley Road, West End Southampton SO3 3JB, GB

Häfner, Prof. Dr. Dr. Heinz,
Director, Central Institute of Mental Health, P.O.Box 5970, D-6800 Mannheim, FRG

Hauser, Professor em. Dr. Philip M.,
Population Research Center, University of Chicago, 1126 East 59th Street, Chicago III., 60637, USA

Heiss, Professor Dr. W.-D.,
Max-Planck-Institut für Neurologische Forschung, Ostmerheimer Straße 200, D-5000 Köln 91 (Merheim), FRG

Henderson, Dr. A. Scott,
Director, National Health and Research Council, Social Psychiatry Research Unit, The Australian National University, Canberra, ACT 2600, Australia

Jones, Dr. R. G.,
The University of Nottingham Medical School, Department of Health Care of the Elderly, 'B' Floor, The Medical School, Queen's Medical Centre, Clifton Boulevard, Nottingham NG7 2UH, GB

Kanowski, Professor Dr. S.,
Freie Universität Berlin FU, Universitätsklinikum Charlottenburg (FB 3), Psychiatrische Klinik (WE 12), Leiter der Abt. Gerontopsychiatrie, Reichsstraße 15, D-1000 Berlin 19, FRG

Kohlmeyer, Professor Dr. Knut,
Leiter der Abt. Neuroradiologie und Röntgen, Zentralinstitut für Seelische Gesundheit, J 5, D-6800 Mannheim 1, FRG

Lehr, Professor Dr. Ursula,
Psychologisches Institut der Universität Bonn, Römerstraße 164, D-5300 Bonn 1, FRG

León, Professor Dr. Carlos,
Director WHO Collaborating Centre for Research and Training in Mental Health, University del Valle Mental Health Dept. Aptda Aero 1418, Cali, Columbia

Loew, Dr. Dieter M.,
Leitung Product Management, Pharmazeutisches Department, Sandoz AG., CH-4002 Basel, Switzerland

Mann, Dr. Anthony H.,
Senior Lecturer in Psychiatry, Royal Free Hospital School of Medicine, University of London, Pond Street, London NW3 2QG, GB

Macfadyen, Dr. David M.,
World Health Organization, Regional Office for Europe, 8, Scherfigsvej,
DK-2100 Copenhagen 0, Denmark

Mechanic, Professor Dr. David,
The State University of New Jersey Rutgers, Faculty of Arts and Sciences, Office of the Dean, 77 Hamilton Street, New Brunswick, New Jersey 08903, USA

Osuntokun, Professor Dr. B. O.
Provost and Medical Director, Aro Neuro-Psychiatric Hospital,
WHO Collaborating Centre for Research and Training in Mental Health,
P.M.B. 2002, Abeokuta, Ogun State, Nigeria

Radebold, Professor Dr. Hartmut,
Gesamthochschule Kassel, Interdisziplinäre Arbeitsgruppe für Angewandte Soziale Gerontologie, Postfach 101380, Mönchebergstraße 19,
D-3500 Kassel, FRG

Strömgren, Professor Dr. Erik,
Institute of Psychiatric Demography, Psychiatric Hospital,
DK-8240 Risskov, Denmark

Svanborg, Professor Dr. Alvar,
University of Göteborg, Dept. of Geriatric and Longterm Care Medicine,
Vasa Hospital, S-411 33 Göteborg, Sweden

Taylor, Dr. R. C.,
2 Lillybank Garden, University of Glasgow, GIZ Glasgow, UK

Veiel, Dr. Hans O. F.,
Zentralinstitut für Seelische Gesundheit, Postfach 5970, D-6800 Mannheim 1, FRG

Table of Contents

4 Biological and Medical Aspects of Aging and Age-Specific Brain Diseases

5 Assessment, Prevention, and Control of Mental Disorders in the Elderly: Biological, Psychological, and Environmental Influences: Prospects for Early Recognition and Intervention

1 Introduction

H. Häfner, G. Moschel, N. Sartorius

The size of the world's population aged over 65 was estimated at about 250 million in 1980; by the year 2025 it is expected to grow to about 760 million (see Hauser, this volume). This sharp increase in life expectancy at birth, in some countries amounting to almost 100% in only a hundred years, has resulted from better nutrition and improved living conditions, hygiene and medical care. Not only life expectancy at birth, but also further life expectancy in advanced age has shown a clear, though more moderate increase.

This increased life expectancy, together with a simultaneous fall in birth rates, has caused the mean age of the world population and, especially, the average age of the population of industrial nations to climb substantially in recent times, a development which will reach its peak only some decades from now.

For these demographic reasons alone, health care authorities will have to devote more attention to the health problems of the elderly. The main task of medical research is to develop improved methods of disease prevention and treatment. Yet, because the full benefits of such research are only realized after many years of work, researchers have already begun to respond to demographic pressures by focussing part of their efforts on the study of illnesses characteristic of old age.

In the last hundred years, medical research has understandably focussed its main interest on the health problems of younger generations. Its greatest achievements have been the development of effective methods for the prevention and treatment of acute, life-threatening diseases, in particular of infectious and communicable diseases. Morbidity and mortality among infants, children, and adults have been reduced on an impressive scale. In contrast, only modest progress has been made toward understanding the etiology of chronic diseases and disabilities and developing methods for their prevention.

By giving priority to the earlier stages of human life and to acute diseases, medicine itself has not only contributed to the increase in mean life expectancies, but also helped to extend substantially the life span and life expectancy of the physically and mentally handicapped. These developments account in part for the increased prevalence of chronic physical and mental illness in later life.

In this context, the World Health Organisation has spoken of a "rising pandemic of chronic ill health and disability". (World Health Organization 1981). Illnesses typical of old age, especially mental disorders in old age, occur with high frequency – epidemiological surveys conducted in developed countries indicate a mean prevalence of about 25% for the segment of the population aged over 65 – and in most cases also lead to disability and the need for care. In particular, progressive mental disorders of old age such as dementia place heavy psychological and financial burdens upon the patients themselves, their families and society as a whole. Moreover, in what has aptly been called an insidious epidemic of dementia (Henderson, 1983), the frequency of mental disorders associated with brain alterations, of which dementia is a prime example, increases sharply in very old age, amounting to 20% – 30% of those over 80 years of age (see Cooper and Beck-Dreßler, this volume).

Psychogeriatric research faces difficulties that make it unlikely for major breakthroughs in elucidating the causes of mental disorders in old age and in developing preventive measures against them to be achieved rapidly. The nexus of social, physical, and psychological factors giving rise to mental disorder is complex and the simultaneous presence in the elderly of several diseases, both mental and physical, is frequent. Moreover, the onset of mental illness in old age may be influenced by processes suffered earlier in life, and their course may in turn be subject to modification through numerous organic and environmental factors. Therefore, the relevant variables are often masked and difficult to detect. Psychogeriatric research requires multilevel approaches, the use of a variety of research methods, and the collaboration of many disciplines – psychiatry, neuropsychology, biochemistry and the social sciences among others – striving to realize common goals. However, despite their shared goals, the various disciplines involved in psychogeriatric research frequently apply strategies of which neighbouring disciplines are unaware.

Immediately before and after the turn of the century, psychiatry experienced a fruitful period of multimethodological research on the important group of psychogeriatric disorders comprised of processes of dementia. Belonging to this period is Alzheimer's discovery in 1907 of argyrophilic tangles and plaques in the nerve cells of patients suffering from forms of senile and presenile dementia associated with cortical atrophy. At that time, brain research relied on morphological and neurohistological techniques, while cognitive deficits and mental states were identified through methods derived from experimental psychology and descriptive psychopathology. The tools used determined the nature and scope of the discoveries, which up to the present moment, have retained their applicability to both the clinical field and the study of the complex questions facing brain research. In the decades to follow, however, researchers' interest in psychogeriatrics and the neuroscience of the aging brain waned.

It is only recently that the tide has turned. Thanks to new paradigms and technologies, psychogeriatrics in general and research on the aging brain in particular have developed into the most promising fields of both basic and clinical psychiatric research. It has also become evident that many research problems relating to mental health in old age can be identified only by overcoming the limitations of individual research methods when they are used singly, without taking into account other approaches or disciplines, and that multimethodological approaches are required in order to provide solutions to these problems. Furthermore, medicine as a whole has directed its attention not only toward increasing the productivity of the worker by preventing or curing diseases that jeopardize it, but also toward improving the quality of life and leisure through disease control and other preventive measures. This process of reorientation has encouraged the notion that quality of life should be an important objective of health care in old age.

The aim of this volume is to provide a broad overview of the most recent developments in the main fields of psychogeriatric research. Scientists of different professional backgrounds from 11 countries, all of whom have made important contributions to psychogeriatric research, were invited to report on current research in their own specialties. The reports were to focus on as yet unanswered questions and point out promising directions for psychogeriatric research in each specialty. It was hoped that the papers, based on a diversity of opinions and approaches, would identify a number of unsolved problems and convey a comprehensive picture of multidisciplinary psychogeriatric research. Ultimately, this may facilitate a better understanding of the relations among the various disciplines and indicate new heuristic approaches.

The volume commences with demographic and epidemiological topics dealing with the effects of aging, illness and impairment on the population as a whole. These reports are complemented by reviews of psychological and biographical studies on aging and the aged based on individual cases and small groups. Following this section are contributions dealing with factors that foster or detract from physical and mental functioning, well-being, and autonomy into advanced old age. The relations between the social problems of the elderly, such as poverty and social isolation, and indicators of physical and mental health, home referrals and mortality are examined next. Complementing the sociopsychological analysis of the role of life events, coping styles and social support is an analysis of the impact of behavioural and physical risk factors and physical ill health on mental health, well-being and mortality in old age.

A substantial part of the volume is dedicated to brain research, brain imaging techniques and findings on glucose, peptide and transmitter metabolism that have become possible through these new technologies. These promising research fields, combining both clinical and basic research, focus on the question of the pharmacological manipulability not only of disorders associated with aging such as Alzheimer's dementia and other disabling diseases, but also of the normal aging process itself.

Because of their special importance for epidemiological and clinical research in psychogeriatrics, the questions of how to evaluate measurement techniques designed for screening and for diagnostic assessment of psychopathology, in particular of the dimensions of cognitive impairment and emotional and behavioural changes, have been dealt with in a special contribution.

Service research, the last main topic, derives its *raison d'être* from a dual concern: the necessity of providing better care for the elderly suffering from mental illness and for others limited in their capacity for self-care and the necessity of assessing the efficiency and cost effectiveness of the care offered. Therefore, issuses concerning the assistance provided by self-help groups and professionals in the form of psychosocial support, instrumental help and nursing are also discussed. The volume closes with papers on the evaluation of domiciliary and residential care, especially as available to the mentally handicapped and demented elderly.

Although a wide range of topics have been covered, it was impossible to include in a single volume all aspects of such a vast subject as mental health in the elderly. The genetic, virological, immunological, and cultural aspects had to be left out. Each of these complex areas deserves an independent treatment not necessarily limited to the aged over 65, as in this volume.

Through this report on current research relating to mental health in the elderly, we do not hope merely to add yet another volume to the many others already available on this important subject. Rather, we have aimed at presenting a mosaic of topics, at once broad-ranging and systematic, from authors actively engaged in fruitful research in their special fields.

Acknowledgments. This volume includes most of the papers presented at the symposium "Research on Mental Health in the Elderly – Present State and Future Prospects" held in Mannheim on 24 – 26 September 1984. They are complemented by two additional contributions requested by the editors to round off the subject matter.

The Central Institute of Mental Health, WHO Collaborating Centre for Research and Training, together with the WHO Mental Health Division, organized the symposium with the support of the Minister of Research and Technology of the Federal Republic of Germany, to report on the present state of knowledge, unsolved problems and promising research approaches in this field. We thank the Minister of Research and Technology for the provision of ample funds to finance the symposium and subsidize the printing of this volume.

We are also thankful to A. Komulainen-Tremmel for her competent and reliable help in editing the volume and to Springer-Verlag for its ready acceptance and prompt publication of the manuscript.

Reference

Henderson AS (1983) The coming epidemic of dementia: Australian and New Zealand Journal of Psychiatry 17:117–127

World Health Organisation (1981) Social dimensions of mental health. Geneva, p. 23

2 Mental Health in the Elderly: Epidemiological Approach

2.1 Aging and Increasing Longevity of World Population

P. M. Hauser

The data are presented for the world as a whole and, in the aggregate, for the MDCs and the LDCs, respectively. This summary is based on a comprehensive paper by the author which also contains data for the 10 United Nations Regions of the MDCs and the 14 United Nations Regions of the LDCs. The paper was published by the Nihon University Population Research Institute in Tokyo (Hauser 1983).

After considering the statistics relating to population aging and to the extension of life, a brief summary is given of trends in mortality and morbidity – the latter being inferred from trends in causes of death.

Population Aging

In 1980, in the world as a whole, there were 4.37 billion persons, of whom 250 million were 65 years of age or older. According to United Nations' projections, by the end of this century the world population will total 6.11 billion and by 2025, 8.20 billion. In 2000 the number of persons 65 years of age and over will be 402.9 million, and by 2025, 760.7 million. With present trends, then, the number of older persons in the world will increase by 57.7% between 1980 and 2000, and will triple between 1980 and 2025 (Table 1).

Of the 4.37 billion persons in the world in 1980, 3.19 billion were in the LDCs (73.0% of the total). By reason of the more rapid increase of population in the LDCs than in the MDCs, they will constitute 79.2% of the world's population in 2000 and 83.2% in 2025. Between 1980 and the end of the century, it is projected that the world population will increase by 40% while the population in the LDCs will increase by 52.0% and that in the MDCs by only 7.6%. While it is projected that the world population will increase by 87.6% between 1980 and the year 2025, the projected figure for the population increase in the LDCs is 94.5% and that for the MDCs, only 16.9%. With present trends, then, the population in the LDCs may almost double between 1980 and 2025.

In 1980 the number of persons 65 years of age and older in the MDCs, at 130.9 million, was greater than that in the LDCs, at 124.7 million. The elderly in the LDCs, in 1980, made up 48.8% of the world's older people. With present trends, however, by the end of the century the number of elderly in the LDCs, at 236.9 million, will greatly exceed that in the MDCs, at 166.0 million. By 2000, the elderly in the LDCs will constitute 58.8% of all old people in the world. The acceleration in the aging of LDCs' populations will generate 530.4 million persons 65 and over by 2025. Older persons in the LDCs will then make up 69.7% of all the elderly in the world.

Table 1. Population aging and extension of life for world, more developed countries (MDCs), and less developed countries (LDCs), 1980–2025 [source: Hauser 1983 (data taken from United Nations Department of International Economic and Social Affairs 1981)]

Item	Year	World	MDCs	LDCs
Aging measurements				
Total population (billions)	1980	4.37	1.18	3.19
	2000	6.12	1.27	4.85
	2025	8.20	1.38	6.82
Population 65 and over (millions)	1980	255.5	130.9	124.7
	2000	402.9	166.0	236.9
	2025	760.7	230.3	530.4
% population 65 and over	1980	5.8	11.1	3.9
	2000	6.6	13.0	4.9
	2025	9.3	16.7	7.8
Median age	1980	22.6	31.7	19.9
	2000	26.1	35.8	24.1
	2025	30.8	38.2	29.5
Aged dependency ratio	1980	10.0	17.0	7.0
	2000	10.5	19.8	7.9
	2025	14.1	26.4	11.8
Aging index	1980	16.4	46.3	9.8
	2000	21.5	62.2	14.7
	2025	37.1	83.9	29.8
Extension of life				
Expectation of life at birth – both sexes (years)	1980	57.5	71.9	55.1
	2000	63.9	73.7	62.5
	2025	70.4	75.4	69.6
Expectation of life at birth – male (years)	1980	56.3	68.4	54.2
	2000	62.4	70.2	61.2
	2025	68.2	72.0	67.7
Expectation of life at birth – female (years)	1980	58.8	75.7	56.0
	2000	65.5	77.5	63.7
	2025	72.6	79.0	71.7
% persons 75 and over of persons 65 and over	1980	32.0	36.3	27.4
	2000	33.7	38.2	30.5
	2025	32.5	38.9	29.8

Succinctly summarizing the trend, the number of older persons in LDCs will considerably more than double between 1980 and the end of the century and will more than quadruple between 1980 and 2025. It may be anticipated that although population aging, as will be shown below, is much more advanced in the MDCs than in the LDCs, the sheer magnitude of older population being generated in the LDCs will increasingly become a matter of major social, economic, and political concern.

Whereas in 1980, persons 65 and over constituted 5.8% of the world population, by the year 2000 they will make up 6.6% and by the year 2025, 9.3% (Table 1).

In 1980 the median age of world population was 22.6 years. By 2000 the median age will have risen to 26.1 years and by 2025 to 30.8 years. The aged dependency ratio (the number of persons 65 and over per 100 persons 15 – 64 years of age taken to represent persons of working age) was 10.0. By 2000, the aged dependency ratio will have risen to 10.5 and by 2025, to 14.1. The aging index (the number of persons 65 and over per 100 persons under 15 years of age) was 16.4 in 1980 and is projected to rise to 21.5 by 2000 and to 37.1 by 2025.

These data for the world as a whole obscure the great differences between the populations in the MDCs and the LDCs. In 1980 the proportion of the population 65 and older in the MDCs, in the aggregate, was 11.1%, as contrasted with 3.9% in the LDCs. By the year 2000 it is projected that the proportion of persons 65 and older in the MDCs will be 13.0% and by 2025, 16.7%. In contrast, by 2000, the projected proportion of persons 65 and over in the LDCs is 4.9%, and by 2025, 7.8%. Thus, the proportion of older people, as defined, almost three times as great in the MDCs than in the LDCs in 1980, is likely to diminish to about twice as great by the year 2025. The decrease in the gap between the proportion of elderly in the MDCs and in the LDCs in the coming decades is attributable, of course, to the acceleration of the demographic transition in the less developed countries and the consequent changes in their age structure, paralleling those changes which occurred earlier in the MDCs.

In 1980 the median age of the population in the MDCs was 31.7 years. This was in contrast with the median age of 19.9 years in the LDCs. By 2000, it is projected that the median age of population in the MDCs will be 35.8 years, as contrasted with 24.1 years for the LDCs, and by 2025, 38.2 years, as against 29.5 years for the LDCs.

In 1980 the aged dependency ratio for the MDCs was 17.0, in contrast with 7.0 for the LDCs. By 2000 it is anticipated that the aged dependency ratio of the MDCs will have risen to 19.8, whereas that of the LDCs will still be relatively low at 7.9. By 2025 the projected respective aged dependency ratios are 26.4 and 11.8, respectively.

Finally, in respect of population aging, in 1980 in the MDCs there were 43.6 persons 65 years and older for each 100 persons under 15 years of age. In contrast, the aging index among the LDCs was 9.8. By the years 2000 and 2025, respectively, it is anticipated that the aging index of the MDCs will increase to 62.2 and 83.9, while that of the LDCs will increase to only 14.7 and 29.8.

The data make it clear that, because of the earlier impact of the demographic transition among the MDCs, their populations are considerably older than those in the LDCs. It is also evident that although population in both the MDCs and the LDCs will continue to age in the coming decades, the gaps between their indexes will continue to diminish. This will come about, because the mortality and fertility rates of the less developed regions will come down more rapidly than the comparable rates in the more developed countries, which, in some respects, may be reaching limits of decline. The relatively high levels of aging of the more developed countries' populations are generating increasing social, economic, and political problems. On the whole, the more developed countries are confronted with a number of difficulties attributable to the aging of their populations, including such problems as the maintenance of adequate income flow in old age and adequate provision for health and medical care, and problems in general requiring increased gerontological and geriatric attention. In the MDCs the need for older people to make serious adjustments in their social, economic, and political life is increasing; and societies as a whole face the necessity of making major adjustments in social, economic, and political policies and programs.

It may be observed that the LDCs, faced with very difficult problems of achieving economic development and higher levels of living for their populations, at least for the time being, are not seriously experiencing the problems of aging. However, the data make it clear that, in the coming century, present trends will produce problems of aging both for individuals and for societies in the LDCs paralleling those now observable in the MDCs.

Extension of Life

In 1980 in the world as a whole expectation of life at birth for both sexes combined was 57.5 years. By the end of the century it is anticipated that life expectation will rise to 63.9 years and by 2025 to 70.4 years. Considerable differences are to be found, of course, between expectation of life in the MDCs and in the LDCs. In 1980 expectation of life at birth in the MDCs was 71.9 years, as contrasted with 55.1 years in the LDCs. By 2000 it is anticipated that life expectation in the MDCs will have risen to 73.7 years, as compared with 62.5 years in the LDCs; and by 2025 expectation of life in the MDCs will have risen to 75.4 years, as compared with 69.6 years in the LDCs. Thus it is anticipated that the gap between life expectation in the MDCs and the LDCs, which was 16.8 years in 1980, will narrow to 11.2 years by the year 2000 and to 5.8 years by 2025.

The expectation of life at birth for females, as is well known, is considerably above that of males. In 1980, for the world as a whole, life expectation at birth for females was 58.8 years, as compared with 56.3 years for males. In the MDCs expectation of life for females was 75.7 years, as compared with 68.4 years for males. In contrast, expectation of life in the LDCs for females was only 56.0 years, as compared with only 54.2 years for males. By 2000 it is anticipated that expectation of life for females for the world as a whole will have risen to 65.5 years and by 2025, to 72.6 years. For males expectation of life by 2000 will have risen to 62.4 years and by 2025 to 68.2 years.

In the MDCs, by 2000, expectaton of life for females will be 77.5 years, as compared with 70.2 years for males; and by 2025 expectation of life for females will have reached 79.0 years, as compared with 72.0 years for males. In the LDCs the expectation of life at birth for females in 2000 will have risen to 63.7 years and in 2025, to 71.7 years. For males it is anticipated that the corresponding years of life will be 61.2 and 67.7 years, respectively.

For the world as a whole it is anticipated that the gap between female and male expected years of life will increase between 1980 and the successive periods 2000 and 2025, respectively. The increase in favor of females would be 21.1 years by the year 2000 and 24.4 years between 2000 and 2025. Among the MDCs the difference between female and male life expectancies will not change very much between 1980 and year 2000 and 2025, respectively. The differences between male and female life expectation of 7.3 years in 1980 would remain 7.3 years in 2000 and decline slightly to 7.0 years by 2025. These data suggest that life expectancies of both sexes in the MDCs will be reaching limits by the end of the first quarter of the next century. In contrast to this situation in the MDCs, it is anticipated that differences between the sexes in life expectancies in the LDCs will continue to increase for some time to come. The difference was 1.8 years in 1980 and is projected to rise to 2.5 years by 2000 and to 4.0 years by 2025. As was the experience among the MDCs, as mortality decreases in the LDCs, over time, the difference between female and male life expectancies will increase.

As the data indicate, it is projected that the differences in expectation of life between the MDCs and the LDCs for each sex will diminish over the coming decades. In 1980 the differences in male life expectation between the LDCs and MDCs was 14.2 years. By 2000 this difference will have decreased to 9.0 years and by 2025 to 4.3 years. Similarly among females, it is projected that the difference between MDCs and LDCs in life expectancies, at 19.7 years in 1980, will diminish to 13.8 years by 2000, and to 7.3 years by 2025. These changes, of course, are attributable to the more rapid decrease in mortality taking place among the LDCs than among the MDCs as mortality rates in the MDCs tend to reach limits.

Young-Old and Old-Old

An index with important social, economic, and political implications is that reporting the proportion of persons 65 years of age and older who are 75 years of age and older. A distinction has been made between the young-old and the old-old. The former includes persons 65 – 74 years of age; the latter, persons 75 years old or older (Neugarten 1974).

In 1980, for the world as a whole, the proportion of the old-old was 32.0%. This proportion is not anticipated to change much by 2000 and 2025 (Table 1). The world averages, of course, obscure differences between the MDCs and the LDCs. In the MDCs in 1980, 36.3% of those 65 and over were 75 years of age or older. It is anticipated that by 2000 this proportion will rise to 38.2% and, by 2025, to 38.9%. In contrast, the proportion of the old-old was 27.4% in the LDCs in 1980, and is anticipated to rise to 30.5% in 2000 and to remain at about the same level, at 29.8%, in 2025.

The proportion of the old-old may dramatically increase in the coming decades. This may be demonstrated by the projections for Japan. In Japan in 2025, projections indicate that persons 75 and older may reach 47.3% of persons 65 and older. As the old-old reach and exceed half of all persons 65 and over, problems of aging – social, economic, and political – are certain to call for basic personal and social changes of an unprecedented character.

Mortality and Morbidity

Because of space limitation, only the briefest outline of trends in mortality and morbidity is possible in this paper. The data on the aging of population and the extension of life are the products, as explained above, of the interaction of fertility and mortality trends over time. The organizers of this conference have asked me to summarize trends in mortality and morbidity. Mortality statistics by cause of death are compiled by the World Health Organization. Trends in morbidity, in the absence of adequate morbidity statistics, are inferred from cause of death data.

In MDCs, which were the first to experience the demographic transition, death rates declined considerably during the latter part of the nineteenth century and during this century. Decreases in mortality first occurred among infants and younger persons as a result of a combination of a number of factors – increased levels of living, public health measures, and advances in medicine. Initial decreases in death rates resulted from declines in contagious, infectious, and communicable diseases.

As the LDCs became subject to the demographic transition, they, similarly, experienced initial declines in the death rates of infants and younger persons and for the same reasons. Although death rates from infectious, contagious, and communicable diseases have fallen in the LDCs, these diseases are, in general, still at relatively high levels.

In the MDCs as the earlier major causes of death were reduced or eliminated, the degenerative diseases – heart and vascular disease, cancer, diabetes, etc. – became the major causes of death. These degenerative causes of death are now also diminishing as modern medicine achieves spectacular breakthroughs. It may be anticipated that the degenerative diseases will become increasingly important in the mortality of LDCs' populations.

In considering extension of life, it is important to distinguish between the "span of life" and the "expectation of life." The span of life is the biological limit of life. The expectation of life refers to the number of years actually lived or expected to be lived within the limits set by the span of life. The span of life at the present time is probably not much different from what it was two millennia ago. Continued research in biology, including genetics, holds the promise of increased life span for the human species. Currently, in the MDCs, expectation of life may be approaching the asymptote imposed by the present span of life; but new knowledge and practices which may increase the span of human life may set in motion additional increases in expectation of life.

Details in trends in mortality and morbidity are available in recent U.N. publications (Coale 1982; United Nations 1982).

References

Coale AJ (1982) A reassessment of world population trends. Popul Bull UN 14:1–16

Hauser PM (1983) Aging of population and labor force for world, more developed and less developed areas and their regions: Population aging 1970–2025; labor force aging 1970–2000. Nihon University, Population Research Institute, NUPRI Research Paper Series, No. 15, Tokyo, Japan, Oct 1983

Neugarten BL (1974) Age groups in American society and the rise of the young-old. Ann Am Acad 187–198, Sept., 1974

United Nations (1982) Levels and trends of mortality since 1950. Department of International Economic and Social Affairs, (A joint study by the United Nations and the World Health Organization), United Nations, New York

United Nations Department of International Economic and Social Affairs (1981) World population prospects as assessed in 1980. Population Studies, No. 78, New York

2.2 Epidemiological Data on the Health of the Elderly [1]

A. M. Davies

Epidemiological studies of the health of elderly populations are in their infancy and current knowledge is based on a collage of information obtained in diverse ways. Many of the data have been collected in order to assess the needs of the elderly for social support, with information on health status being based on responses to questionnaires. And while summaries of causes of death, of greater or lesser validity, are available for many countries, accurate morbidity data based on population samples are available from very few (WHO Technical Report Series, No 706 1984).

The paper reviews briefly the kinds of epidemiological information available, their limitations and the conceptual and methodological problems that arise, together with the new indicators and end points that might be used in future studies.

Mortality

Mortality in general, and of the elderly in particular, continues to fall in many industralized countries (WHO Technical Report Series, No 706 1984; Grundy 1984; Lopez and Hanada 1982; Siegel and Hoover 1982), as illustrated by Fig. 1, based on data from England and Wales (Grundy 1984). In many countries, the group aged 80 and over is the fastest growing and will double in size by the end of the century. In the more developed countries three-quarters of deaths in people over 65 are attributed to cardiovascular diseases and cancer, with ischaemic heart disease and malignant neoplasms contributing about a quarter each (Lopez and

1 Part of the material given in this review (in chapter 2.2) is taken from a lecture to the International Epidemiological Associations 10th Scientific Meeting in August 1984, subsequently published in the International Journal of Epidemiology (1985) 14:9–19.

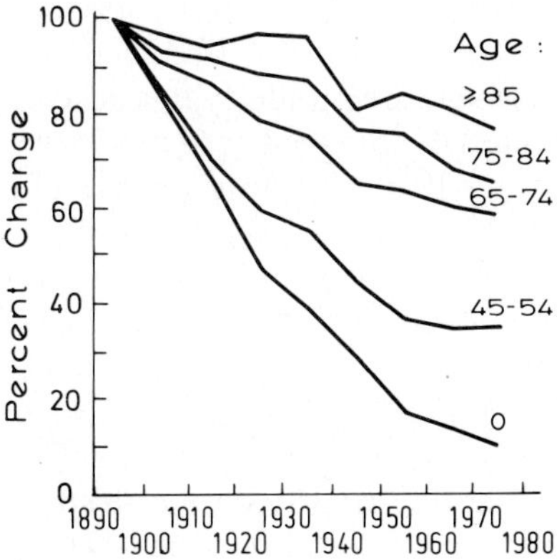

Fig. 1. Percentage fall in age-specific death rates (England and Wales, 1891–1980)

Table 1 Age specific death rates for ischaemic heart disease and stroke (direct and indirect causes). White males in the US, 1968–1977. Rates per 100 000 [8][a]

Cause of death	Age	1968	1977	1977:1968
Ischaemic heart disease	<65	162.8	123.1	0.76
	65 – 74	2465.1	1960.2	0.80
	75 – 84	5308.4	4410.9	0.83
	85 +	10525.8	8984.9	0.85
Stroke	< 65	32.3	22.4	0.69
	65 – 74	723.1	512.8	0.71
	75 – 84	2226.2	1664.9	0.75
	85 +	5001.5	3828.8	0.77

[a] After Manton (1982)

Hanada 1982). There is considerable variation, however, in the proportion of deaths ascribed to each specific cause in different countries.

Deaths from cardiovascular diseases have been falling in recent decades in some industrialized countries, e.g. Australia, Belgium, Finland and USA, although not in others, e.g. Sweden, and mortality from cerebrovascular diseases is declining, albeit at a different rate and with the exception of Eastern Europe (Lopez and Hanada 1982; Siegel and Hoover 1982; Havlick and Feinleib 1979; Garraway et al. 1979).

Manton (1982) has combined direct and underlying causes of death for a sample of U.S. death certificates for the years 1968 and 1977 as a way of estimating the total burden of defined diseases. His data for ischaemic heart disease and stroke for white males, shown in Table 1, illustrate the continued importance of these causes of death at the highest ages. The table also shows that the oldest groups shared equally in the fall in IHD and stroke mortality in the decade following 1968. Data for non-white males showed similar trends.

Mortality in the elderly from neoplastic diseases is on the increase in about half of the industrialized countries studies by Lopez and Hanada (1982) but is falling in the other half. When there is an increase it is mainly explained by breast cancer in women and lung cancer in men.

For those over 75, "senility" and ill-defined causes of death are recorded more frequently depending on local custom, while the rarity of autopsies in the very old makes reliable information sparse. A recent, careful analysis of 1000 French death certificates of persons over 65 shows that senility as a direct or underlying cause of death was recorded in 2% – 3% of certificates at ages 70 to 89 but rose to 25% at age 90 and over. The overall rate for those over 65 was 10.6% but was given as the leading cause in only 3.6%; in most cases it was possible to use ICD coding rules to classify the cause of death satisfactorily (Table 2). The most prevalent causes of death were diseases of the cardiovascular system (41% of men and 45% of women), neoplasms (28.6% and 17.5% respectively) with injuries and poisoning, diseases of the digestive system and ill-defined signs and symptoms each acounting for 5.3% ± 1.1% of male deaths and 7.2% ± 0.5% of female deaths.

This ability to classify the cases by main cause of death begs the whole question of the effect of coding rules on certification practice and on reported statistics in

Table 2. Main causes of death as recorded in 1000 certificates of persons aged 65 and over, France, 1983 (percentages)

ICD coding	Women (n=518)	Men (n=482)
Circulatory system	45.0	40.9
Neoplasms	17.5	28.6
Injury and poisoning	7.7	4.2
Digestive system	7.3	6.4
Symptoms, signs, ill defined	6.7	5.6
Respiratory system	5.8	6.0

[a] Unpublished data from WHO "Study of the term senility or equivalent terms on medical certificates of cause of death" DES/ICD/C/84.7, 1984

the face of multiple organ disease: other series have shown higher proportions of deaths ascribed to senility. In the Gothenburg study where cohorts of 70-year-olds are carefully examined and followed up, as many as a third of those dying are deemed to die of "old age", with considerable difficulty in ascribing death to failure of any single organ system (Svanborg et al. 1982).

Morbidity

Increasing survival brings increasing frailty and morbidity, mainly from chronic disease (Gruenberg 1977; Brody 1982). The elderly sick live longer and because of this, in developed countries, there are more cases of disease that are managed or controlled rather than cured (Rice and Feldman 1983).

The patterns of morbidity in the elderly have many facets and each of the sources of information currently available illuminates a different one.

All sources, self-reporting, health service statistics and health surveys, confirm that total morbidity increases with age and at any given age is greater for women than men. An attempt to summarize the available information, however, reveals many problems of definition, measurement and enumeration.

Accurate morbidity data based on population samples are available from only a handful of developed countries and even here comparisons are difficult due to lack of methodological standardization. Grimley Evans (1982) makes the point that "normal aging can neither be defined nor measured and there is an abundant literature on the confused and heterogeneous nature of conditions that society or professions find it convenient to call disease". Without agreement on definitions, let alone cut-off points, it is too much to expect comparative data on the prevalence of disease.

Symptoms in the elderly are often less clear-cut than in younger people and may not cause them to seek care or to receive it when they do. Many symptoms may be regarded by the elderly (and by their doctors too) as normal or expected in the old and thus not be investigated seriously. Others may interpret the decrements of aging as disease and overtreat (WHO Technical Report Series, No 706 1984; Svanborg et al. 1982). These factors are further affected by the cost, availability and accessibility of health services which affect utilization statistics more for this group than perhaps for any other.

The data available, however, to permit a number of generalizations and the various indicators of morbidity all increase with age. In one Scottish study, annual visits to the doctor rose from 4.4 at ages 65–74, to 7.0 at ages 75–84 and to 7.9 at age 85 and above (Bond and Carstairs 1982). The same trends have been observed in Manitoba, Canada (14) and in England and Wales (Owen 1977), among others. It should be noted, however, that 18% of those over 65 in Manitoba, 25% in the United States (Kovar 1982) and 36% in England and Wales did not see their doctor at all during the study year.

Admissions to short stay hospital increase even more steeply with age. In the United States in 1977–1979 there were 265 discharges per 1000 aged 65–69, rising to 430 at 75–79 and 499 at 85 and over (Kovar 1982). Days of care and average length of stay also increased in parallel. Israeli (Davies 1984), Canadian (Department of National Health and Welfare 1983) and Danish (Agner et al. 1982) series, among others, show the same trend. The most prevalent diagnoses in the US data were diseases of the circulatory system (one-quarter to one-third of all admissions of the elderly), followed by diseases of the digestive system, neoplasms, diseases of the respiratory system and accidents.

Not surprisingly, disease prevalence was quite different in general practice statistics. In England and Wales in 1970–71 the ranking was respiratory diseases, diseases of the circulatory system, symptoms and ill-defined conditions, diseases of the musculoskeletal system and diseases of the nervous system and sense organs (Owen 1977). The frequency was higher in women and higher at older ages; the ranking remained.

Morbidity patterns derived from surveys are again different and the number and frequency of conditions recorded vary from survey to survey, as do definitions and methods (WHO Technical Report Series, No 706 1984). Svanborg's study of a cohort of 70-year-olds in Gothenburg showed angina pectoris or probable myocardial ischaemia in 21% of men and 14% of women, hypertension in 23% and 48% respectively and chronic bronchitis in 18% and 9% (Svanborg et al. 1982). Forty-six per cent complained of dyspnoea, which was frequently combined with moderate hypertension and increased heart volume. This triad could well be physiological at this age but was taken as evidence of heart failure and treated as a disease. Moreover, 60% of those with electrocardiographic evidence of previous myocardial infarction had never experienced precordial pain or been aware of their condition.

If the findings of a specific cross-sectional survey, such as the US National Health Survey, are taken at face value, a model of morbidity from chronic diseases at each age may be constructed and compared with a curve of mortality (Fig. 2). The distance between the curves indicates the length of life with illness before death. On the basis of the 1980 mortality rates and the findings of the 1978 survey, half of American women born in 1980 may be expected to reach the age of 68 without significant chronic disease.

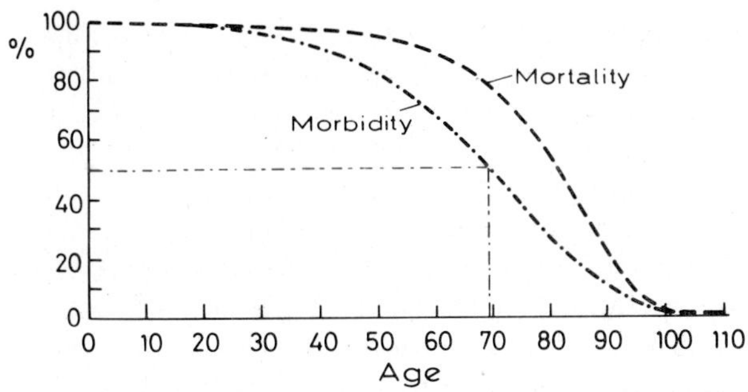

Fig. 2. Morbidity and mortality survival curves (United States, women, 1980 (After WHO 1984)

When the elderly are asked "In general how do you feel?" or "How do you rate your health?", most answer "well" or "very well" and "good" or "very good". In the WHO 11 countries' study, 78% of men aged 60–64 rated their health as good, and although this decreased with age, it was still 58% for the 85–89 group (Heikkinen et al. 1983). Responses of the same age – sex groups in different countries, however, showed considerable variation, suggesting a marked cultural effect on the response; those in East European countries rated their health relatively poorly.

None of these measures of morbidity give a reliable idea of the ability of an individual to cope in his daily life. A diagnosis of "bronchitis" or "heart failure" gives no indication of severity or the degree of incapacity produced by the disease. Moreover, different individuals react quite differently to the same disease of (as far as one can judge) the same severity. In addition, disorders of mobility, hearing, seeing and chewing, among others, are of special significance to the elderly but might not be perceived as morbidity. These impairments are common and their frequencies increase with age although, here too, there are wide differences in reported prevalences even with standardized questionnaires (WHO Technical Report Series, No 706 1984; Heikkinen et al. 1983). The results from one fairly representative study in Jerusalem (Davies and Fleishman 1981) are given in Table 3. These impairments are of particular importance as early detection and treatment can prevent much misery to the eldery person as well as preventing a chain of undesirable consequences.

Oral pathology is particularly frequent and neglected in all groups where examinations have been made. Of subjects in different centres of the WHO study,

Table 3. Percentage of elderly reporting disabilities. Baka, Jerusalem, 1979

Age	60 – 64	70–74	80+
Hearing	14	34	50
Seeing	44	54	69
Chewing	33	39	48
Walking	20	29	62
Talking	6	9	22

12% – 60% reported difficulty in chewing (Heikkinen et al. 1983). In Jerusalem the overall percentage was 39; nearly three-quarters of them had dentures, mostly ill fitting and often painful. Almost all were found to be in need of urgent oral care (Fleishman and Peles 1983).

Other distressing conditions that are prevalent but frequently neglected in the aging, include problems with feet and varicose veins, aches and pains in the joints and, of special significance, depression and deficiencies in control of the sphincters (Svanborg et al. 1982; Bond and Carstairs 1982; Owen 1977). Williamson gave the following estimates of *non*-reporting: urinary symptoms 30%, locomotor 31%, feet 70%, dementia 54% and depression 19% (Williamson 1981).

Impairments and Disabilities

Not all of those ill or impaired are disabled. In a British survey in 1971 over a third of those aged 75 and over showed impairments of one kind or another due to defined disease, but only 9.2% were handicapped (WHO Regional Office for Europe 1982), as shown in Table 4. In spite of the prevalence of such impairments the majority of elderly continue to lead independent lives. Even in the richest countries fewer than 8% are in long-term care facilities, including nursing homes.

For the elderly themselves and for their families, neighbours and the social services who may need to support them, a diagnosis of the presence of pathology,

Table 4. Impairment and disablement at age 75 and above (selected causes, United Kingdom 1971) [24]

Disease	Percent impaired	Percent severely disabled
Osteoarthrosis	10.6	2.7
Circulatory	5.1	1.0
Respiratory	2.1	0.3
Stroke	2.0	1.2
All conditions	35.4	9.2

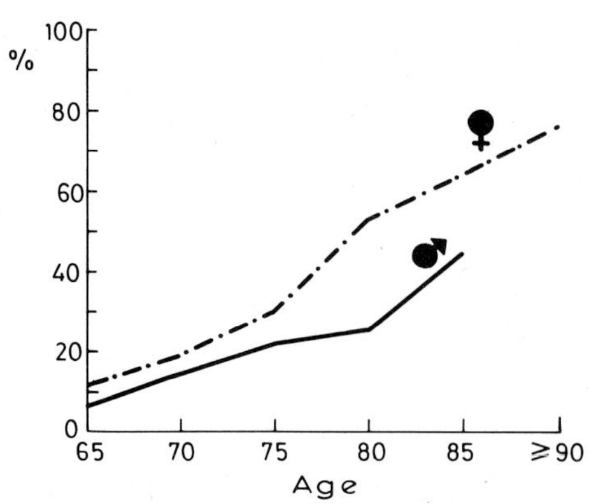

Fig. 3. Defined functional incapacity (per centage by age and sex, Scotland, 1982)

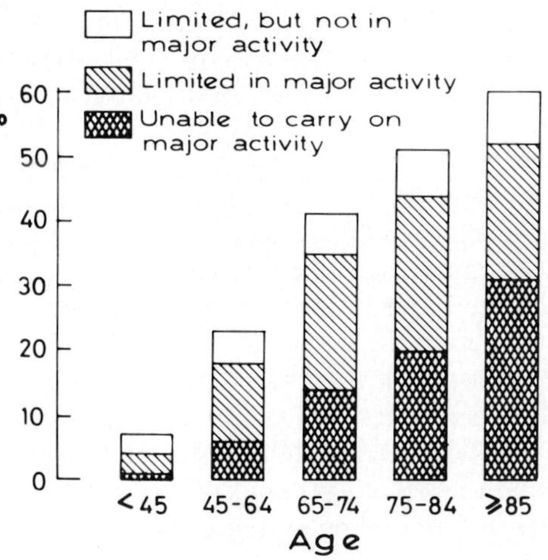

Fig. 4. Percent with limitation of activity due to chronic condition by age group and type of limitation (United States, 1978)

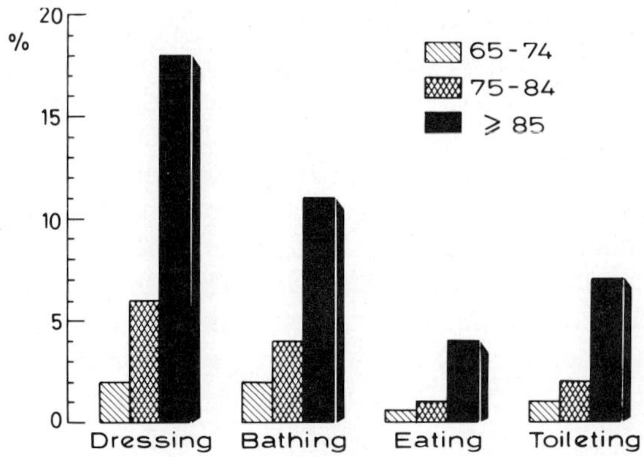

Fig. 5. Percent needing assistance in activities of daily living by age group (United States, 1978)

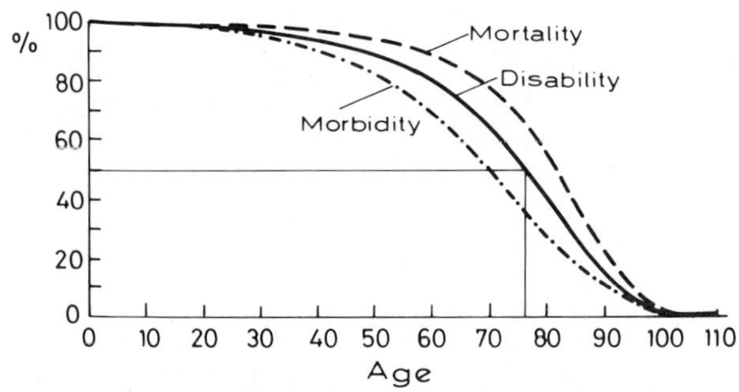

Fig. 6. Morbidity, disability and survival curves (United States, women, 1980)

unless curable, is of limited value. What is important is the ability to cope with daily life in spite of chronic morbidity and the degree to which the elder may need assistance to continue to do this even at decreased levels of activity. Such functional activity is widely measured by indices of activities of daily living (ADL). The most common index, developed and standardized by Katz and his colleagues (1963), includes the basic needs of mobility, bathing, dressing, using the toilet, eating and getting out of bed or chair. Functional incapacity increases with age, the rates being higher in women than in men (Fig. 3), but here too, there is considerable variation from place to place (Heikkinen et al. 1983). Figure 4, based on the US National Health Survey, shows the percentage of the population at different ages who needed assistance with specific activities of daily living, while Fig. 5 shows the need to quantify the degree of limitation. Using different measures of disability, curves can be drawn which will extend the model described above and indicate the time, in populations, from morbidity to the onset of disability and the durations of disability before death. Such a model is shown in Fig. 6.

Toward a Measurement of Health

Given these different measures, morbidity, subjective health, limitation of activity, use of services and index of ADL, do we have the beginnings of an index of health of the elderly? Not yet. A comparison of four measures in elderly men in a community survey in Jerusalem (Gofin 1982) shows the expected increase with age for each measure although each clearly measures something different (Fig. 7). Note the cross-over of the upper curves in the oldest group, the survivors being rated more healthy by the physician. The coefficient of agreement between doctors' appraisal and self-appraisal of health was only 22% and a similar poor correlation has been reported by others. The same general trends also obtained for women in this community (Gofin et al. 1981), with women considering

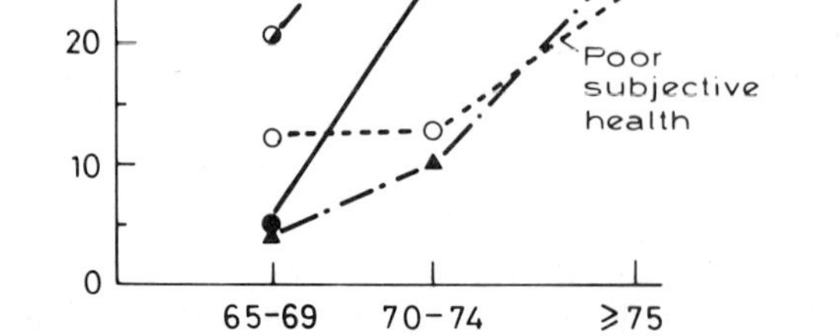

Fig. 7. Indices of subjective and objective health (217 males, Jerusalem, 1969–71)

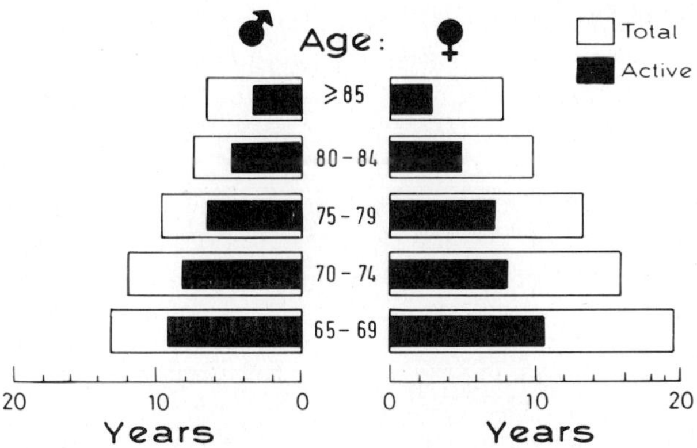

Fig. 8. Average expectation of life, total and active (Massachusetts, 1974) (After Katz et al. 1983)

themselves less well than men of the same age but having fewer problems with ADL. Ratings were thus affected by age and sex. Subjective appraisals were also affected by income and by social class: the poorer people were, the more pessimistic their view.

Self-appraisal of health proved to be a better predictor of mortality than doctor's appraisal in a large Canadian study (Mossey and Shapiro 1982). As a predictor of 5-year mortality in the Jerusalem study, doctor's appraisal of the presence of moderate or severe illness had a sensitivity of 44% and a specificity of 75% while self-appraised limited capacity or inability to work had a higher sensitivity of 64% but a lower specificity of 63% (Abramson et al. 1982).

Expectation of life at different ages is clearly of limited value without a measure of its quality: expectation of active life is a step nearer to the kind of measure that is needed for the planning of services and, for the time being, might serve as a proxy for the measurement of health status. Figure 8, based on data from Massachusetts, shows such an index (Katz et al. 1983). Men have a shorter life expectancy but a more independent one and similar indices based on a recent French survey show the same trends (Robine and Colvez 1984).

Autonomy

In the current state of knowledge we cannot prevent the majority of the diseases and impairments of old age, but if we are to make a start it will be necessary to study the epidemiology of these conditions and measure the risk factors. This will involve the epidemiology of the specific diseases prevalent in the elderly: osteoarthrosis, cardiovascular diseases, osteoporosis, senile dementia, senile cataract and the like. In addition, it will involve study of the aggravating factors which change disease to impairments and impairments to handicaps. The application of the epidemiological method requires a defined and measurable end point. I suggest that the end point we seek is loss of autonomy. If we agree that the purpose of health and social services is not only to prolong life but to maintain quality of life for as long as possible, then that quality requires a degree of

Table 5. Groups of elderly at risk of illness and breakdown

Age over 80
Recently discharged from hospital
Minimum income
Live alone
Childless
Socially isolated
Single/divorced/separated
Recently widowed
Recently moved
Social class v

Source: Owen (1977)

independence that we must be able to define. The amount of health care and social support needed to achieve some acceptable minimum quality of life in those handicapped to various degrees could then be computed and epidemiology fill its essential role in the planning and evaluation of services.

In a stimulating review earlier this year, Grimley Evans (1984) examines the implications of this approach. He suggests that autonomy "be operationalized primarily by measures of capability of achieving culturally appropriate objectives".

The variables involved are much broader than those usually considered in relation to pathological change and cover the whole range of human activity. It is already possible to define risk factors in the economic environment and social support (widowers living alone have a greatly increased chance of being admitted to hospital), the physical environment (accidents and poor housing), the degree of social support (depression in those left alone) and the attitudes of society (provision of services), to name but a few. Table 5 shows risk categories of the elderly found to be of practical value in a study in Scotland (Owen 1977). Some of the risk factors can be modified, others cannot but serve to alert people and services to avoidable outcomes.

Future Studies: Methodological Considertions

Current information on population groups, as has been pointed out, has been collected mainly as a guide to the planning of services or to their workings. The data are usually based on assessment of functional status of groups of individuals and, as Fillenbaum (1984) points out: "The number of multidimensional assessment measures specifically designed to assess functional status which are intended to be relevant to the total older population and which meet acceptable standards of validity and reliability (indeed in which there has been any concern to establish validity and reliability) is small."

The problems of assessment and of validation of questionnaires in studies of the elderly is well discussed in Fillenbaum's review and in the Kanes' excellent monograph (1981), which also covers the much neglected populations in receipt of long-term care. A short description of the approaches developed in Britain can be found in the introduction to the classical Clackmannan (Scotland) survey (Bond and Carstairs 1982). The methodological problems which so frequently prevent extrapolation of survey information are primarily those of epidemiological research, generally intensified when applied to older populations. A reliable introduction to survey methodology is given in the monograph of Abramson (1983); some of the special problems are highlighted below.

The Questions

A major source of confusion in the interpretation of existing data is the lack of clearly defined purpose of the particular survey and the translation of that purpose into clearly stated sub-objectives against which the validity of the questions and measurements is tested. The effects of education and culture on response to questions are well-known pitfalls in the interpretation of all social survey data. The phrasing of the question may be all-important. For instance, answers to "How do you rate your health in general?" will give a different distribution on a five-point scale from "Compared to others of your age, how do you rate your health?". Similarly, "Can you prepare your own meals?" is different from "Do you cook your own meals?". This problem becomes particularly acute in cross-national studies, when translated questions may have a slightly different meaning in a different language.

The Data Collectors

Different interviewers asking the same questions of the same subjects will obtain different results. The same is true of any measurement, biochemical or clinical, so that inter-observer variation is a fact of life and must be taken into consideration. Variations can be minimized by standardizing the question or the test as much as possible, by training the observers and by regular supervision. Relatively unskilled personnel, when trained, often perform more consistently than physicians or nurses! The extent of inter-observer variation and, indeed, intra-observer variation, should be measured and the investigator must decide the degree of rigidity which the study demands (WHO Technical Report Series, No 706 1984; Fillenbaum 1984; Abramson 1983).

The Population Studied

It is difficult to obtain complete information on total populations or representative samples of the elderly, particularly in the highest age groups, because of the difficulty of identifying the subjects and the variability of their response. Reliable information on the identity and residence of the elderly may not be available and the investigator may have to do his own census. Decisions as to sampling and the choice of appropriate methods require special expertise (Abramson 1983) and cannot be discussed here. The point to be stressed is that the population easily reached and responding to a study may well differ in many ways from that difficult to contact or refusing to collaborate.

In a survey in Jerusalem (Davies and Fleishman 1981) a complete questionnaire was administered to 77% of an elderly population and partial information could be obtained for a further 20%. There was a decrease with age in the population responding and a deficit particularly in the oldest group of women. Non-respondents tended to be sicker, more limited in their mobility and more likely to have been recently discharged from hospital. In the 11-country study (Heikkinen et al. 1983), the response rate ranged from 30% – 40% for the oldest groups in one area to 93% – 100% in others. In the former area, the results cannot be extrapolated to the whole population; for the latter, the response rate is so good as to raise questions about the sampling methods used. Completion rates of 75% – 85% for surveys of the elderly are considered to be satisfactory by some investigators (cf. Svanborg et al. 1982). The definition of satisfactory, however, will vary with the purpose of the survey (Abramson 1983). In a study of the prevalence of, say, senile dementia in a population over 65 with an expected prevalence of 6% of cases of moderate and marked severity, half or more of the cases could be included in the 15% – 25% of non-responders. The extent and significance of such a bias needs to be investigated for each condition studied in each population. It will be easier to miss cases of depression than fractures of the neck of the femur.

The length of the interviews is another important variable as old people can tire rapidly. Responses toward the end of the interview may be less consistent than those at the beginning and attempts should be made to keep examinations short. Place of testing is also critical, the response rate to an invitation to visit a clinic or hospital for an examination being lower, with selection bias towards the healthy and the worried.

Longitudinal Studies

For the near future there will be no alternative to epidemiological studies based on cross-sectional data and much valuable information is to be obtained by this approach. However, those alive at any particular time are survivors of earlier ages and much of the age difference observed in many variables may be due to selection mortality of those with different characteristics. Moreover, measures of physiological and behavioural changes with age may differ from generation to generation (WHO Technical Report Series, No 706 1984; Svanborg et al. 1982) so that the 80-year-old cohort of tomorrow may differ from that of today. Particularly for the study of antecedents and causes of disease and disability and for the measurement of risk factors, it will be necessary to study representative cohorts of populations and follow them up by periodic examination. This approach requires very long-term commitments by investigators and providers of funds. A combined approach which yields results more quickly, is that of Svanborg and his colleagues in Gothenburg, Sweden (Svanborg et al. 1982), who have undertaken cross-sectional studies of successive representative samples of 70-year-old populations with a continuing follow-up of cohorts recruited at 5-year intervals.

Conclusions

The epidemiological approach provides a powerful tool for the measurement of attributes of health of elderly populations, for basic research as well as for estimation of the need for services. Such studies, however, are time consuming and expensive. Although they seem deceptively simple, they are fraught with pitfalls and need the same scientific rigidity that is applied in other forms of investigation.

References

Abramson JH (1983) Survey methods in community medicine: an introduction to epidemiological and evaluation studies. Churchill, London

Abramson JH, Gofin R, Peritz E (1982) Risk markers for mortality among elderly men – a community health survey in Jerusalem. J Chronic Dis, 35:565–572

Agnes E, Damm P, Hansen PF, Schroll M (1982) Causes of hospitalization in different age intervals. Dan Med Bull 29:140–144

Bond J, Carstairs V (1982) Services for the elderly. Scottish Health and Service Studies No. 42. Scottish Home and Health Department, Edinburgh

Brody JA (1982) Life expectancy and the health of older persons. J Am Geriatr Soc 30:681–683

Davies AM (1984) Epidemiology and services for the elderly. In: Epidémiologie et médecine communautaire. Proceedings of the France-Israel symposium on epidemiology and health services, Paris, 12–15 Dec 1983, INSERM

Davies AM, Fleishman R (1981) Health status and the use of health services as reported by older residents of the Baka neighbourhood, Jerusalem. Isr J Med Sci 17:138–144

Department of National Health and Welfare, Ottawa (1983) Fact book on aging in Canada

Fillenbaum GG (1984) The wellbeing of the elderly: approaches to multidimensional assessment. Geneva, World Health Organization (Offprint Series No. 84)

Fleishman R, Peles D (1983) Indicators of oral health among the elderly. Brookdale Institute of Gerontology and Adult Human Development in Israel, Jerusalem. Discussion paper D 89

Garraway WM, Whisnant JP, Kurland LT, O'Fallon WM (1979) Changing pattern of cerebral infarction 1945–1974. Stroke 10:657–663

Gofin R (1982) The health status of elderly men: a community study. Public Health 96:345–354

Gofin J, Kark E, Mainemer N, Kark SL, Abramson JH, Hopp C, Epstein LM (1981) Prevalence of selected health characteristics of women and comparisons with men. A community health survey in Jerusalem. Isr J Med Sci 17:145–159

Grimley Evans J (1982) Review symposium. Interdisciplinary gerontology: success or failure? Ageing and Society 2:118–119

Grimley Evans J (1984) Prevention of age-associated loss of autonomy: epidemiological approaches. J Chronic Dis 37:353–363

Gruenberg EM (1977) The failures of success. Milbank Mem Fund Q 55:3–24

Grundy E (1984) Mortality and morbidity among the old. Br Med J 288:663–664

Havlick RJ, Feinleib M (cds) (1979) Proceedings of the conference on the decline in coronary heart disease mortality. US Department of Health, Education and Welfare, Public Health Service, NIH Publication No. 79–1610, Bethesda, MD

Heikkinen E, Waters WE, Brzezinski ZJ (1983) The elderly in eleven countries. A sociomedical survey. Copenhagen, WHO Regional Office for Europe (Public Health in Europe, No. 23)

Kane RA, Kane RL (1981) Assessing the elderly: a practical guide to measurement. Lexington Books, Lexington, Mass.

Katz S, Ford A, Moskowitz R, Jackson B, Jaffe M, Cleveland MA (1963) The index of ADL: a standardized measure of biological and psychosocial function. JAMA 185:914–919

Katz S, Branch LG, Branson MH, Papsidero JA, Beck JC, Greer DS (1983) Active life expectancy. N Engl J Med 309:1218–24

Kovar MG (1982) The public health impact of an increasing elderly population in the United States of America. World Health Stat Q 35:246–258

Lopez AD, Hanada K (1982) Mortality patterns and trends among the elderly in developed countries. World Health Stat Q 35:203–224

Manton KG (1982) Changing concepts of morbidity and mortality in the elderly population. Milbank Mem Fund Q 60:183–244

Mossey JM, Shapiro E (1982) Self-rated health: a predictor of mortality among the elderly. Am J Public Health 72:800–808

Owen F (1977) Profiles of the elderly 4. Their health and the health services. Age Concern Publications, Mitcham, Surrey

Rice DP, Feldman JJ (1983) Living longer in the United States: Demographic changes and health needs of the elderly. Milbank Mem Fund Q 61:362–396

Robine JM, Colvez A (1984) Espérance de vie sans incapacité et ses composantes: de nouveaux indicateurs pour mesurer la santé et les besoins de la population. Population 1:27–46

Roos NP, Shapiro E, Roos LL (1984) Aging and the demand for health services: which aged and whose demand? Gerontologist 24:31–36

Siegel JS, Hoover SL (1982) Demographic aspects of the health of the elderly to the year 2000 and beyond. World Health Stat 35:133–202

Svanborg A, Bergström G, Mellström D (1982) Epidemiological studies on social and medical conditions of the elderly. Copenhagen, WHO Regional Office for Europe, 1982 (EURO Reports and Studies, No. 62)

WHO Regional Office for Europe (1982) Preventing disability in the elderly: report on a WHO Working Group Copenhagen (EURO Reports and Studies, No. 65)

WHO Technical Report Series, No. 706 (1984) Uses of epidemiology in the study of the elderly: report of a WHO scientific group

Williamson J (1981) The preventive approach. In: Kinnaird J, Brotherston J, Williamson J (eds) The provision of care for the elderly. Churchill Livingstone, Edinburgh London, p 131

2.3 Epidemiology of Mental Illness

A. S. Henderson

Behind the etiological and public health functions of epidemiology is the heuristic value it offers in leading to a style of thinking. For any professional working with the elderly, there is so much to be gained by thinking in terms of the denominator. So, whatever the clinical issue, it very frequently helps to ask oneself, "What is the true population out of which this particular problem has emerged?" In this paper I shall try to review the present state of knowledge about the two main mental disorders in older persons: depression and dementia. Because of their overwhelming importance, I shall focus only on these but this is no way denies the importance of the epidemiology of anxiety states, hypochondriasis, alcohol abuse, or personality disorder in this age-group. I shall then go on to identify the major tasks which lie ahead for an advancement of knowledge and for public health.

Depression

Over the years there have been a number of reports from community studies on depressive illness in the elderly (Henderson and Kay 1984), but here I want to focus on some recent developments. These point to two things: the value of standardized case-finding methods and the identification of risk factors. Using the Comprehensive Assessment and Referral Evaluation (CARE) instrument, Gurland et al. (1983) have recently reported prevalence rates for community samples in New York and London. For the class called Pervasive Depression, the rates were 13.0% and 12.4% respectively. Blazer and Williams (1980), using DSM – III criteria for major depression in Durham County, USA, found a rate of 3.7%. Weissman et al. (1985), using the Diagnostic Interview Schedule on a sample of 2,588 persons aged 65+ years in New Haven, reports a 6 month prevalence of 1.7% for major depression. Cooper and Schwarz (1981) in a study in Mannheim, used a modification of the Clinical Psychiatric Interview Schedule (CPIS). (Goldberg et al. 1970) and found a 2-week prevalence of depressive disorders of 7.1% in their sample of 312.

In Hobart, Tasmania, Kay and ourselves (Kay et al., 1985) have applied both DSM – III and the Gurland criteria to data obtained from interviewing a community sample of 274 persons aged 70+ years. We found rates of 16.1% for pervasive depression, not significantly different from New York or London; but using DSM – III criteria for major depression, we obtained a rate of 10.2%, which is much, much higher than the Weissman or Blazer findings. We do not know why this might be. It is unlikely to be due to a fault in our algorithm.

These and further reports of prevalence rates are of little value unless there are hypotheses to test, an issue to which we shall shortly return. One area which has seemed promising for etiological factors in depression is the level of social support available in a person's environment. This has become an area of great interest, though the methodology and interpretive problems are quite difficult (Henderson 1984).

In the Hobart study, which was deliberately only cross-sectional as a prelude to a prospective survey being designed, we examined the association between depression and certain social variables. These included social support as measured by the Interview Schedule for Social Interaction (ISSI) (Henderson et al. 1981). The main findings were: The elderly had fewer social relationships than younger adults, but were as or more content with those they did have. Elderly women had more affectional ties than elderly men. Having offspring in the same town increased the number of both close ties and more diffuse relationships, especially for men. Rates for both dementia and depression on DSM–III criteria and on other measures increased with age. Persons in the community with an established dementia declared themselves as having too little social interaction for their needs. Those with depression reported having markedly less social interaction than the mentally healthy elderly. These associations are known not to be due to confounding by sociodemographic variables (Henderson et al., 1986).

Prevalence of Dementia

We have recently examined 20 surveys of dementia conducted in Scandinavia, Northern Europe, Japan, and North America (Henderson and Kay 1984; Henderson 1985, 1986). These confirm the summary by Mortimer et al. (1981) that about 5% of persons aged 65+ years, but 20% of those aged 80+ years, have a moderate or severe dementia. Al least 80% of all cases are in the community rather than institutions. Preston (1984) has recently made a useful comment about the frequent assertion that prevalence rates are not readily comparable because of the wide variation in casefinding methods, diagnostic criteria, and the demography of the denominator. Using age-specific prevalence data from a recent survey in New Zealand (Campbell et al. 1983), Preston derived the following simple regression equation to relate age to the prevalence one should expect in other surveys, including those we ourselves reviewed. The fit was highly satisfactory: there was close agreement between the observed and the expected age-specific rate, calculated from the formula

$$P_e = \exp[0.1258\ (a - 42.1008)]$$

where Pe is the expected prevalence (%) and a is the lower level of a 5-year age range. This work suggests that the reliability with which cases of moderate or severe dementia are identified is much greater than has been inferred in recent reviews, including our own. This is an issue which will be confirmed or refuted when standardized case-finding procedures are used in several geographical regions.

Diagnosis of Dementia in Field Surveys

It is believed that about 60% of cases of dementia are of Alzheimer type (SDAT) and a further 20% have both SDAT and MID. Here, though, is a problem of great importance for epidemiological research: studies of risk factors or etiology are in serious methodological trouble if this dependent or outcome variable is a mixture of dementias. The importance of SDAT, both scientifically and for public health, greatly exceeds that of the other dementias. Yet SDAT is a neuropathological diagnosis which can be made during life only by inference. It can probably not be reliably diagnosed in community surveys, particularly where these are only cross-sectional. We do not yet know how seriously this problem may retard progress in knowledge about etiology. It could at worst obscure, through a dilution effect, the identification of risk factors or causal variables.

Incidence. Data on incidence are scarce, yet they are much more valuable for etiological studies. Relative or attributable risk can be calculated only from these, whereas prevalence data allow one to calculate the odds ratio (Schlesselman 1982). By far the best known incidence data come from the work of Hagnell and his colleagues (Hagnell et al. 1981, 1983), who have reported incidence rates in the same population over 25 years. The cumulative probability of developing a dementia of mild, moderate, or severe degree rises to about 0.45 by age 89. As many of you know, the reported drop in incidence over the 25 years has since been shown by them to hold both for SDAT and for MID.

The Tasks Ahead

It is of paramount importance that the research community pauses to give careful thought to what questions should now be asked in epidemiological studies. I have listed ten:

1. Are the currently available diagnostic criteria adequate for dementia, for SDAT, and for depressive disorders in the elderly, adequate for them to be studied in community samples?
2. Are there internationally used instruments for reliably obtaining the data for these criteria, or their successors?
3. Is there confusion about a typology of depressive disorders, particularly in the elderly, and does it matter?
4. What proportion of cases of dementia or depression are not so recognized by their general practitioner?
5. Assuming that satisfactory screening instruments were available, would they be used in primary care and in general hospitals or nursing homes?
6. Does case-recognition benefit the patient or the family?

Now to some basic scientific questions about dementia:

7. Can SDAT be reliably diagnosed in field studies? If it cannot, we then need to know how damaging that is to a search for risk factors. There may be no point in setting up large and expensive longitudinal studies if we are insecure about

the diagnostic homogeneity of the dependent variable. This is an issue I think worth discussing thoroughly.

8. What risk factors for SDAT can be identified, additional to the four we have already (age, having Down's syndrome, a family history, and head injury or boxing)? The new risk factors may be some attribute of the individual, or some exposure in earlier life. In this search, it will be important to bear in mind that recent findings point to there being at least two syndromes within SDAT (Selzer and Sherwin 1983; Rossor et al. 1984). This is important in our search for etiological clues.
9. Do all cases of mild dementia in the community progress? This question in turn calls for a satisfactory set of diagnostic criteria for mild dementia, and a suitably efficient instrument for its reliable detection.
10. What characterizes those who survive to extreme old age without developing an age-related dementia? (Gruenberg 1978).

Criteria. For the first three of these questions on criteria, it must be apparent that the psychiatric research community needs a common language and a common method for deciding, in particular, who has a dementia, and what its severity is. The priority is therefore that diagnostic criteria be established for dementia and, within that group, for SDAT. This will then provide a basis for an instrument which will reliably obtain at least the core information for a diagnosis and a grading of severity. In this task, WHO has already made a beginning, strongly supported by a specific recommendation from its Global Advisory Committee on Medical Research.

This initiative is none too soon. The available diagnostic criteria for dementia are inadequate. While ICD – 9 lacks the detailed specification necessary for it to be practiced with reliability for this diagnostic group, DSM – III is also regrettably deficient. For instance, the second criterion for DSM – III dementia is simply "Memory Impairment," without further specification. A third set of criteria, by Gurland et al. (1983), give different rates. They are also idiosyncratic and their validity uncertain. Criteria for mild dementia are even more of a problem. To our knowledge the best available are those of Hughes et al. (1982), who rightly emphasize their provisional nature. Criteria for diagnosing dementia of Alzheimer type are indeed set out in DSM – III but may be hard, or even impossible, to apply in epidemiological fieldwork. This has implications, as I said above. I must set aside the validity and utility of the various classifications of depression.

Instruments. There is already a wide choice of standardized instruments: The original GMS (Copeland et al. 1976), which has a community survey version and for which Copeland will shortly have a computer algorithm for making ICD – 9 type diagnoses. There is the CARE, used in the US – UK cross-national study and subsequently in New York. Then there is the Canberra version of the GMS, which has some CARE implants and demonstrated reliability (Henderson et al. 1983). Next is the psychogeriatric version of the CPIS, as used by Cooper and his colleagues here in Mannheim (Cooper and Schwarz 1981). Lastly, there is the DIS or its WHO version, the CIDI. But its only cognitive component is the Mini Mental State Examination (Folstein et al. 1975) which has been grafted on to the end of the instrument. I doubt if Folstein ever intended that the MMSE be used to make a diagnosis. From the MMSE score, one can make a statement about the *probability* that the respondent has cognitive impairment, or a dementia, or a delirium, but that is all. I have just heard that Wing has developed a new instrument, the SCAN, which contains a revision of the PSE and includes provision for assessment of cognitive function, with an algorithm for DSM–III criteria for dementia. I do not know about other instruments, such as those being used in the ECA surveys in the United States.

I think there is one problem with the instruments I have mentioned: for reliable and valid case-identification, particularly of mild dementia, self-reported information is unsuitable, or at best insufficient. Neuropsychological tests can offer much better coverage of relevant cognitive functions used in daily living; and they are more systematic. Yet to my knowledge, the interviews mentioned offer at best only a rather coarse approximation of a neuropsychological test, with no systematic sampling of diverse cognitive functions. Next, as the GMS and CARE instruments do provide for, there should be an interview with an informant.

For *screening instruments*, a great deal has to be done and, as Cooper and Bickel (1984) have justifiably asserted in their recent review, the probable cases so identified present a considerable problem in requiring costly further investigation, with no guarantee that it helps the individual or family. The choice of instruments is wide. We have been impressed with the performance of the MMSE in Hobart. It gave 85% sensitivity and 92% specificity against a criterion of DSM–III dementia defined by us as moderate or severe. For Gurland's pervasive depression, the values were 90% and 93%. However, it does very poorly in screening for mild dementia.

To conclude, I have indicated some of the recent findings in field surveys before listing the issues which are now being faced. Of these, the most pressing are, I personally believe, diagnostic criteria for dementia and particularly mild dementia; and the construction of a composite instrument, including neuropsychological tests and an informant's section, for field use in prospective longitudinal designs. Meanwhile, the search has already started for risk factors and clues to etiology. This need not wait for perfect instruments. Any contribution from epidemiology towards an understanding of dementia will be a worthwhile contribution to public health.

References

Blazer D, Williams CD (1980) Epidemiology of dysphoria and depression in an elderly population. Am J Psychiatry 137:439–444

Campbell AJ, McCosh LM, Reinken J, Allan BC (1983) Dementia in old age and the need for services. Age and Ageing 12:11–16

Cooper B, Bickel H (1984) Population screening and the elderly detection of dementing disorders in old age: A review. Psychol Med 14:81–95

Cooper B, Schwarz R (1981) Psychiatric case-identification in an elderly urban population. Social Psychiatry 17:43–52

Copeland JRM, Kelleher MJ, Kellett JM, Gourlay AJ, Gurland BJ, Fleiss JL, Sharpe L (1976) A semi-structured clinical interview for the assessment of diagnosis and mental state in the elderly: The Geriatric Mental State Schedule. I. Development and reliability. Psychol Med 6:439–449

Folstein MF, Folstein SE, McHugh PR (1975) 'Mini-mental state.' A practical method for grading the cognitive state of patients for the clinician. J Psychiatr Res 12:189–198

Goldberg DP, Cooper B, Eastwood MR, Kedward HB, Shepherd M (1970) A standardized psychiatric interview for use in community surveys. Br J Prev Soc Med 24:18–23

Gruenberg E (1978) Epidemiology. In: Katzman R, Terry RD, Bick KL (eds) Alzheimer's disease: senile dementia and related disorders, Raven, New York (Aging, vol 7)

Gurland B, Copeland J, Kuriansky J, Kelleher M, Sharpe L, Dean L (1983) The mind and mood of aging. Croom Helm, London

Hagnell O, Lanke J, Rorsman B, Öjesjö L (1981) Does the incidence of age psychosis decrease? A prospective longitudinal study of a complete population investigated during the 25-year period 1947–1972: The Lundby Study. Neuropsychobiology 7:201–211

Hagnell O, Lanke J, Rorsman B, Ohman R, Öjesjö L (1983) Current trends in the incidence of senile and multi-infarct dementia. Arch Psychiatr Neurol Sci 233:423–438

Henderson S, Byrne DG, Duncan-Jones P (1981) Neurosis and the social environment. Academic Press, Sydney

Henderson AS, Duncan-Jones P, Finlay-Jones RA (1983) The reliability of the Geriatric Mental State Examination. Acta Psychiatr Scand 67:281–289

Henderson AS, Kay DWK (1984) The epidemiology of mental disorders in the aged. In: Kay DWK, Burrows G (eds) Handbook of studies in psychiatry and old age. Elsevier, North-Holland, Amsterdam

Henderson AS (1984) Interpreting the evidence on social support. Soc Psychiatr 19:49–52

Henderson AS (1985) Developments in the epidemiology of senile dementia. In: Tansella M (ed) L'Approccio Epidemiologica in Psichiatria. Boringhieri, Torino

Henderson AS (1986) The epidemiology of Alzheimer's disease. Brit Med Bull 42:3–10

Henderson AS, Grayson DA, Scott R, Wilson J, Rickwood D and Kay DWK (1986) Social support, dementia and depression among the elderly living in the Hobart community. Psychol Med 16: in press

Hughes CP, Berg L, Danziger WL, Coben LA, Martin RL (1982) A new clinical scale for the staging of dementia. Br J Psychiatry 140:566–572

Kay DWK, Henderson AS, Scott LR, Wilson J, Rickwood DJ, Grayson D (1985) Dementia and depression among the elderly living in the Hobart community: the effect of the diagnostic criteria on the prevalence rates. Psychol Med 15:771–788

Mortimer JA, Schuman LM, French LR (1981) Epidemiology of dementing illness. In: Mortimer JA, Schuman LM (eds) The epidemiology of dementia. Oxford University Press, New York, pp 3–23

Preston GAN (1984) The prevalence of dementia: estimates and interpretations in Australia Research report, National Institute of Gerontology and Geriatric Medicine, Melbourne

Rossor MN, Iversen LL, Reynolds GP, Mountjoy CO, Roth M (1984) Early and late onset types of Alzheimer's disease are neurochemically distinct. Br Med J 288:961–4

Schlesselman JL (1982) Case-control studies: Design, conduct, analysis. Oxford University Press, New York

Selzer B, Sherwin I (1983) A comparison of clinical features in early- and late-onset primary degenerative dementia. Arch Neurol 40:143–146

Weissman MM, Myers JK, Tischler GL, Holzer CE, Leaf PJ, Orvaschel H, Brody JA (1985) Psychiatric disorders (DSM–III) and cognitive impairment among the elderly in a U.S. urban community. Acta Psychiatr Scand 71:366–379

2.4 Mental Illness, Disability and Social Conditions among Old People in Mannheim [1]

B. Cooper

Introduction

Both the absolute numbers of old people and their proportion in the general population have increased sharply in all developed industrial countries during the present century. In the Federal Republic of Germany and its predecessor, the German Reich, the proportion of persons aged over 65 years grew during the period 1880–1980 from 5.0% to 15.4%. Here, as in most European countries, one must reckon with a further proportionate rise, especially among the very old, over the next several decades (WHO 1979). These major demographic changes have given rise to a variety of economic, social and public health problems. Because mental illness is one of the most important causes of chronic disability and handicap in the elderly, the care of mentally impaired old people has become an increasingly urgent sociopolitical issue. In order to obtain the comprehensive, reliable morbidity data required for service planning, epidemiological research into the mental disorders of old age is called for.

This is a fairly new field of research and the available data are still scanty. Statistics from psychiatric hospitals or case registers are of only limited value here, since at any point in time the great majority, even of severely mentally impaired old people, in the population will not be in contact with psychiatric services (Kay and Bergmann 1980). Most of the immediately relevant data are derived from a handful of psychiatric field studies, which have focused on the age groups over 65 (cf. Table 1). Apart from providing estimates of the prevalence of different forms of mental disorder, these projects have also supplied such information as is available on their biological and social concomitants in the elderly population. Here again, it must be said that there is a paucity of firmly established knowledge on the subject. Grad de Alarcon (1971), in a succinct review, concluded that:

> ...the relationship between social processes and mental disorders remains an area rich in speculation, generalizations and hypotheses. No clear causal effects of social deprivation on mental illnesses have been found, and some social factors thought to be causal are more likely consequences of the illness.

The present report summarizes some findings of a field study carried out in the West German city of Mannheim which made use of a standardized psychiatric interview for purposes of case identification and clinical assessment; it also enquired systematically into the physical health status and social situation of the

---

1 This research project, which formed part of Special Research Programme 116 (Psychiatric Epidemiology), based at the University of Heidelberg, was supported financially by the German Research Association (Deutsche Forschungsgemeinschaft).

Table 1. Prevalence of mental disorder in the population aged over 65: estimates from field studies

Authors	Survey area	Persons (*n*)	Organic psychoses (%)	Milder organic syndromes (%)	Functional psychoses (%)	Neuroses and personality disorders (%)	Total[a] (%)
Sheldon (1948)	Wolverhampton, U.K. (urban)	369	3.9	11.7	–	12.6	28.2
Primrose (1962)	N. Scotland (rural)	222	4.5	–	1.4	12.6	–
Nielsen (1962)	Samsø Island (rural)	978	3.1	15.4	3.7	6.8	29.0
Kay et al. (1964)	Newcastle, U.K. (urban)	443	5.7	5.7	2.4	12.5	26.3
Parsons (1965)	Swansea, U.K. (urban)	228	4.4	–	2.6	4.8	–
Dilling et al. (1984)	Upper Bavaria, FRG (semirural)	295	——— 8.5 ———		3.4	10.2	23.1
Cooper and Sosna (1983)	Mannheim, FRG (urban)	519	6.0	5.4	2.2	10.8	24.4

[a] Totals given include only cases in the four broad categories listed. In the Samsø and Newcastle surveys higher prevalence estimates are also given, which include various borderline groups

old persons in order to establish the relevance of these characteristics for mental health. The report draws on findings which have already been published in German (Cooper and Sosna 1983; Sosna and Wahl 1983; Cooper et al. 1984).

Research Design and Method

Mannheim is an industrial city with a largely working class population of just over 300 000, of whom at present 16% are over the age of 65. Seven widely contrasting urban districts were selected, containing in all one-fifth of the population, and in each district, a 5% random sample of elderly persons living in private households was drawn, using an updated residents' list. The seven districts, taken as a group, proved to be highly representative for the city as a whole in respect of a number of demographic indices. For old people in long-term care, a different approach was required, since as a rule their names had been deleted from the local lists. After completion of the community survey, therefore, a search was made in the two psychiatric institutions which provide long-term care for Mannheim patients, as well as in the city's 27 geriatric and old people's homes. The institutional sample was made up of all elderly hospital patients, and one-half of the elderly home residents, who had been admitted from addresses in the seven survey districts.

All members of both samples were interviewed twice, with the exception of the small minority who were too severely demented for systematic questioning. Mental health status was assessed by a psychiatrist, using the Clinical Psychiatric

Interview (Goldberg et al. 1970) in a German translation and supplemented for use with the elderly (Zintl-Wiegand et al. 1980; Cooper and Schwarz 1982). The interview schedule focuses on the individual's current mental state, as gauged both from reported symptoms and from abnormalities observed during the interview. Criteria for case identification have been established on the basis of the interviewer's ratings. Because physical examination, to say nothing of special investigations, could not be systematically undertaken on the basis of a home interview, the assessment of physical health was limited to taking a brief medical history, enquiring into any current treatment and checking for any pronounced physical or sensory impairments, as well as for disabilities in everyday activities (Cooper et al. 1982).

The social investigation, also based on an interview of known reliability (Sosna 1980), dealt with the old person's living conditions, socio-economic status and pattern of family and social contacts. Information on old persons who were severely demented, deaf or aphasic was obtained to a greater or lesser extent from relatives or nursing staff. Social class was rated in terms of the occupational prestige classification of Kleining and Moore (1968). A number of different indices of social isolation were derived from the interview (Sosna 1983). In particular, a distinction was drawn between 'objective' isolation, rated from the number and quality of current contacts, and 'subjective' isolation, rated on the basis of attitude scores and reported feelings of loneliness (Sosna and Wahl 1983).

Two sets of point prevalence estimates were computed: one for old people living in private households and one for the total elderly population. In computing the latter, appropriate weightings were given to each subgroup in accordance with the sampling quotas; namely, one for the hospital patients (100% sample), two for the home residents (50% sample) and 20 for the persons living in private households (5% sample).

Research Findings

Representativity of the Sample

The survey population of 10 005 elderly persons comprised 20.2% of the Mannheim elderly population at the beginning of 1978 (49 545). Of 503 persons whose names were drawn from the residents' list, 418 (83.1%) proved to be still alive and living in private households. Social interviews were completed with 350 (83.7%) and psychiatric interviews with 343 (82.1%) of this at-risk sample. Those interviewed were broadly representative of the survey population, apart from containing a small relative excess of persons aged over 75 years.

The numbers living in geriatric or old people's homes was not so readily ascertainable, since no central register exists. Altogether, 339 admitted from the survey districts were identified, corresponding to 19.8% of all old persons in such homes in Mannheim. Of 167 who were included in the 50% sample, it was possible to investigate 146 (83.0%). Finally, all but two of the 32 elderly psychiatric hospital patients who had been admitted from the survey districts (corresponding to 19.9% of the total number) could also be examined.

Prevalence of Psychiatric Illness

Of the 343 community residents, 80 satisfied the operational criteria for a psychiatric case. Assuming an equal frequency among the non-contacts and refusers, this number corresponds to a point prevalence of 23.3% among old people in private households, or 22.3% of the total elderly population. The overall frequency among the home residents was much higher; 61 of a total of 146 investigated persons (41.8%) were identified as psychiatric cases. A large disparity in this respect was found between the geriatric home residents, of whom 57.0% fulfilled the case criteria, and those in old people's homes, of whom only 23.9% – virtually the same proportion as among the community residents – did so. Finally, all 30 hospital patients were confirmed to be suffering from severe or moderately severe mental disorders. The total point prevalence, based on all persons aged over 65, was computed as 24.4%. In table 1, prevalence estimates for the main diagnostic categories are compared with those reported from a number of other field studies of elderly populations.

The age distribution of psychiatric cases, summarized in Table 2, indicates a sharp increase in prevalence after the age of 80, accounted for entirely by the organic psychosyndromes. The frequency of functional mental disorders appears actually to decline with increasing age, but this finding can be explained in terms of the hierarchical relationship between the two categories, as analysed in this study. When cases of organic mental illness are removed from the sample, the frequency of functional mental illness among the remainder is constant over all age groups: 14%–15%.

Comparison between the sexes shows the prevalence of psychiatric illness to be higher among women than among men, the point prevalence being 28.7% for the former and 16.4% for the latter. The difference can be explained only partially by the higher mean age for women, since it is present in some degree for all age groups over 65. The difference in age trends already noted between organic and functional mental illness was found to apply to each sex: whereas the frequency of organic psychosyndromes rose with advancing age, that of functional mental disorders remained constant with age among men and declined slightly among women.

Table 2. Prevalence of psychiatric illness among the elderly living in the community (per 100 persons aged over 65)

Age group	65–69	70–74	75–79	80+	65+
Organic mental disorders	5.0	4.8	13.1	23.8	10.2
Functional mental disorders	13.8	13.6	13.2	11.1	13.1
All psychiatric illness	18.8±3.9	18.4±3.8	26.3±5.1	34.9±6.0	23.3±2.3
Number in interview sample	101	103	76	63	343
Registered population of the survey districts aged over 65	3456	2971	1983	1595	10005

Mental Illness, Physical Impairment and Disability

Severe or moderately severe impairment of vision was found in 17.2% of the community sample, of hearing in 13.1% and of mobility in 25.6%. On the basis of combined ratings, 9.6% of the sample were rated as severely and a further 25.4% as moderately physically impaired. The distribution of mental illness in the sample was found to be positively associated with that for physical impairment ($\chi^2 = 55.18$; df=2; $P < 0.001$), and this association held good for both the organic and the functional mental disorders. It was also found in both sexes and in all age groups over 65.

As could be expected, the physical impairment ratings correlated highly with scores for disability in self-care and, in the case of women, for disability in carrying out household tasks. Table 3 shows that the distribution of mental illness in the sample was closely related to that for disability in self-care and, once again, that this association existed for both organic and functional forms of mental disorder. Further analysis revealed that this relationship too was present in both sexes and in the age groups both over and under 75 years.

Table 3. Distribution of disability for self-care, psychiatric cases and others ($n=343$)[a]

Mental health status	Self-care score		
	0 (unrestricted) (%)	1–3 (mildly restricted) (%)	4+ (severely restricted) (%)
Normal	83.9	59.0	20.0
Psychiatric cases	16.1	41.0	80.0
Organic	4.9	27.9	33.3
Functional	11.2	13.1	46.7
Total	100.0	100.0	100.0
Probands (n)	267	61	15

[a] χ^2 (normal/psychiatric) = 58.13; $df=2$; $P<0.001$

The frequency of physical impairments was generally much higher among the institutional residents than in the community sample. Of the former group, 42.0% were rated as severely and a further 22.7% as moderately physically impaired. The association between mental and physical impairment appeared to be much weaker than in the community sample; indeed, it did not reach the 5% level of significance ($\chi^2 = 2.27$; df=2; $P > 0.05$). The reason for this discrepancy is unclear. Since, however, the institutional group as a whole constitutes only some 4% of the elderly population of Mannheim, the latter finding does not cast doubt on the validity of the general association between mental and physical impairment in the elderly.

Mental Illness and Housing Conditions

Various aspects of the housing situation were rated as unsatisfactory if they were judged inadequate to the old person's needs and unfavourable for maintaining an independent existence. The proportion thus rated differed a great deal, as between individual items of the rating scale:

1. Subtenancy only	2.9%
2. No running hot water	30.5%
3. Outside W.C. only	4.6%
4. No bath or shared with other tenants	14.6%
5. No central heating	50.3%
6. No telephone in apartment or on same level	23.1%
7. Living space inadequate[1]	15.5%
8. Shared use of kitchen with other tenants	0.9%
9. Apartment not on ground floor; no lift	55.2%

Housing conditions were rated as good or adequate (0–2 points) for 232 respondents (66.3%), as relatively poor (3–4 points) for a further 78 (22.3%) and as very poor (5–9 points) for the remaining 40 (11.4%). In view of the high proportion with unsatisfactory housing, it is noteworthy that only a single respondent was found to be living in squalor, while a further 30 (8.3%) were found in untidy or mildly neglected surroundings. Self-neglect in personal hygiene and clothing was observed in only ten instances (3.5%). It is, of course, entirely possible that these proportions would have been higher had the non-responders (16.3% of the sample) also been available for investigation.

Among persons with inadequate or poor housing conditions, the proportion classified as mentally ill was 32.5%, compared with 18.6% in the remainder of the sample ($\chi^2=7.56$; df=1; $P<0.01$). A similar positive association was noted between unsatisfactory housing and the frequency of physical impairments. Of the respondents in inadequate or poor housing, 45.3% were rated as severely or moderately physically impaired, compared with 32.2% in the remainder of the

1 operationally defined as less than 40 sq. metres for a single-person household, less than 50 sq. metres for a couple and less than an additional 15 sq. metres for each additional member of the household.

Table 4. Frequency of psychiatric illness in the community sample according to physical status and quality of living conditions ($n=343$)[a]

Mental status	No or only mild physical impairment; living conditions good (%)	Physical impairment (severe or moderate) *or* poor living conditions (%)	Physical impairment (severe or moderate) and poor living conditions (%)	Unknown (%)
Normal	87.0	80.9	55.7	2
Psychiatric cases	13.0	19.1	44.3	2
Total	100.0	100.0	100.0	4
Persons (n)	108	152	79	4

[a] $\chi^2=27.70$; $df=2$; $P<0.001$

sample ($\chi^2=4.33$; df=1; $P<0.05$). Since both physical impairment and poor housing conditions can give rise to handicaps in daily life (as with an old person with limited mobility on an upper floor of a building with no lift), the association with mental health was tested for both factors in combination. Table 4 reveals that mental disorders were in fact diagnosed most frequently among physically impaired old people who lived in poor housing conditions.

Mental Illness, Physical Impairment and Socioeconomic Status

The frequency of mental illness was found to vary inversely with social class. This association, however, was due entirely to a steep social class gradient among persons with organic mental disorder, who congregated in the lower status groups of the elderly population. (Since allocation to a social class category was based on previous occupation, this finding could not be attributed to an illness-linked loss of status in late life). A similar inverse relationship was found between social class and frequency of physical impairment. In order to examine the relative contributions of physical health and social class to psychiatric risk, a three-way table was prepared (cf. Table 5).

When the proportion of psychiatric cases was examined for each grade of severity of physical impairment, no linear trend with social class was observed. The frequency of mental illness was in each instance highest in the lower middle class group, but the interclass differences as a whole were no longer significant. It seems that, if the degree of physical impairment is held constant, the association between psychogeriatric disorder and social class virtually disappears. The significance of social class for mental health in old age may thus have less to do with a direct sociogenic effect than with the increased risk of bodily ill health and

Table 5. Frequency of psychiatric illness, by social class and physical impairment score ($n=339$)[a]

	Social class according to Kleining and Moore (1968)								
	Middle class[b] weighted impairment score			Lower middle class[c] weighted impairment score			Working class[d] weighted impairment score		
	0–1 (none or only mild) (%)	2 (moderate) (%)	3–4 (severe) (%)	0–1 (none or only mild) (%)	2 (moderate) (%)	3–4 (severe) (%)	0–1 (none or only mild) (%)	2 (moderate) (%)	3–4 (severe) (%)
Normal	90.1	82.4	42.9	84.5	57.1	28.6	88.5	63.3	33.3
Psychiatric cases	9.9	17.6	57.1	15.5	42.9	71.4	11.5	36.7	66.7
Total	100.0	100.0	100.0	100.0	100.0	100.0	100.0	100.0	100.0
Probands (n)	71	17	7	71	21	7	78	49	18

[a] No information available on social class of four probands
[b] $\chi^2=11.48$; $df=2$; $P<0.01$
[c] $\chi^2=14.94$; $df=2$; $P<0.001$
[d] $\chi^2=26.25$; $df=2$; $P<0.001$

disability in the lower social classes, which in turn puts them at increased risk for psychiatric disorder.

A negative association between psychiatric prevalence and the level of household income was found. The frequency of mental illness rose from 12.6% among those with over DM 1200 net monthly income, to 31.2% among those with less than DM 800 monthly. Within this range, no 'threshold' was found, such as might stress the significance of poverty or material hardship in absolute terms. However, the mean household income for this sample was under DM 1500 monthly, and the distribution suggested that very few indeed of the old people concerned could be regarded as affluent. It may be that extension of the survey to include a larger middle class population would have yielded evidence of such a threshold.

Mental Illness, Physical Impairment and Social Isolation

Neither organic nor functional mental disorders were found more commonly among old persons living alone than among those who lived in household groups. Furthermore, no general association could be demonstrated between psychiatric prevalence and the index of 'objective' social isolation, even though a raised frequency of mental illness was present in the subgroup with the highest rating for this variable. By way of contrast, a highly significant association could be shown between psychiatric prevalence and 'subjective' social isolation: Table 6 reveals a fourfold difference in this respect between the subjects with high and low isolation scores. Old persons who during the interview complained of severe loneliness or whose scores on the attitude scale were thought to indicate marked alienation from group norms ('anomia') had high rates of psychiatric diagnosis.

The research findings with regard to physical impairment and social isolation are essentially similar. Here also, the index of 'objective' isolation is of little discriminatory power ($\chi^2=10.54$; df=6; $P>0.05$), whereas that for 'subjective' isolation differentiates quite well between persons with and without severe impairment ($\chi^2=22.12$; df=4; $P<0.001$). Moreover, the same patterns of association were found in the sample of residents of geriatric and old people's homes (Cooper et al. 1984). In general, therefore, the survey data suggest that,

Table 6. Frequency of psychiatric illness in the community sample, according to the degree of 'subjective' social isolation ($n=343$)[a]

Mental health status	Rating for subjective social isolation		
	0 (not at all) (%)	1 (mildly) (%)	2 (severely) (%)
Normal	88.4	79.9	54.8
Psychiatric cases	11.6	20.1	45.2
Total	100.0	100.0	100.0
Persons (n)	86	184	73

[a] $\chi^2=27.18$; $df=3$; $P<0.01$

while objective and subjective aspects of isolation are to some extent interrelated in the elderly population, they are not infrequently found to be separate and, moreover, have considerably different implications for mental health.

Discussion

Social disadvantage, as indicated by inadequate housing standards, low social class and low household income, appears to be associated with increased risks both for mental and for physical impairment and disability among the elderly. Since the latter characteristics are also highly intercorrelated, all the evidence points to a concentration, in certain subsections of the elderly population, of multiple health and social factors, which tend to result in handicap and loss of the capacity for independent living. Relatively objective measures failed to confirm any general association between social isolation and the frequency of mental disorder, though this negative finding certainly in no way implies either that social isolation is never a causal factor of such disorder or that isolation among the elderly is not a serious problem in its own right.

Social class, as assessed on the basis of previous occupation, influences both the level of household income and the quality of housing in old age. Members of higher social status groups are, as a rule, in a position to acquire houses or apartments of a satisfactory standard while they are still actively earning. Moreover, the social insurance system in the German Federal Republic, as in many other countries, favours the extension of social inequality into old age, since pensions are based largely on the level of earnings prior to retirement. Nevertheless, the associations found between these variables are not so strong that they justify using social class – or any other single variable – as an accurate indicator of the standard and quality of life of elderly individuals: rather, it would seem politic in survey research of this kind to make use of a number of different socio-economic indices.

Comparison of the Mannheim findings with those of psychogeriatric field studies in other countries indicates quite good agreement with respect to prevalence ratios (cf. Table 1) and also to the distribution by age group. There is, however, no consensus as regards the significance of social conditions. Two other surveys which examined the relationship of social class to psychiatric prevalence came to differing conclusions. Kay et al. (1964) in Newcastle found no association, whereas Lowenthal and Berkman (1967) in San Francisco reported an inverse relationship similar to that observed in Mannheim. Kay et al. (1964) did note that low income and poor housing quality were more commonly found among the mentally ill subgroup of their community sample, but thought that this was probably due to a deterioration in old age, linked to the failing health of those affected.

Survey findings as regards the role of social isolation have also been somewhat inconclusive. Neither Nielsen (1962) nor Kay et al. (1964) found any general association between isolation and the frequency of mental illness. Lowenthal (1964), who in her San Francisco survey explored this issue in much greater detail, concluded that, while a lifelong habitual pattern of social isolation was not a risk factor for old age mental disorder, a relative degree of isolation commencing in late life could be so.

The causal significance of the variables included in this study cannot be assessed on the evidence of cross-sectional data alone. The findings reported here suggest some tenable working hypotheses which ought, however, to be tested by means of prospective longitudinal studies and also, where feasible, by controlled evaluative research. More immediately, they suggest that it is possible to identify high-risk subgroups of the elderly population who could benefit from programmes of social support.

Acknowledgment. I am indebted to the members of the project team who cooperated in this work, in particular, to H. Bickel, G. Glettler, B. Mahnkopf, U. Sosna and H.-W. Wahl.

References

Cooper B, Schwarz R (1982) Psychiatric case-identification in an elderly population. Soc Psychiatry 17:43–52

Cooper B, Sosna U (1983) Psychische Erkrankung in der Altenbevölkerung: eine epidemiologische Feldstudie in Mannheim. Nervenarzt 54:239–249

Cooper B, Glettler G, Abt H-G (1982) Psychiatric disorder, physical impairments and disability among the elderly in an urban community. In: Magnussen G, Nielsen J, Buch J (eds) Epidemiology and prevention of mental illness in old age. Hellerup, Denmark

Cooper B, Mahnkopf B, Bickel H (1984) Psychische Erkrankung und soziale Isolation bei älteren Heimbewohnern: eine Vergleichsstudie. Z Gerontol 17:117–125

Dilling H, Weyerer S, Castell R (1984) Psychische Erkrankung in der Bevölkerung. Enke, Stuttgart

Goldberg DP, Cooper B, Eastwood MR, Kedward HB, Shepherd M (1970) A standardized psychiatric interview for use in community surveys. Br J Prev Soc Med 24:18–23

Grad de Alarcon J (1971) Social causes and social consequences of mental illness in old age. In: Kay D, Walk A (eds) Recent developments in psychogeriatrics. Royal College of Psychiatrists Special Publication no 6, London pp 75–86

Kay D, Bergmann K (1980) Epidemiology of mental disorders among the aged in the community. In: Birren JE, Sloane RB (eds) Handbook of mental health and aging. Prentice-Hall, Englewood Cliffs, pp 34–56

Kay D, Beamish P, Roth M (1964) Old-age mental disorders in Newcastle-upon-Tyne. Part 1: a study of prevalence; part 2: a study of possible social and medical causes. Br J Psychiatry 110:146–158, 668–682

Kleining G, Moore H (1968) Soziale Selbsteinstufung: ein Instrument zur Messung sozialer Schichten. Köln Z Soziol Sozialpsychol 20:502–552

Lowenthal MF (1964) Social isolation and mental illness in old age. Am Sociol Rev 29:70–95

Lowenthal MF, Berkman PL (1967) Aging and mental disorder in San Francisco. Jossey Bass, San Francisco

Nielsen J (1962) Gerontopsychiatric period-prevalence investigation in a geographically delimited population. Acta Psychiat. Scand 38:307–330

Parsons PL (1965) Mental health of Swansea's old folk. Br J Prev Soc Med 19:43–47

Primrose EJR (1962) Psychological Illness: a community study. Tavistock, London

Sheldon JH (1948) The social medicine of old age. Report of an inquiry in Wolverhampton. Oxford University Press, London

Sosna U (1980) Empirical measurement of social isolation in relation to mental disorders of the elderly. In: Strömgren E, Dupont A, Nielsen JA (eds) Epidemiological research

as basis for the organization of extramural psychiatry. Acta Psychiatry Scand 62 [Suppl 285]:220–229
Sosna U (1983) Soziale Isolation und psychische Erkrankung im Alter. Campus, Frankfurt
Sosna U, Wahl H.-W. (1983) Soziale Belastung, psychische Erkrankung und körperliche Beeinträchtigung im Alter: Ergebnisse einer Felduntersuchung. Z Gerontol 16:107–114
World Health Organization (1979) Psychogeriatric care in the community. Public Health in Europe No 10. WHO, Copenhagen
Zintl-Wiegand A, Cooper B, Krumm B (1980) Psychisch Kranke in der ärztlichen Allgemeinpraxis: eine Untersuchung in der Stadt Mannheim. Beltz, Weinheim

2.5 Physical Factors in Mental Health in the Elderly: Gerontological and Internal Medical Aspects

J. G. Evans

The interactions between physical and mental illness and disability are complex at any age, but particularly so among the old. Recognition of this led some years ago to the creation in Britain of psychogeriatric assessment units under the joint care of psychiatrists and physicians. For reasons unconnected with the pattern of patients' needs, enthusiasm for these joint units has waned and psychogeriatrics has evolved into a psychiatric specialty. However, it is only the solution that has changed; the problem remains the same.

At one level of discussion, at once both profound and trivial, the distinction between physical and mental illness is necessarily false. 'Mind' is a term conventionally used to comprise certain functions and activities of the human organism (Ryle 1949). These activities and functions are largely regarded as directly dependent upon the activities of the neocortex but both neurophysiological and clinical studies indicate the involvement of other neurological structures in 'mental' functions. The possibility that mentally mediated behaviour may have non-neurological precipitating causes is so familiar to physicans working among the elderly that its implications, perhaps of eschatological magnitude, have long since ceased to command attention. This is not an aspect that could usefully be considered further here but has been invoked to encourage an appropriately broad and unified view of 'mind' and 'body' and of psychiatry and internal medicine.

Aging, from a gerontological standpoint, is characteristically a time-dependent loss of adaptability of an individual organism. Homeostatic mechanisms become slower, less sensitive, less accurate and less well-sustained although the age at which such changes become detectable or functionally significant varies with the organ or tissue under examination and with environmental demands. A change in the parameters of homeostatic processes have their effects magnified by interactions with other homeostatic processes. This underlines the observation of Shock (1979) on the greater age-associated decline in complex than in simple physiological processes and also explains the demonstrably earlier age-associated decline in function of the organism as a whole (as indicated by age-associated mortality rates) than in some components of total body function, e.g. renal function.

Strictly, aging can only be assessed by longitudinal study, but in practice age-associated changes are usually inferred from cross-sectional observations which are also affected by factors and processes other than aging. Table 1 sets out sources of difference between young and old people as they may emerge from a cross-sectional population study. True aging refers to those changes within an individual as he or she grows older. These changes may be intrinsic in the sense of being directly genetically or constitutionally determined while extrinsic processes are those due to the environment. Interactions between environmental factors and

Table 1. Differences between young and old

True aging	
Primary:	Intrinsic
	Extrinsic
Secondary:	Species
	Individual
Non-aging	
Cohort phenomena	
Aggravated aging	
Selective survival	

genetically determined susceptibilities must also be anticipated, one of the clearest animal models of this being the interaction between sodium intake and hypertension in certain strains of rats (Meneely and Battarbee 1976).

Table 1 also postulates a distinction between primary and secondary aging, the latter comprising adaptive or compensatory responses to aging. At a species level, the human menopause may be an evolved response, in the specific context of a family social structure, a cumulative culture and a prolonged pre-maturity phase, to an age-associated decline in the reproductive efficiency of the female. There will come a time in the female's life when it will be more profitable in biological terms for her to give up increasingly unsuccessful attempts to produce viable offspring of her own, each containing 50% of her genes, and to contribute instead to the survival of her grandchildren, each containing 25% of her genes. The male makes a much smaller biological investment in unsuccessful pregnancies and so will not experience a corresponding selection pressure towards sterility in later life. A crucial prediction of this hypothesis is that a menopause, in the sense of a permanent programmed loss of fertility at an age well below the maximum lifespan, will not occur in species where grandparents do not contribute to the survival of grandchildren. So far the menopausal phenomenon appears to be uniquely human. With the well-established exception of osteoporosis its effect on morbidity appears to be neutral or in some diseases, notably breast cancer, beneficial. The long-assumed influence of the menopause on mental health appears to be non-specific and more a consequence of culturally determined perceptions of its significance than of its physiological effects (Wood 1979).

The hypothesis that there also be secondary aging processes within the individual organism is of profound interest since a basic biological enigma is the lack of repair of aging damage. It has been suggested that an increase in sensitivity of hypothalamic osmoreceptors with age may be an adaptation to a decline in renal function (Helderman et al. 1978), but this has not been unequivocally established and other explanations are at least equally plausible.

In addition to these true aging processes, differences between old and young can arise from other sources which need to be recognised. Differential mortality is a process more often invoked than actively researched, and one can wonder whether, in economically advanced societies, it can have much effect on the characteristics of older age groups. There is certainly evidence that differential mortality from extrinsic causes contributes to the age-associated change in sex-ratio through mortality in late middle age (Evans 1981). It is not clear whether more subtle effects occur as the force of mortality increases in old age; as will be discussed below, it is usually difficult to establish correlates of morbidity and mortality at late ages whose distribution might be changed through selective mortality.

In cohort effects successive generations acquire characteristics early in life which, in rapidly developing cultures, may become increasingly environmentally inappropriate as society changes. Although cohort phenomena are most likely to be mistaken for aging when cultural changes are improving the health or performance of younger generations, they may appear to produce 'negative' aging when societies are deteriorating. There is a hint in the work of Schaie and Strother (1968) that the assumption that verbal abilities decline with age later than other skills may be biassed by a decline in literacy since 1900 among successive generations of the English-speaking peoples. Cohort effects are most apparent in the field of mental functioning but can also be anticipated in important physical variables, nutritional habits for example.

Age-associated changes may be exaggerated by aspects of social organisation that impose more severe environmental challenges on the elderly than are presented to the young. Poorer housing and relative poverty are two specific examples that are easily documented (Wroe 1973) and poorer quality of medical services provided to older patients, particularly mentally impaired older patients, is probably more pervasive than we like to think. A Newcastle study showed that mental impairment was a powerful predictor of death following proximal femoral fracture (Evans et al. 1979), but this effect was aggravated by features of the treatment offered at one of two hospitals to which patients were admitted (Evans et al. 1980). Ironically, most of the patients with mental impairment were admitted to the hospital providing the worse care for them.

There are technical problems in establishing connections between physical and mental disease in old age that reflect a more general epidemiological unpredictability of morbidity and mortality among the elderly (Evans 1984). Some of the factors that lead to this state of affairs can be briefly summarised:

1. Most diseases of relevance in the elderly are multifactorial and are therefore final common pathways of a variety of antecedent causal chains. In old age both environmental and genetic causes (Hamilton 1966) may be expected to accumulate, so that the proportional contribution from any one causal mechanism can be expected to diminish with age. Against a background of incidence or prevalence rates that rise with age, of course, the absolute contribution of a single causal mechanism may nonetheless increase (Evans and Rose 1971).

2. The variance of most variables will increase with age. This is partly an increase in inter-individual variance due to age-associated changes occurring at different rates and to different degrees but there is also an increase in intra-individual variance due to impaired homeostatic mechanisms and also, in some situations at least, to increased error variance. Increase in intra-individual variance has the effect of reducing precision and predictive power.

3. Independent variables in epidemiological studies are often not the factors that are of actual interest but correlates (metameters) of them. A classic example of this is sphygmomanometric blood pressure taken as a metameter of intra-arterial

pressure. The relationship between the metameter and the variable of interest may change with age.
4. Differential mortality will tend to remove from a population those individuals susceptible to a specific baneful influence which may therefore be expected to become less important apparently with age. As already noted, there is no direct evidence that this is an important effect in advanced societies.
5. Cohort effects, as discussed earlier, may lead to differences in the relationship between a risk factor and a specific outcome through modulating interacting variables.
6. Probably the most important reason for an underestimation of the effects of environmental factors on morbidity and mortality in old age lies with the use of current values of a risk factor rather than some more accurate measure of past cumulative exposure. The remoteness of some of the determinants of morbidity in the elderly can be illustrated from the epidemiology of cerebrovascular stroke in which obesity in early adult life appears to be a determinant of stroke in old age, although obesity in old age is not (Evans 1982). The same explanation may underlie the association between a past diagnosis of diabetes and stroke which is not matched by any association between glucose intolerance and subsequent stroke in old age (Peacock et al. 1972). More poignantly, the barbaric privations imposed by the Japanese on their prisoners of war are now being recognised as a cause of both physical and mental illness in British and Australian victims 40 years later.

A number of studies have shown a relationship between mental impairment in the elderly and subsequent mortality (Britton 1984). This appears to be a remarkably robust finding and has recently emerged in one of our population studies on the incidence of stroke. A very crude series of questions (Prudham and Evans 1981) aimed at detecting evidence of temporal disorientation were significantly associated with subsequent mortality over a 4- to 5-year follow-up. The work of Vaillant (1979) showing a relationship between mental health and subsequent physical health during middle life (not attributable entirely to alcohol and tobacco use, or to obesity) may or may not be analogous. The implication that good mental health in middle life leads to good physical health is not a necessary conclusion; it is perhaps more plausible to suggest a cognate relationship, although the nature of the common antecedents remains obscure.

Efforts, largely unsuccessful, have been made to identify specific physical factors related to subsequent mental health in the elderly. Physical impairments, not surprisingly, lead to affective reactions, and many drugs given for physical illness may produce depressive reactions as well as delirium. We also have to be aware of the action of Berkson's bias in producing associations between disorders that are not biologically based (Sackett 1979). One theme that recurs in the literature is an association between blood pressure and mental test functioning: the higher the blood pressure the more frequent the evidence of mental impairment. Medication is a complicating factor, and not all studies have been able to replicate the finding; it was not present in our own data although, as emphasised, our mental test score was extremely crude.

Although blood pressures may be unusually high in the course of some depressive illnesses, the conventional postulated explanation for these observations has been a deleterious effect of hypertension on cerebral function. Specific cognitive defects occur as a result of stroke, and this pattern of impairment, rather than a global deficit, has emerged in some studies. Implicit in the work of Tomlinson and colleagues (Blessed et al. 1968; Tomlinson et al. 1970) on the neuropathology of dementia is the concept of a threshold whereby damage from a variety of causes may accumulate to produce a clinical picture of dementia. One corollary is that those subjects with poorer mental endowments to begin with will cross the threshold of dementia earlier. Although in pure multi-infarct dementia approximately 50 – 100 ml of cerebral substance has to be lost before dementia becomes clinically apparent, it is conceivable that more subtle changes in the cerebral microcirculation may contribute to the genesis of mental impairment even though rarely sufficient in themselves to produce the full dementia syndrome. The pathogenic processes linking hypertension with such micro-impairments are not established except in gross cases of hypertensive encephalopathy. The mechanism may lie in faults in autoregulation, perhaps associated with reflow phenomena in which capillaries that have been closed down by arteriolar constriction fail to become re-perfused when constriction ceases.

The plausibility of such a haemodynamic contribution to mental impairment is increased by the observations of the effect of polycythaemia and hyperviscosity on cerebral function (Thomas et al. 1977). Within the ordinary range of haematocrit and blood flow it can be anticipated that an inverse relationship will lead to a constant oxygen supply to the brain. At increased levels of haematocrit, however, owing to a disproportionate effect upon viscosity, blood flow may fall more steeply than is appropriate to oxygen delivery, and impairment of mental function results. This observation does suggest that, under some circumstances at least, reduction of blood flow short of total ischaemia producing irreversible brain damage may impair cerebral function. It does seem to be well established that there is a range of oxygen tensions at which neuronal cells will be alive but not able to synthesise neurotransmitters or to function.

The threshold model of dementia has analogies in early work in the psychology laboratory. It was found that the learning ability of some experimental animals was impaired proportionally to the amount of cerebral tissue removed and there appeared to be little evidence of cerebral localisation and specific deficits corresponding to specific parts of the brain. This ancient debate has recently been reviewed (Phillips et al. 1984). There is now evidence that there may be some specific association between damage to certain parts of the brain and affective status following stroke. Robinson and colleagues (Robinson et al. 1984) have shown in a series of patients that in cerebrovascular accidents affecting the dominant hemisphere the severity of depression correlated significantly with proximity of the lesion on CT scan to the frontal pole. Conversely, patients with lesions in the right hemisphere showed the reverse trend in that those with posterior lesions were more depressed than patients with anterior lesions, who, indeed, tended to be unduly cheerful and apathetic. Robinson et al. suggest that this relationship may be explicable in terms of specific biogenic amine containing pathways in the cerebral cortex. If this work is replicable it would appear to offer important opportunity for exploring mechanisms linking physical and mental phenomena.

Useful research opportunities in this area surely also lie in the elucidation of mechanisms of delirium. The identification and management of delirium is an important component of medical and nursing practice among elderly patients. The phenomenology of delirium is described in terms of component features that can be more or less well established from clinical observation of an individual patient (Lipowski 1980). But clinical descriptions are Procrustean devices and like any other manifestation of cognitive control may impose a false pattern. Even when the descriptive distinction between agitated and quiet delirium is drawn, the implication remains that what is being described is a unitary state and that all the infective, metabolic and pharmacological causes of delirium act through a final common pathway which, if we could identify it, would be pathognomic for the condition. There are hints in the literature, as in clinical practice, that the pharmacological and physiological mechanisms underlying delirium may be highly varied. We should perhaps speak not of delirium but of the deliria. One possible basis for a sub-classification that would have implications for rational therapy lies with derangement of specific neurotransmitter systems. The association of anticholinergic medication with delirium is well documented particularly in the postoperative situation (Tune et al. 1981). Conversely, the delirium tremens of alcoholics appears to be associated with catecholamine (Griacobini et al. 1960) and possibly steroid (Bannan et al. 1984) release. Defects in cholinergic neural systems are established as associated with dementia of Alzheimer's type, at least in elderly patients [in cases with younger onset there may be more diffuse neurotransmitter abnormalities (Rossor et al. 1984)], and exogenous adrenergic drugs are reported to have caused delirious states. Propranolol, a beta-adrenergic blocker which readily crosses the blood – brain barrier, has been reported as a cause of delirium (Kuhr 1979) and also as an effective treatment in some cases of delirium (Petrie and Ban 1981).

A complicating factor in considering the catecholamines and some other neurotransmitters is that they are also vasoactive. Their mechanism of action on brain function may lie in modulation of cerebral autoregulation, leading to delirium through generalised or localised hypoxia of cerebral tissue (Loach and Benedict 1980). There has recently been a suggestion that alcohol may also have a direct cerebral vasoconstrictive action (Altura et al. 1983). There is evidence that impairment of cerebral autoregulation may be more common in the elderly than at younger ages and may be a factor that underlies such phenomena as transient localised neurological signs (Wollner et al. 1979) and symptoms associated with minor falls in systemic blood pressure, as well as the increased susceptibility to the effects of hypotensive medication (Jones and Graham 1978). In the latter case there may be problems with the decline in sensitivity of the baroreflexes (Floras and Sleight 1982) and presumably other systemic cardiovascular reflexes.

If this approach has virtue, more work needs to be done on characterising the biochemical characteristics of delirious patients on an individual basis with a view to matching medication to identified abnormalities. The poverty of our current pharmacotherapeutic approach to delirium is exemplified by a recent review of delirium which is 21 pages long but has slightly under 16 lines on medication in treatment (Liston 1982). Earlier in this review the author comments that doctors and nurses usually only concern themselves seriously with the agitated type of delirium, leaving the less disturbing quietly delirious patients to follow the natural course of their illness. This may perhaps explain the popularity of haloperidol in the treatment of delirium, which by its powerful sedating and dystonic effects will effectively quieten a patient whatever the cause of his disturbed behaviour. Use of such drugs, essentially as a means of restraint rather than as rational treatment, might be seen as raising issues other than the pharmacological.

One would also postulate on the basis of hints in the literature that deliria not only reflect the effects of short-term imbalance between neurotransmitter systems but may also be caused by longer term modifications in receptor numbers. Such processes could explain, for example, the surprisingly long clinical course of deliria due to benzodiazepine withdrawal (Fruensgaard 1976). There is animal work to suggest that in certain experimental situations at least prolonged administration of drugs modifying neural action may lead to modification of receptor numbers (Smith et al. 1981). Such processes may also underlie the growing evidence of the effect of personality in predisposing to delirium.

References

Altura BM, Altura BT, Gebrewold A (1983) Alcoholic induced spasm of cerebral blood vessels. Relation to cerebral accidents and sudden death. Science 220:331–333

Bannan LT et al. (1984) Effect of alcohol withdrawal on blood pressure, plasma renin activity, aldosterone, cortisol and dopamine betahydroxylase. Clin Sci 66:659–663

Blessed G, Tomlinson BE, Roth M (1968) The association between both quantitative measures of dementia and of senile change in the cerebral grey matter of elderly subjects. Br J Psychiatry 114:797–811

Britton PG (1984) Cognitive change in the elderly. In: Evans J Grimley, Caird FI (eds) Advanced geriatric medicine, 4. Pitman, London, pp 83–89

Evans J Grimley (1981) The biology of human ageing. In: Dawson AM et al. (eds) Recent advances in medicine, 18. Churchill Livingstone, London, pp 17–38

Evans J Grimley (1982) "Stroke" predictors. In: Sarner M (ed) Advanced medicine, 18. Pitman, London, 288–301

Evans J Grimley (1984) Prevention of age-associated loss of autonomy: epidemiological approaches. J Chron Dis 37:353–363

Evans J Grimley, Rose GA (1971) The epidemiology of hypertension. Br Med Bull 27:37–41

Evans J Grimley, Prudham D, Wandless I (1979) A prospective study of fracture proximal femur: factors predisposing to survival. Age Ageing 8:246–250

Evans J Grimley, Wandless I, Prudham D (1980) A prospective study of fractured proximal femur: Hospital differences. Public Health 94:149–154

Floras JS, Sleight P (1982) The lability of blood pressure. In: Amery A (ed) Hypertensive cardiovascular disability: Pathophysiology and treatment. Nijkoff, The Hague, pp 104–117

Fruensgaard K (1976) Withdrawal psychosis: A study of 30 consecutive cases. Acta psychiatr Scand 53:105–118

Giacobini E, Izikowitz S, Wegmann A (1960) Urinary norepinephrine and epinephrine excretion in delirium tremens. Arch Gen Psychiatry 3:289–296

Hamilton WD (1966) The moulding of senescence by natural selection. J Theor Biol 12:12–45

Helderman JH et al. (1978) The response of arginine vasopressin to intravenous ethanol and hypertonic saline in man: the impact of aging. J Gerontol 33:38–477

Jones JV, Graham DI (1978) Hypertension in the cerebral circulation and its relation to the elderly. Am Heart J 96:270–271

Kuhr BM (1979) Prolonged delirium with propanolol. J Clin Psychiatry 40:198–199
Lipowski ZJ (1980) Delirium. Acute brain failure in man. Thomas, Springfield
Liston EH (1982) Delirium in the aged. Psychiatr Clin North Am 5(1):49–66
Loach AB, Benedict CR (1980) Plasma catecholamine concentrations associated with cerebral vasospasm. J Neurol Sci 45:261–271
Meneely GR, Battarbee HD (1976) High sodium – low potassium environment and hypertension. Am J Cardiol 38:768–789
Peacock PB et al. (1972) The Birmingham stroke epidemiology and rehabilitation study. In: Stewart GT (ed) Trends in epidemiology. Thomas, Springfield, pp 231–341
Petrie WM, Ban TA (1981) Propranolol in organic agitation. Lancet I:324
Phillips CG, Zeki S, Barlow HB (1984) Localization of function in the cerebral cortex. Brain 107:327–362
Prudham D, Evans J Grimley (1981) Factors asociated with falls in the elderly. Age Ageing 10:141–146
Robinson RG et al. (1984) Mood disorders in stroke patients. Importance of location of lesion. Brain 107:81–93
Rossor MN et al. (1984) Neurochemical characteristics of early and late onset types of Alzheimer's disease. Br Med J 288:961–964
Ryle G (1949) The concept of mind. Hutchinson, London
Sackett DL (1979) Bias in analytic research. J Chron Dis 32:51–63
Schaie KW, Strother CR (1968) A cross-sequential study of age changes in cognitive behaviour. Psychol Bull 70:671–680
Shock N (1979) Systems physiology and aging. Fed Proc 38:161–162
Smith RC et al. (1981) Aging, receptors and neuroleptic drugs. In: Enna SJ, Samorajski T, Beer B (eds) Brain neurotransmitters and receptors in aging and age-related disorders. Raven, New York, pp 231–244
Thomas DJ et al. (1977) Effect of haematocrit on cerebral blood flow in man. Lancet II:941–943
Tomlinson BE, Blessed G, Roth M (1970) Observations on the brains of demented old people. J Neurol Sci 11:205–242
Tune LE et al. (1981) Association of postoperative delirium with raised serum levels of anticholinergic drugs. Lancet II:651–652
Vaillant GE (1979) Natural history of male psychologic health. N Engl J Med 301:1249–1254
Wollner L et al. (1979) Failure of cerebral autoregulation as a cause of brain dysfunction in the elderly. Br Med J I:1117–1118
Wood C (1979) Menopausal myths. Med J Aust 1:496–499
Wroe DCL (1973) The elderly. Soc Trends 4:23–34

3 Psychological and Social Aspects of Mental Well-Being and Mental Health in the Elderly

3.1 Aging as Fate and Challenge: The Influence of Social, Biological and Psychological Factors

U. Lehr

"Our life expectancy is dependent on our life-style. Life expectancy does not only mean length of life, but also quality of life. It does not count how old one will become, but how one will become old." (Schaefer 1979)

Individuality and Multidimensionality of Aging Processes

Many recent studies point to a broad range of interindividual differences within age groups in terms of level of biological, psychological, and social functioning (Thomae 1976, 1983; Lehr 1972, 1982a,c; Birren and Schaie 1977; Baltes and Labouvie 1973; Baltes and Schaie 1976). The view that a general and universal decline, i.e., a decrease in capacity, affects all people in all their areas of functioning is radically contradicted by findings of international basic research in gerontology. These studies have highlighted individual differences and the multifactorial determination of changes in old age and have led to the concept of "differential gerontology" (Thomae 1976). They have proved that the behavior of elderly people is flexible and can be influenced, and have taught us to regard concepts such as "age decay" or "age norm" as largely relative.

Introduction

The demographic transition, the decline in mortality followed with some lag by a decline in fertility and diminished population growth rates, has profoundly altered the age structure of human populations and has greatly increased longevity. Two interrelated but distinguishable consequences are manifest in the more developed countries (MDCs) and are becoming increasingly evident in the less developed countries (LDCs). The first is the accelerated aging of population and the second is increased extension of life. The aging of population is measured by a number of indexes relating to the population of a nation as a whole. The increase in longevity is measured by indexes relating to years of life lived or expected to be lived; and, in this paper, by the age structure of elders. Although both fertility and mortality trends and their interaction are involved in population aging and in increased longevity, the aging of a population is more the result of decreases in fertility, whereas extension of life is more the result of decreases in mortality.

The indexes of population aging which are used in this paper include the following: the proportion of the population 65 years of age and older, median age, the aged dependency ratio, and the aging index. The indexes of increased longevity include the expectation of life at birth and the proportion of the population 65 years of age and older which is 75 years of age and older. The data utilized in this paper are drawn from estimates and projections of population published by the United Nations (United Nations, Department of International Economic and Social Affairs 1981).

The necessity for a differential approach to gerontology is obvious in the light of the growing evidence of the effects that education, health, housing conditions, socioeconomic status etc. have on processes of aging. Interindividual variability is not only apparent in comparisons of the *state of the aged*, but also in *comparisons of the processes or the sequences of change in different individuals in different areas of behavior*. Especially longitudinal studies (Palmore 1970, 1974; Thomae 1976, 1983; Helander and Thomae 1982) have reported different interindividual patterns of intraindividual processes, pointing out the processes of aging in which individuals differ from each other.

These patterns are determined by the interaction between a variety of variables. The behavior and awareness of a person 70, 75, or 80 years of age (or older) is in part determined by biological factors, but also by social, economic, and ecological factors. *Aging, however, is a cohort-specific fate.* Historical events – like war, economic depression or boom, and political revolutions – are major determinants of the state of the aged and the processes of aging. Aging is determined by the life-history; aging is a biographical fate. (But it is not a fate to which we are exposed as passive beings or have to suffer in a passive manner. *Aging is a fate we have to deal with; it is a challenge which we have to cope with; it is a fate that must be mastered.*)

Briefly, the course of life is multifactorially determined. All these factors also determine directly the present life situation of the aging individual – and also future orientation is naturally contingent upon his or her present and, of course, past. *Consequently it is necessary to view a person's life at any one point as a crossroad between past, present, and future.*

Health and Aging

Health may serve as our first example, since it is particularly obvious that health status at any juncture can only be understood in terms of past history (any medical examination starts with the anamnesis). The present status of health will influence the present quality of life and also the processes of future development.

Since ancient times it has been known that the way of life and everyday behavior and habits are important determinants of wellbeing in old age [for example: Hippocrates (460–377 B.C.), Galen of Pergamum (129–199 A.D.) (cited in Stendel 1962), but also van Swieten (1700–1772) and Hufeland (1762–1836)]. Similar references to a lifelong preparation for old age which begins in childhood and adolescence and is related to the physical as well as to the mental sphere can be found in Plato's Republic and Cicero's *Cato the Elder on old Age*. Recent medical studies (e.g., on risk factors, especially for cardiovascular diseases) strongly support this position (for references see Lehr and Thomae 1979/80). Similar findings have also been made in respect of gastrointestinal diseases, particularly by Eitner and his staff (Eitner and Tröger 1968; Eitner et al.

1971; Eitner et al. 1975). They have pointed out that diseases in older age groups are correlated with life-style during the whole life span. Thus people who suffered from stomatological problems had disregarded many simple rules of eating behavior and everyday hygiene (care of the teeth and going to the dentist if necessary). Behavioral patterns preventing good health were evident among those of middle and higher social status more often than among those of lower status, among urban people more often than among rural people and in younger age groups more often than in older ones (which may reflect epochal or secular influences). In other words, rural, lower status people, older age groups, and women more easily become victims of irreversible trends owing to their way of life, which is *not only* affected – and this must be stressed – by their financial situation, in view of the availability of free medical and dental services. (In the Federal Republic of Germany as well as in Austria and some other European countries, most persons have to pay nothing for medical and dental services, hearing aids, glasses, and other prothetic instruments; these are paid by health insurance or social aid.) Rosenmayr (1976a), too, has pointed out similar behavior patterns in aged people of lower socioeconomic status (SES), especially in the rural area: Many of them avoided dental treatment; they refused hearing aids and spectacles or if they used spectacles or hearing aids, these were obsolete (see also Lehr 1976).

Our gerontological longitudinal studies in Bonn (the BLSA) were started in 1965 and concluded after seven measurement points in 1981. The original sample (see Thomae 1976) consisted of 220 men and women, born in the years 1890–95 and 1900–05. This sample – now 87–92 and 77–82 years of age – is reduced to 51 persons (in 1978, at the 6th measurement point, 81 subjects could be tested and interviewed). At the seven measurement points a large set of demographic, social, psychological, and medical variables were assessed, adding up to about 1000 data per person and measurement point (Thomae 1976). These data were obtained from a weekly testing program (including very extensive interviews, intelligence and personality tests, and a general health rating by a specialist of internal medicine).

We obtained data on "objective health" (as assessed by the geriatrician on the basis of physical and laboratory examinations) and "subjective health" (as rated by the report given by our subjects on their health problems). Self-rated health is a summary statement about the way in which numerous aspects of health (both subjective and objective) are combined within the perceptual framework of the individual respondent.

As expected, *objective health* was correlated with lower SES of family of origin ($P<0.002$), with lower level of schooling of both parents (father $P<0.007$; mother $P<0.002$), and with occupation of the father ($P<0.01$). Level of schooling of the subjects themselves showed a significant positive relationship to objective health only among women ($P<0.009$). However, subsequent occupational development, characterized by less continuity, was correlated with lower objective health in old age ($P<0.003$) in the male group (among whom less satisfaction with occupational development was reported).

An economically more stressful experience after World War II (1945–48) correlated with health status in old age in men ($P<0.01$) but not in women; this was especially true for our younger age group of men, born between 1900 and 1905 ($P<0.004$). Problems in marital life and in the housing situation during this time (1945 – 1948) had a greater impact on the health status of women ($P<0.02$), again especially those born between 1900 and 1905 ($P<0.006$), than on that of men.

Passing from biographical conditions to correlates of the *present situation* of our 220 subjects in 1965 (cross-sectional analysis), the objective health status showed a correlation with marital and socioeconomic status as well as with housing conditions: single persons were in worse health than married ones ($P<0.045$), women had a poorer objective health status than men ($P<0.02$), and subjects of lower SES ($P<0.004$) and living in small cities or rural areas ($P<0.087$) were in poorer health than middle class subjects and subjects living in urban areas. In the younger group of women, but not in the older one, poorer health was also correlated with stress in housing conditions ($P<0.034$) and with stress situations in the family and partnerships ($P<0.026$) during the years after World War II.

In the younger group of women and men and in the older group of women a correlation between health and present economic situation could be demonstrated.

The objective health status is mainly correlated with achievement-related behavior as measured by mental and psychomotor tests ($P<0.001$). This is true for the cross-sectional as well as the longitudinal analysis. Of the survivors from measurement points 1 – 7, 41.5% remained consistent, 19.5% showed a decline in objective health status, while 39% displayed better health than 15 years ago (according to the physician). Those who showed a decrease in their health status during the 15 years also showed a decisive decrease in their psychomotor and mental test performances. Especially some subtests of the WAIS (digit symbol test and picture completion test, which measure the ability to concentrate, the degree of focussing, abstraction, etc.) were most sensitive to health problems. Those subjects with decreasing health status also had declining adjustment scores and a reduction in self-confidence during this time.

As mentioned above, we also obtained data on the *"subjective" health status.* There are many indications of a considerable divergence between "subjective" and "objective" health. As we can see in Table 1, in 1965 24.52% of the 220 subjects

Table 1. Self-rating of health in relation to medical assessment (figures are percentages)

Assessment	Whole group	Men			Women			Men and women	
		60–65 years	70–75 years	Both age groups	60–65 years	70–75 years	Both age groups	60–65 years	70–7 year
Subjective worse than objective	24.52	26.78	15.25	20.87	29.52	24.52	26.21	28.18	18.5
Same as the physician's assessment	26.44	26.78	23.75	25.22	35.19	26.44	34.95	30.91	28.7
Subjective better than objective	49.04	46.44	61.00	53.91	35.19	49.04	38.84	40.91	52.7

rated their health worse than was to be expected from their medical assessments; only 24.44% rated their health in agreement with the doctor, and 49.4% perceived their health as better than the doctor's assessment. Men rated their health better more often than women (the correlation coefficient between objective and subjective health was 0.31 for men and 0.25 for women).

We could find no significant correlations between the subjective health status and biographical data such as the SES of the family of origin, level of schooling, and the life situation after World War II.

In 1965 the subjective health of men was better than that of women ($P<0.007$). Subjective health was not correlated to mental test scores but was highly related to many personality variables: those who perceived themselves as more healthy were more secure ($P<0.001$), more active ($P<0.002$), more responsive ($P<0.087$), better adjusted ($P<0.09$), in a better state of mind ($P<0.003$) and had more self-control ($P<0.009$). Future time perspective was also more related to subjective than to objective health. Those who felt subjectively healthier – even if diagnosed as being in poor health by the doctor – also showed a higher level of interest ($P<0.02$) in their environment, greater activity, less boredom and loneliness, and a less restricted future time perspective.

In this context we may refer to a finding of our longitudinal analysis of "survivors" and "nonsurvivors" (Lehr and Schmitz-Scherzer 1976). According to this analysis, "longevity" in terms of survivorship was more closely related to subjective health than to objective health. This may be explained by the higher activity of the subjectively more healthy subjects: activity showed the highest correlation with longevity.

Processes of Aging, Personality, and Cognitive Functioning

We have seen that age status and processes of aging are determined by the objective as well as the subjective health status, but they are also influenced by personality variables and intellectual functioning.

Intelligence, as mentioned above, was measured in the BLSA with the Wechsler Bellevue and the Raven tests, while psychomotor performance was measured by the Mierke (*"Kieler Determinationsgerät"*) pursuit rotor, and Beck tests. By contrast, our measures of personality were questionnaires (Riegel inventories, scales on self-concept, etc.), projective techniques (Rorschach, Behn-Rorschach, Wilde, TAT), and most of all intensive and extensive semistructured interviews related to the past (data on life history from childhood onward – we inquired systematically about the time during and after World War II), the present, and the future. An overview is given in the first report of the study (see Thomae 1976).

The major dimensions of personality referred to in this paper are activity and mood (which is high correlated with satisfaction in the present life situation); changes in these areas are often seen as "typical signs of aging."

Intelligence

With regard to intelligence, today is agreement that level of schooling, occupation, SES, ecological conditions and certain secular events determine the level of intellectual functioning during the entire course of life, and especially during old age. Consequently, chronological age in itself does not play a major role during adulthood and old age, but its importance in earlier stages of development has also been questioned. Recent empirical studies confirm that there is neither a general nor a universal decline in cognitive functioning in old age (Baltes and Labouvie 1973; Baltes and Willis 1979; Horn 1978; Labouvie-Vief 1977; Lehr 1972; Rudinger 1974a; Rudinger and Lantermann 1980; Schaie 1980; Thomae 1968, 1976).

In the *cross-sectional* analysis of the BLSA data chronological age accounted for not more than 4.5% of the total variance in general intelligence (verbal part: 1%, performance part 6%–7%). Health accounted for between 8% and 10%, level of schooling for about 19% (verbal part 21%, performance part 13%–14%) and the (former) occupational level in the male group for 20%. Sex accounted for 6% – 8.5% of the variance in the intelligence scores.

The *longitudinal analysis* (Rudinger and Lantermann 1980) showed a complex structure of conditions which are accepted to have an effect on intelligence in old age. This analysis turned particularly to the socioeconomic conditions with their stimulating or depriving attributes. Subjects of higher SES did not show a significant decline in mental abilities during these 12 or 15 years. Persons who had a higher level of schooling showed an increase in the "crystallized" intelligence during this time. A decline in the "fluid intelligence" over this period was correlated with a decline in the objective health status. Finally, residents of rural areas showed a greater decline of intelligence scores over time than the urban population, possibly because of reduced intellectual and cultural stimulation in rural settings (see also Rudinger 1974b; Charles 1973; Schoenfeld 1973).

Personality and Aging: Activity

One of the important signs of aging by which people are judged as "younger" or "older" is the extent, intensity and quality of their activities. Looking first at the findings on women, we find that in the birth cohort 1890–1905, women from lower SES families of origin were more active in old age than women from higher families of origin ($P<0.025$). There is also a highly significant correlation between a higher level of schooling and a lower degree of activity: women with only 8 years of schooling were more active in their sixties and seventies ($P<0.001$). Somewhat to our surprise, older women with lower schooling were rated as more active than those with better education ($P<0.001$). This apparent paradox may be at least partly explained by the fact that middle-class daughters, who were the only ones who had the chance of enjoying partial high-school education, were destined to use their faculties in feminine passivity and obedience as family-centered housewives. They were, according to sex role stereotypes, not allowed to take outside employment; rather, they had to stay in their families of origin and wait to get married. In contrast to middle class women, lower status women at the beginning of this century in Germany were allowed – or forced – to contribute by outside employment to the economic maintenance of both the family of origin and later their family of procreation. In Germany, the very few women of higher status who were permitted to graduate from high school and enter a college and were admitted to a profession in the first quarter of this century in our country were not represented in our sample, which included only lower and middle class people. In this respect we can observe cohort-specific socialization practices resulting in different life-styles from young adulthood into old age.

On the other hand, men of the same birth cohort (1890–1905) show a clear and positive relationship between higher SES of parents ($P<0.001$), as indexed by level of education of fathers ($P<0.01$) and – in a stronger form – of mothers ($P<0.001$), and higher present activity level. More active men reported greater economic ($P<0.005$) and occupational stress ($P<0.04$) after World War II., but also more satisfaction with their occupational choice ($P<0.009$).

The *longitudinal analysis* shows clearly that more than a half of the subjects (51.8%) had a surprising stability and sometimes even an increase in level of activity over the 12/15-year-period of investigation. A declining level of activity was more frequently found in men than in women ($P<0.035$), possibly due to the loss of occupational role and the concomitant reduction in environmental stimulation.

In this connection it may be mentioned that persons living in larger households showed the greatest decline in activity during the 12/15 years: people living in small households (including one-person households) showed stability and frequently even an increase in activity level ($P<0.003$). This may be explained by the fact that these single people had a broader range of interests and more extrafamilial social contacts, which increased during the years of observation; the extrafamilial contacts of married people very often showed a decrease during the 7th to 9th decade of life.

Fooken's (1980a,b) study of the female group of BLSA population showed that unmarried women and women who had become widows or divorcees at a relatively early age (our sample includes a group of war widows) were more active in their sixties, seventies, and eighties than women who had been married all the time or who had become widows during their seventies or eighties. This decline in activity (which very often correlates with decreasing subjective health status and increasing negative mood or depressive reactions), was especially frequent in strongly family-centered women who had not developed any other interests, involvements, or extrafamilial social participation during their former lives. However, more independent women, i.e., women who had worked outside of their home during their middle age and women who were less family-centered in their interests and activities, sometimes perceived the loss of their husband as an extension or expansion of their "life-space", and this was often reinforced by an extended future time perspective.

An additional important finding was that stable or even increasing activity during old age is nearly always contingent on subjectively experienced intensive and positive contacts with friends ($P<0.001$) (see also Thomae 1983). This finding was even stronger than the parallel finding of a correlation of stable or increasing activity with an effort to maintain ($P<0.008$) or extend ($P<0.007$) social contacts; this was true for men and women and for the "younger" as well as for the "older" group of our sample. A positive state of mind or morale ($P<0.001$) and a higher score on responsiveness ($P<0.002$) also correlated with higher activity level in old age.

In our research on social-psychological correlates of longevity (Lehr and Schmitz-Scherzer 1976; Lehr 1982a), higher level of activity was one of the best predictors of survivorship.

Personality and Aging: Mood

In addition to activity, mood is regarded as an indicator of the aging processes. We did not find any significant correlation between SES of the family of origin, educational level, and occupation of parents and mood. Compared with men, women had a more negative mood if they had higher education. This difference was larger in the 1890–95 cohort ($P<0.001$) than in the 1900–05 cohort ($P<0.02$).

In another of our biographical studies (Lehr 1969) we found that women born before 1900 who had to adjust to the conditions of World War I at the age of 14–24 years were much more "emancipated" than those 10–15 years younger. Due to the adverse economic conditions of the 1920s, the women of these cohorts (1900–1915) did not include an occupational career in their plans for the future. Therefore today they very often have more adverse living conditions and more often belong to a problem group of elderly people than those born 10–15 years earlier.

In the female group of the BLSA sample the level of education was not correlated with mood in old age, whereas in the male group a high correlation ($P<0.001$) existed between a better education and more positive mood; in addition, a higher degree of satisfaction with the chosen occupation was correlated with more positive mood ($P<0.04$).

Generally, mood is apparently less influenced by the family of origin and the development in childhood than by specific experiences in later adolescence and adulthood. We found a close relationship between the perception of the situation after World War II and mood in old age. Those men who had a more negative mood in old age reported significantly more stress in the financial ($P<0.01$) as well as in the occupational area ($P<0.03$). Women with a more negative mood more often reported stress and conflict in the relationship with their partners in the period following World War II ($P<0.008$) than did those with a more positive mood.

As far as the *present life situation* was concerned, perceived stress in the family ($P<0.006$) and a larger household ($P<0.01$) correlated with negative mood in men and women. On the other hand – and contrary to our expectations – we did not find any relationship between negative mood and lower SES or higher stress in the financial situation or housing conditions.

The *longitudinal analysis* demonstrated that 45.6% of the subjects were stable or showed an improved mood during the 12 years of observation, while 54.4% displayed a deterioration in mood. This change to a more depressive mood was found more frequently among women than men ($P<0.01$). A deterioration in mood correlated with the perceived unchangeability of their personal situation ($P<0.017$). However, in respect of experienced stressful situations in the areas of "objective" health, ecology and financial situation, we found no significant difference between the subjects at the more depressed pole of the variable "mood" and persons whose scores remained consistent or had moved toward the more positive pole. Only stressful situations in the family were experienced more intensively by the more depressed ($P<0.05$). Subjects who lived in larger households ($P<0.002$) and engaged more in partnership activities ($P<0.02$) reported the most stressful experiences as residing in the partner role. An increasingly positive mood was positively correlated with less activity in the parent role ($P<0.02$) and greater and positively experienced activity in social contacts ($P<0.002$). A more positive mood was related to efforts to broaden the range of personal interests ($P<0.03$), whereas a more negative mood showed a relationship with "impact of narrowing the range of interests" ($P<0.02$).

According to the findings of Fooken (1980a), a deterioration in mood was more frequently reported by married women than by singles ($P<0.06$). A deterioration in positive mood was correlated with growing dissatisfaction and growing stress situations in the family role. These findings may explain why married women in a better financial situation significantly more often showed a deterioration in mood than married women in a worse financial situation ($P<0.02$). Increasingly positive mood was more often found in singles and was correlated with increasing activity in extrafamilial roles, with an increasing range of interests, and with a change to a more positive subjective health status.

Conclusion

The findings reported here represent only a small percentage of the data collected in the detailed biographical studies carried out in Bonn since 1955. We thought that data referring to social background and particularly those pertaining to parameters of the family of origin would be of special interest.

While sociologists tend to draw from such data generalizations about processes of socialization, we tried to show that identical parameters and events may have different consequences in life span development for groups of individuals who differ on other dimensions such as cohort "belongingness" and physical and psychological characteristics. Sex or gender identity introduces, especially in interaction with factors of secular change, new sources of variation. In the final analysis it appears that in addition to norms of aging there exist forms of aging or "patterns of aging." Individual coping styles, that is the way in which an individual tries to come to grips with the vicissitudes of life presented to him by his environment and history, are apparently at the core of these patterns of aging. In any case, life span development is undoubtedly to be viewed as a result of multiple interactions of a variety of social, biological, and psychological effects on the experience of the individual.

References

Baltes PB, Labouvie GV (1973) Adult development of intellectual performance. In: Eisdorfer C, Lawton MP (eds) The psychology of adult development and aging. APA, Washington D.C., pp 157–219

Baltes PB, Schaie KW (1976) On the plasticity of intelligence in adulthood and old age. Am Psychol 31:720–725
Baltes PB, Willis SL (1979) The ciritical importance of appropriate methodology in the study of aging. In: Hoffmeister F, Muller C (eds) Brain function in old age. Springer,Berlin Heidelberg New York, pp 164–187
Birren JE, Schaie KW (1977) Handbook of the psychology of aging. Van Nostrand, New York
Charles DC (1973) Explaining intelligence in adulthood. The role of life history. In: Baltes PB (ed) Life-span models of psychological aging. A symposium. Gerontologist 13:483–488
Cicero (1981) Cato major de senectute (Cato der Ältere über das Alter). dtv, Munich
Eitner S, Tröger A (1968) Soziale Risikofaktoren im Aspekt der gerohygienischen Konzeption. Z Alternsforschung, 21:1–19
Eitner S, Tröger A, Masius E (1971) Schwerarbeit und Alter im mehrdimensionalen Aspekt. Z Alternsforschung 25:139–150
Eitner S, Rühland W, Siggelkow H (eds) (1975) Praktische Gerohygiene. Steinkopff, Dresden
Fooken I (1980a) Frauen im Alter – eine Analyse intra- und inter-individueller Differenzen. Lang, Frankfurt
Fooken I (1980b) Biographische Faktoren des Alterserlebens lediger und langjährig verwitweter Frauen. Z Gerontol 13:475–490
Hippokrates (1962) Prognostikon. Translated by Diller H, Hippokrates, Schriften
Horn JL (1978) Human ability systems. In Baltes PB (ed) Life-span development and behavior, vol. 1. Academic New York, pp 212–257
Hufeland CW (1958) Makrobiotik oder die Kunst, das menschliche Leben zu verlängern, 10th edn. (Ist edn, 1796)
Labouvie-Vief G (1977) Adult cognitive development. Merrill Palmer Q 23:227–263
Lehr U (1969) Die Frau im Beruf – eine entwicklungspsychologische Analyse der weiblichen Berufsrolle. Athenäum, Frankfurt
Lehr U (1972) Psychologie des Alterns. Quelle & Meyer, Heidelberg
Lehr U (1976) Zur Frage der sozialen Benachteiligung älterer Menschen. Medizin, Mensch und Gesellschaft 1:207–214
Lehr U (1982a) Social-psychological correlates of longevity. Annual Review of Gerontology and Geriatrics, III, Springer, New York, pp 102–114
Lehr U (1982b) Subjektiver und objektiver Gesundheitszustand im Lichte von Längsschnittstudien. Medizin, Mensch und Gesellschaft 7:242–248
Lehr U (1982c) Alternsformen statt Altersnormen – psychologische und soziale Aspekte des Alternsprozesses. Schweiz Z Vormundschaftswesen 37:81–100
Lehr U, Thomae H (1979/80) Psychologische Grundlagen der Rehabilitation Herz-Kreislauf-Kranker. Angiokardiologie 2:293–319
Palmore E (ed) (1970) Normal aging, vol. 1. Duke University Press, Durham N.C.
Palmore E (ed) (1974) Normal aging, vol. 2. Duke University Press, Durham N.C.
Rosenmayr L (1976a) Die soziale Benachteiligung alter Menschen. In: Doberauer W (ed) Scriptum Geriatricum. Urban & Schwarzenberg, Munich, pp 203–219
Rosenmayr L (1976b) Schwerpunkte der Soziologie des Alters (Gerosoziologie). In: König R, Rosenmayr L (eds) Handbuch zur empirischen Sozialforschung vol. 7, Enke, Stuttgart, pp 218–406
Rosenmayr L, Rosenmayr R (1978) Der alte Mensch in der Gesellschaft. Rowohlt, Hamburg
Rudinger G (1974a) Eine Querschnittuntersuchung im Altersbereich 20–90 Jahre. Z Gerontol 7:323–333
Rudinger G (1974b) Psychologische Auswirkungen von Dauer des Heimaufeinhalts und sozialer Schicht. Aktuel Gerontol 4:33–38
Rudinger G, Lantermann ED (1980) Soziale Bedingungen der Intelligenz im Alter. Z Gerontol 13:433–441
Schaefer H (1979) Plädoyer für eine neue Medizin. Piper, Munich
Schaie KW (1980) Intelligenzwandel im Erwachsenenalter. Z Gerontol 13:373–384

Schoenfeldt LF (1973) Life history subgroups as moderators in the prediction of intellectual change. In: Jarvik LF, Eisdorfer C, Blum JE (eds) Intellectual functioning in adults. Springer, Berlin Heidelberg New York

Steudel J (1962) Alter Altersveränderung und Alterskrankheiten – historischer Abriß. In: Kaiser H (ed) Der Mensch im Alter. Umschau, Frankfurt, pp 9–12

Swieten G van (1978) Rede über die Erhaltung der Gesundheit der Greise. Wien

Thomae H (1968) Psychische und soziale Aspekte des Alterns. Z Gerontol 1:43–55

Thomae H (ed) (1976) Patterns of aging – findings from the Bonn Longitudinal Study of Aging. Karger, Basel

Thomae H (1983) Alternsstile und Altersschicksale – ein Beitrag zur differentiellen Gerontologie. Huber Bern

3.2 Social Factors Affecting the Mental Health of the Elderly

D. Mechanic

Throughout the developed world, elderly persons are a growing proportion of the population, and in many countries the number of very old persons is increasing markedly. In the United States, for example, the number of elderly increased 55% between 1960 and 1980 to almost 30 million. By the year 2000 we expect and elderly population of more than 36 million (Rice and Feldman 1983). More dramatic and important for health policy, however, is that between 1960 and 1980, persons over 85 years of age increased 174% (Rice and Feldman 1983). The population over 85 is expected to increase by 110% between 1980 and 2000 (Rice and Feldman 1983). By the year 2000 one-quarter of the elderly population will be older than 80. These trends toward an aging population are even more pronounced in various European nations (Crystal 1982). Social expenditure as a proportion of Gross Domestic Product has grown remarkably in all European nations between 1960 and 1981 and has brought about reassessments and retrenchment affecting the elderly (Markham 1984).

The age structure of the population is a product of the fertility of various population cohorts in the past and improving longevity throughout the life course. The increasing numbers and proportions of the elderly of various ages reflect the fact that fertility has remarkably decreased in developed nations with more education, changing family norms, and contraceptive technologies; while improved social conditions, life-styles, and medical interventions have extended the expected life span and period of effective functioning.

The age structure of populations, and the number of people in successive cohorts, have important impact on the opportunities and frustrations experienced by the individuals who make up these cohorts. As the proportion of retired elderly increases in a population relative to those working, a smaller proportion of the population must support the social security, medical care, and welfare benefits of the retired or nonworking population. As these demands fall on smaller segments of populations, potentialities arise for inadequate provision for the elderly and increased conflict among generations. Such problems are not inevitable. They depend on the strength of the economy, the values of the society, and the political power of the elderly, among other factors (Estes 1983b).

In examining the health and welfare of the elderly, and their psychological vulnerability, one must differentiate between age and historical cohort (Riley et al. 1982). Each age cohort faces unique social, economic, and health issues over the life span that shapes personal development, coping resources, and physical functioning. In relation to health, for example, it is abundantly clear that a person of age 65, 75, or even 80 is much more likely than in the past to remain healthy, to live an active and satisfying life, and to retain skills and social effectiveness (Feldman 1983). The artificial dichotomy of those above and below age 65, although socially important because of retirement policies, pension rights and social security benefits, have little scientific relevance for understanding vulnerability and risk. Moreover, health outcomes of past cohorts, when used to project the future burden of illness, health care needs and dependency, while informative, must be used with sensitivity and care.

While aging is not the same as morbidity or loss of capacities it is significantly correlated with such risks. While we remain uncertain as to whether increasing length of life will be relatively free of serious disease until the approach of death (Fries 1980), or marked by high rates of illness burden, incapacity, and dependence over some considerable time (Schneider and Brody 1983), the fact is that with increased scientific knowledge, improved technology, high expectations among the elderly, and their growing political influence, demands for health and social security programs will become a difficult challenge for most developed societies.

While we often think of the aged as a frail subgroup, the majority of aged persons are resilient (National Research on Aging Planning Panel 1982). In part this reflects selective mortality and in part the fact that many of the same social, environmental, and personal factors that promote effective functioning in young adulthood and middle age continue throughout the lifespan. High quality epidemiological data are limited, and major problems involving measurement and nosology persist, but most studies suggest that the incidence of psychiatric impairments, in contrast to chronic physical illness, is modest in the elderly relative to other age groups (Dohrenwend and Dohrenwend 1969; Dohrenwend et al. 1980; Veroff et al. 1981). The prevalence, of course, may be higher because of the longevity of patients with intractable mental disorders that occur at younger ages but persist or recur in later life. Organic brain syndromes, and particularly SDAT, pose major challenges in old age (Kay and Bergmann 1980) both in appropriate diagnosis and the provision of human care.

The factors promoting vulnerability and risk of psychiatric disorder among the elderly are similar to those among younger populations, but various risk factors, or those affecting the course of disease, may be more exaggerated among the elderly. One of the most consistent factors associated with psychiatric morbidity, for example, is deprived socioeconomic status, and in most nations the elderly are at greater risk of deprivation of income and a valued social position. Given the large differential in mortality by sex, large numbers of widows in single-person dwellings must struggle to make ends meet. Socioeconomic deficiencies may affect the quality of shelter, nutrition, social participation, household assistance, and acquisition of needed medical care. Although the economic position of the elderly has been enhanced enormously by improvements in social security and by various health and social programs, many elderly still experience considerable deprivations that interact with other social and biological factors contributing to distress and disorder. One irony is that as income improves, elderly persons choose to live alone, an this decision makes it less likely that they will have an adequate living standard or the assistance that helps functioning in the community (Crystal 1982).

Most studies show that elderly persons continue active relationships with children and kin, but that these relationships are increasingly independent of multigeneration households. While elderly persons living by themselves receive assistance and nurturance from loved ones, such assistance is relatively uncertain as friends, relatives, and even children themselves confront life problems, age, and die. What may have once been an effective and strong source of help and social support may erode with the aging process, and the elderly, if they are to retain their independence and avoid institutionalization, may require formal community and home care services that are too often fragmentary, underdeveloped, and unresponsive.

Residence of the elderly depends on their income, cultural attitudes toward household composition, housing availability, number and geographic mobility of children, and beliefs about financial responsibility of children who themselves may be retired or approaching retirement. In developed countries, children of the elderly, and the aged themselves, see the primary responsibility for the economic welfare of the aged as resting with government and the social security system. Between 1957 and 1974, the proportion of the public considering children responsible for income support of the elderly in the United States decreased from 53% to 10%, and the elderly themselves have even lower expectations (Crystal 1982). Similar patterns are found in other Western countries, as in Holland, where one survey found that less than 10% of old people considered children responsible for financial support of the elderly. In some developed countries, for example Japan, the elderly are much more likely to live with their children, but even this pattern appears to be weakening with relief of housing shortages and changes in attitudes and work force participation.

Good physical health, of course, is a major asset, and when combined with adequate economic resources and social support, provides the basis for a continuing life of satisfaction and well-being among the elderly. Chronic physical illness than induces disability and restricts desired activity, in contrast, is a source of dissatisfaction, depression, and diminished well-being. Moreover, medication for chronic conditions, and their multiple interactive effects, may further diminish a sense of vitality. Recent studies suggest hypersensitivity of the elderly to many drugs, and that elderly suffer from both overmedication and poor compliance. Recent studies in the United States indicate that almost three-quarters of the elderly population received a prescription outside the hospital in 1977. The elderly who received at least one prescription averaged 14.2 prescriptions during the year (Lee and Lipton, 1985).

While certain physical and perceptual capacities diminish with aging, many studies suggest that the stereotype of a downward course in cognitive and social performance is simplistic and ignores both the heterogeneity of the aged and the range of judgmental and coping skills that develop over the life course (Schaie 1980; Riley et al. 1983). Many elderly persons continue to develop their social and coping capacities and others suffer decrements due as much to social and community attitudes as incapacities to perform. Older persons tend to be less physically strong, slower in response, and more cautious and concerned about responding correctly but may counterbalance these with more mature judgment and broader experience. The social response, however, is frequently impatient and may reinforce and stigmatize small deficits that undermine self-esteem, confidence, and a desire for continued participation. These in turn may adversely affect satisfaction and well-being.

The importance of activity and continued participation for maintaining individual skills and overall competence cannot be overemphasized. One of the important conclusions derived from many studies of mental patients is that inactivity and withdrawal promote secondary disabilities that may be more profound than the initial problem (Wing 1978). Inactivity is a significant risk factor for the deterioration of the elderly, and one of the significant preventive insights that can be derived from the literature is the importance of encouraging continued functioning. Experiments involving the elderly that allow their own choices, decision making, and responsibility are associated with enhanced well-being. In contrast, institutional settings, and even community attitudes and responses, commonly encourage dependence and helplessness among many elderly persons. It would be sad to forget a lesson learned so painfully over many decades in the care of the chronic mental patient and persons with significant physical impairments and illnesses. It is through continued activity that individuals maintain their skills and sense of social value (Mechanic 1977).

There is much evidence, as well, that involvement in and commitment to a community or system of cherished values promotes health and well-being (Mechanic 1982). Individuals more closely integrated into family, neighborhood, and community, and who are less alienated and anomic, live longer and express greater well-being. There are many ways in which modern societies make the elderly feel redundant and prematurely limit their options for meaningful activities. Correction of discrimination and stigmatization of the aged can do a great deal to enhance well-being.

Coping effectiveness and self-confidence in part depend on confronting familiar challenges that have been mastered successfully in the past. Various epidemiological studies suggest that rapid social change and social instability pose readjustment problems that all individuals, and perhaps the elderly most of all, find difficult. In the current conceptualization, instability is measured by adverse life events, and there is mounting evidence that such events, in the absence of strong coping skills and social supports, may overwhelm the individual resulting in distress and behavioral dysfunction, physical illness, or both (Dohrenwend and Dohrenwend 1981). Among the elderly, such results are seen particularly in males following the death of their spouses although widows appear to cope more effectively and do not show comparable adverse effects. Disorientation and increased mortality also appear to be associated with moving elderly persons from familiar to unfamiliar environments such as from home to institution, or from one institution to another. While we have yet to identify the specific intervening variables that increase risk, studies of many populations, using diverse methods and approaches, support the general hypothesis that rapid change, even if it brings positive and valued benefits, may have negative consequences for physical functioning and health.

The types of broad influences I have described, such as material welfare, the maintenance and enhancement of coping skills, the nurturance of intimacy and social ties, involvement in and commitment to a system of cherished values, and social stability may affect health directly but also influence such essential psychological dispositions as hope and optimism, self-esteem and confidence, and motivation for maintaining participation in activities. These attitudinal and behavioral dispositions, in turn, affect perceptions of physical health and well-being, complaints of depression, anxiety and somatic discomforts, and use of medical, psychological, and social services (Mechanic 1978). They also increase vulnerability to illness and disability, delay recovery from serious physical illness, surgery and hospitalization, and may also adversely influence essential health behavior and self-care including nutrition, use of alcohol and palliative drugs, and exercise and physical activity important for health maintenance.

Social Factors Affecting the Care of the Elderly

The ability of the elderly to live in the community, to receive appropriate medical and social care, and to avoid institutionalization depends on social security and health entitlements, the organization of families and households, cultural values, and the preferences of the aged themselves. In the last several decades there have been substantial improvements in social security and welfare systems that have allowed people to leave the work force earlier in their lives and, with increased longevity, have led to a much longer span of retirement prior to death (Fuchs 1984). The growth of state sponsored medical insurance for the elderly has substantially increased their share of the funds invested in medical care and access to medical services.

In the United States, public funding for medical care for the elderly and the poor, and the incentives implicit in the Medicare and Medicaid programs, greatly influenced patterns of care for the elderly and forces toward institutionalization. The availability of new funding through these programs, introduced in the mid-1960s, encouraged a substantial growth of nursing home beds and a narrow medical and institutional orientation to the health problems of the aged. Elderly with longstanding psychiatric problems and those developing new problems of disorientation and incapacity were particularly affected since existing programs were overwhelmingly directed to care for services provided in institutions, but severely restricted payments for out-of-hospital mental health services (Steering Committee on thc Chronically Mentally Ill 1980). Because of the financial incentives implicit in these programs, the nursing home became a convenient solution not only for the disoriented or incapacitated elderly but also for many younger chronic mental patients who had limited alternatives for appropriate care.

In the period 1975–77, of the 1.3 million nursing home beds, approximately 750 000 were occupied by persons with mental impairments (Goldman et al. 1981). Approximately 350 000 were persons with a primary or secondary mental health diagnosis based on the ICD, and 400 000 diagnosed as suffering from senility without psychosis. In contrast to the 150 000 chronic patients in mental health institutions, the nursing home was the hidden but primary system of chronic mental health care for patients of all ages. While there were strong doubts that the restrictive and inactive atmospheres of these institutions, their low levels of professional staffing, and their dependence on sedation to manage patients, was a good strategy for care of chronicity (Stotsky 1970), this pattern emerged because existing programs paid for such care and not for alternatives. While most analysts concede that such care is neither cost-effective in the individual case, nor the best available system for caring for many of the patients involved, the advantage of the system relative to alternatives is that it has implicit built-in financial protections. The typical elderly person does much to resist institutionalization, and the nursing home becomes the last resort when other informal mechanisms to retain independence fail. The fear among financial analysts is that a more cost-effective but attractive home care alternative would enlist many more elderly leading to substantially increased aggregate costs.

As we look to the future, it is clear that we need a better way of developing community care structures for the elderly and the chronically mentally ill. Such alternatives are particularly difficult to develop and administrate and to finance under existing health and welfare programs. But they offer better opportunities to promote continued functioning and to avoid dependence, and to provide a wide range of social-medical services better fitted to the needs of the elderly. The medicalization of long-term care encourages unrealistic curative efforts, overuse of technologies that often contribute to the further incapacity of many frail elderly, and inappropriate heroic efforts (Gillick 1984). While the appropriate margins of medical activity are not well defined, and good medical care has an indispensable role in the overall pattern, the medical dominance of long-term care and a narrow medical approach can be a real disservice to meeting the health needs of the elderly.

As we confront new demographic realities in the coming decades, there is much we can do to enhance the quality of life of the elderly and to facilitate their continued involvement and contributions to the community. The development of a sound system of social security has been the single most significant factor affecting the welfare of the aged in the United States during this century. While the system faces financial problems at various points in time because of changing demography and economic circumstances, rates of taxation for social welfare benefits are comparatively low in the United States relative to many European nations. Government spending relative to the Gross Domestic Product was only 33.2% in 1980, as compared with 40.7% in Canada, 46.2% in France, 46.9% in Germany, and 66.7% in Sweden (Estes 1983a). There is little doubt that the United States can finance an adequate social security system. The seeming alarm is as much a crisis of values as an issue of economic viability.

The foregoing is not to suggest that the changing demographic structures of developed nations do not pose serious problems of equity among varying age cohorts with changes in the dependency ratio between the working population and the elderly. In the United States, for example, there were approximately nine workers for each elderly person in 1930, approximately four expected between 1980 and 2010 (National Research on Aging Planning Panel 1982), and approximately two in 2030 if present trends continue. A substantial improvement in the economic status of the elderly has occurred during this period, closing the gap in economic deprivations between the elderly and other age groups. When one considers need and other nonincome transfers to the aged, they may even be better off economically than some other age groups. But the elderly population is not homogeneous and includes subpopulations that suffer considerable privations.

While the dependency ratio relative to the elderly has been increasing, declining fertility has reduced the total dependency ratio relative to what it was in 1970 (Ball 1982), and in the aggregate it is expected to decline during the next century. While the economic resources necessary to support an elderly person relative to a child are more substantial, it is increasingly asked whether more of the economic care for the aged should be assumed by their children. The facts that the aged's children are themselves increasingly elderly and that the public perceives the aged as a national responsibility make it questionable whether a significant solution can be found in transferring significant costs to their children.

Given the concerns about the growing proportions of elderly relative to the working population, it is ironic that we provide few incentives for the young elderly who retain their motivation and vitality to remain in the work force. Both our social security and tax systems do little to encourage continued participation in work and relatively few efforts are made to utilize the skills, experience, and wisdom of the elderly in voluntary activities. The elderly population constitutes a large untapped reservoir of skill and potential productivity that we have not been particularly imaginative about. Current knowledge suggests that using this resource would also contribute in many ways to the health and vitality of the elderly as well.

In much of the world, we can do a great deal to capitalize on the desire of the elderly themselves to retain function and avoid dependence and particularly institutionalization. Elderly persons commonly tolerate many privations and difficulties to retain residence in their households and to avoid institutional dependency. Entry into a nursing home or comparable facility often follows major illness and disability, death or major illness of a spouse or primary caretaker, or other major breakdowns in social supports. Institutionalization is resisted and typically is a last resort when individuals can no longer manage by themselves.

The foregoing suggests that sound social policy regarding the aged would make accessible the types of home care and supports that assist the elderly person's struggle to maintain independence and control over their lives. Innumerable studies show that home care is preferred by the elderly and cost-effective on an individual basis. In the aggregate, home care has threatening financial implications because the negative perceptions of nursing homes result in many needy elderly struggling along without services, and the unattractiveness of this alternative effectively operates to ration services and expenditures. The fear is, and it is supported by some evidence, that should more attractive options be available, the demand will rise substantially. Such financial concerns are not trivial, but it would be more appropriate and humane to develop better quality assessment and screening devices for access to long-term care services than to pursue solutions whose primary advantage is that the character of the service itself deters demand.

A second important area for action as well as research is the design of incentives that encourage isolated elderly to live together, substantially increasing their financial resources and social supports. While present trends are toward increased single person households (Crystal 1982), and many elderly prefer this, creative joint housing arrangements that allow communal living but preserve privacy as well might influence individual decision making. Moreover, much more could be done to help the elderly identify compatible living partners, and to socially legitimize such household arrangements. We also need to develop more effective structures that capture the energies of the more vigorous elderly to contribute to those more frail or to the society more generally.

Developed societies that anticipate an increasing elderly population have grave concerns about the growing possibilities and costs of medical care, the increasing burden of financing long-term care, and the decreasing proportion of persons in the labor force in relation to the elderly. In the United States in 1980, the 11% of persons over 65 accounted for 31% of personal health expenditures. Much of these costs are expended during the last year of life, and of these expenditures almost half in the two months prior to death (U.S. Department of Health and Human Services 1984). While it is difficult to anticipate who will live and who will die, there is substantial agreement that the pattern of high technology medicine at the end of life does not use available resources to maximize the social welfare of the elderly.

We must evolve a better method of balancing the allocation of available resources between hospital based medical care, home based social-medical care and appropriate long-term care where the medical model is not so dominant. One way of achieving this is by developing organizations in the community that assume responsibility for the entire spectrum of services on a capitated basis, that either maintain or contract for all necessary services on behalf of the elderly, and that make determinations of appropriate patterns of care given various needs, inclinations, and tastes of those for whom they are responsible. Such community structures face formidable political and technical barriers and much effort would be necessary to develop appropriate criteria and quality assurance measures and to build the organizational structures necessary to bridge the array of professional and supportive services required.

In the United States, at present, research and demonstration projects are directed to studying a broad range of alternative approaches to the provision and financing of long-term care. One exciting alternative is the Social Health Maintenance Organization Program (SHMO), a capitated delivery system for the elderly and disabled. This concept attempts to overcome the fragmentation of financing and categorical services by a single system responsible for acute hospital and nursing services, ambulatory medical care, and such personal care support services as homemaker, home health, and chore services. Other services include emergency psychiatric care, meals, counseling, transportation, etc. The provider organization takes on all financial, programmatic, and case decision responsibility within the capitation constraint (Hamm et al. 1982).

The challenges ahead in the care of the aged are not easy. They make clear the limitations of our resources, the inadequacies of our knowledge, and the fragmentation of our social policies and politics. How we respond to the challenge to provide humane and responsive care for our elderly, and the quality of life and function we allow them in their remaining years, will say much about Western societies and the integrity of their systems of values and behavior.

References

Ball R (1982) The financial condition of the social security program. Study Group on Social Security, New York

Crystal S (1982) America's old age crisis: Public policy and the two worlds of aging. Basic Books, New York

Dohrenwend BP, Dohrenwend BS (1969) Social status and psychological disorder: a causal inquiry. Wiley-Interscience, New York

Dohrenwend BS, Dohrenwend BP (eds) (1981) Stressful life events and their contexts. Rutgers University Press, New Brunswick, NJ

Dohrenwend B, Dohrenwend B, Gould M, Link B, Neugebauer R, Wunch-Hitzig R (1980) Mental illness in the United States: Epidemiological estimates. Praeger, New York

Estes C (1983a) Fiscal austerity and aging. In: Estes C, Newcomer R et al. (eds) Fiscal austerity and aging: Shifting government responsibility for the elderly. Sage Publications, Beverly Hills, Ca, p 25

Estes C (1983b) Social Security: The social construction of a crisis. Health Soc 61:445–472

Feldman J (1983) Work ability of the aged under conditions of improving mortality. Health Soc 61:430–444

Fries J (1980) Aging, natural death, and the compression of morbidity. New Engl J Med 303:130–135

Fuchs V (1984) Though much is taken-reflections on aging, health and medical care. Health Soc 62:143–166

Gillick M (1984) Is the care of the chronically ill a medical prerogative? New Engl J Med 310:190–193

Goldman H, Gattozzi A, Taube C (1981) Defining and counting the chronically mentally ill. Hosp Community Psychiatry 32:21–27

Hamm L, Kickham T, Cutler D (1982) Research demonstrations and evaluations. In: Vogel R, Palmer H (eds) Long-term care: Perspectives from research and demonstrations. U.S. Dept Human Serv, Health Care Financing Admin, Washington DC, pp 167–253

Kay D, Bergmann K (1980) Epidemiology of mental disorders among the aged in the community. In: Birren J, Sloane RB (eds) Handbook of mental health and aging. Prentice Hall, Englewood Cliffs, NJ, pp 34–56

Lee P, Lipton HL (1985) The role of drugs and the U.S. pharmaceutical industry in health care. In: Goldberg T (ed) Review, discussion and implications of state drug substitution laws. National Center for Health Services Research (DHHS), Hyattsville, Md.

Markham J (1984) Europe, too, feels the social program pinch. New York Times, Feb 19, Sec E, p 3

Mechanic D (1977) Illness behavior, social adaptation, and the management of illness: a comparison of educational and medical models. J Nerv Ment Dis 165:79–87

Mechanic D (1978) Medical sociology, 2nd edn. The Free Press, New York

Mechanic D (1982) Disease, mortality, and the promotion of health. Health Aff 1 (3):28–32

National Research on Aging Planning Panel (1982) Toward an independent old age: a national plan for research on aging. U.S. Dept Health Human Serv, Washington DC, NIH Pub No. 82–2453

Rice D, Feldman J (1983) Living longer in the United States: demographic changes and health needs of the elderly. Health Soc 61:362–396

Riley M, Abeles R, Teitelbaum M (eds) (1982) Aging from birth to death, vol II. Sociotemporal perspectives. Westview Press, Boulder, pp 1–26

Riley M, Hess B, Bond K (eds) (1983) Aging in society: Selected reviews of recent research. Lawrence Erlbaum Assoc, Hillsdale, NJ

Schaie WW (1980) Intelligence and problem solving. In: Birren J and Sloane RB (eds) Handbook of mental health and aging. Prentice Hall, Englewood Cliffs, NJ, pp 262–284

Schneider E, Brody J (1983) Aging, natural death, and the compression of morbidity: Another view. New Engl J Med 309:854–855
Steering Committee on the Chronically Mentally Ill (1980) Toward a national plan for the chronically mentally ill. Dept Health Human Serv, Washington, DC
Stotsky BA (1970) The nursing home and the aged psychiatric patient. Appleton-Century-Crofts, New York
U.S. Department of Health and Human Services (1984) Health – United States, 1983. National Center for Health Statistics (PHS), Washington, DC 84–1232, p 15
Veroff J, Kulka R, Douvan E (1981) Mental health in America: Patterns of help-seeking from 1957–1976. Basic Books, New York
Wing JK (1978) Reasoning about madness. Oxford University Press, Oxford

3.3 Social Support and Mental Disorder in Old Age: Overview and Appraisal

H. O. F. Veiel

In recent years "social support" has become an increasingly important concept in social epidemiology and community psychology and psychiatry. The notion that social conditions and processes influence mental and physical well-being is an old one, however. At the end of the last century, Durkheim (1897) emphasized the connection between social alienation ("anomie"; cf. Merton 1938) and suicide, and social isolation came to be recognized as a major determinant of mental illness (e.g., Faris 1934; Jaco 1954; Leighton 1959). A more elaborate framework for the study of pathogenic influences of social structures was later provided by so-called network theory (e.g., Barnes 1972), which distinguished between different *types* of social connectedness. The concept of social support has emerged from these traditional areas of sociological research, and during the last 10 years it has assumed a prominent position in theories of mental illness. In contrast to the sociological concepts of "anomie" and "social network," however, which were at least initially applied to social aggregates, the social support concept reflects a greater emphasis on individual conditions and needs, and on the adequacy of social relationships and transactions in fulfilling these needs. It is therefore not surprising, that, in addition to the approaches mentioned above, a number of other traditional areas of social research have influenced current thinking in the field. Attachment theory (cf. Bowlby 1969, 1973) and related approaches, for instance, have contributed a great deal to theoretical formulations on social support. They emphasize the necessity of close social bonds for normal psychological development and for maintaining mental health. Weiss (1974), for example, who is often referred to in theoretical treatments of the subject (e.g., Brown and Harris 1978), discussed a number of individual needs that have to be fulfilled by social relationships, such as "attachment," "social integration," "nurturance," "assurance of worth," "alliance," and "guidance". Another area of social research that has influenced the field is coping and psychotherapy research, which tends to emphasize the role of social support as crisis help and coping aid (cf. Gottlieb 1981). Broadhead et al. (1983), in a recent review, even stated that "the internal determinants of social support are, in fact, coping strategies" (p. 531). In contrast, the sociological approaches mentioned above were not specific about the mechanisms by which social factors influence mental health, and attachment theory seems to regard the social context as an independent and immediate determinant of human well-being, rather than as a moderator of stress. The different roots of current social support research, and the divergent conceptualizations and methodological paradigms it comprises, would make one expect conceptual incongruities and empirical contradictions. Nevertheless, there now exists a large body of research documenting the usefulness of the social support concept.

Some Empirical Results

The beneficial effects of social relationships and transactions on mental and physical health have been documented in an impressive number of empirical studies. Social contacts have been reported to lower general mortality (e.g., Berkman and Syme 1979; Blazer 1982), to protect against depression (e.g., Billings and Moos 1981; Brown and Harris 1978) and against mental illness and psychological distress in general (e.g., Williams et al. 1981; Lin et al. 1979; Miller and Ingham 1976), to reduce pregnancy complications (Nuckolls et al. 1972; Norbeck and Tilden 1983), and to prevent or alleviate a host of other ailments and disorders.

Despite the enormous number of recent studies in the field, few were concerned with the specific situation of the elderly. Among these few, moreover, the results were inconsistent. On the one hand, Lowenthal and Haven (1968) reported that the presence of intimate relationships was associated with good mental health and even compensated for the otherwise generally deleterious effects of low levels of social interaction. Similarly, Stephens et al. (1978) showed that alienation and depression increase monotonically with decreasing levels of social support, and Blazer (1982) found increased mortality rates in a subgroup of elderly subjects with very low social interaction and perceived support. Gurland et al. (1980), on the other hand, found no overall effect of social support variables on mental health in an elderly sample in New York, and Kay et al. (1964b) data suggest at most a weak relationship between indices of isolation and functional mental disorders. Nielsen (1962) also reported onla a weak association between social isolation and mental disorder, and Murphy (1983) found no evidence that an intimate relationship protected against relapses of depression. Sosna (1983), in a large-scale survey of elderly inhabitants of the city of Mannheim, found mental health to be associated with only some of a number of social support indices. These were, moreover, empirically or conceptually related to feelings of alienation and reduced extrafamiliar contacts, which are *symptoms* of poor mental health (cf. Blazer 1983).

The mixed evidence of beneficial effects of social support on mental health in the elderly stands in contrast to the abundant evidence of such effects in general populations. One probable reason for this discrepancy is the reduced variation of social support variables in samples of old people: A number of studies show that the number of social contacts and relationships tends to decrease with age (e.g., Blau 1961; Phillips 1957; Sosna 1983; Stephens et al. 1978; Townsend 1957; Tunstall 1961), and one can assume that the variation of these and other social support variables decreases correspondingly. The lower the variation of variables, the more difficult it becomes to establish empirical associations. It is probably no accident that Stephens et al. (1978), who found social support to be clearly associated with mental health in their elderly sample, report that "relatively few of the aging people studied score low on the social support system..." (p. 37).

A second likely reason is the selection process in communities whereby mentally disturbed people without social support are more likely to be removed to institutions than those with intact social support systems (Sosna 1983). Field studies of mental health in the elderly, therefore, have to deal with selected populations in which the distribution of social spport and mental health is biased against finding associations between them. Similar selective mechanisms exist, of course, for younger subjects, buth these are more likely to be integrated in a functional nexus (e.g., work rules) that provides normative structures and cognitive guidance, and that makes them go on in the community despite being depressed, anxious, etc., even when no emotional or help-giving support system exists.

Another cause of the inconsistent empirical results lies in the differences between the various measures of social support. While Kay et al. (1964b) and Nielsen (1962), for example, used single items (marital status, living conditions) as indicators of social support or social isolation, Gurland et al. (1980) used composite indices of social contacts and relationships, and of need fulfilment. None of these investigators found substantial general associations between social support and functional mental disorders. The one approach may have missed important aspects of the social context, the other may have buried them under many irrelevant variables. Multidimensional studies which systematically vary conceptual and empirical dimensions of social support are completely lacking. The practice of separately calculating the effects of single items such as marital status or living cnditions is no viable substitute for systematically examining different support dimensions. While it may reveal differential effects, such a strategy depends for its success on the accidents of item selection and item definition, and allows few systematic generalizations.

A further cause of the inconsistency and lack of clarity of the results lies in the neglect of motivational and personality variables except in a general and indirect way through indices of "satisfaction" with social contacts (e.g., Henderson et al. 1981) or of "loneliness" (e.g., Sosna 1983), which causes methodological problems (see below). Gurland et al. (1980) reported that voluntarily isolated old people were not worse off than socially integrated ones, and that only the *involuntarily* isolated showed worse mental health. Lowenthal (1964) similarly found a subset of elderly subjects in her community sample with a lifelong pattern of isolation who were, as a group, not more impaired than the more socially integrated subjects.

A related issue concerns the decreased relevance of some of the usual indicators of social support for the elderly. Normative expectations change in old age, and whereas, for example, being married is (or was) the expected state of affairs for middle age and young adulthood, this is no longer the case in old age, when spouses are increasingly likely to have died. While not being married in middle age may signify a generalized pattern of normative deviance with a concomitant higher risk of mental disorder, the proportion of such individuals among the unmarried elderly is bound to be smaller. Hence, to the extent that the detrimental effects of not being married on mental health in general population samples is related to general normative deviance, they will be more difficult to demonstrate in older populations[1].

Lastly, the causes of mental disorders in old age are different from those relevant for younger populations. The increased prevalence of age-related

1 This and the following point were suggested by Prof. H. Häfner

degenerative processes, not always evident, leads to a concomitantly reduced proportion of functional disorders which are, by definition, more responsive to psychosocial influences. The association of support factors with indices of overall mental health can therefore be expected to be lower in the elderly.

Taken together, the above considerations would let one expect difficulties in empirically demonstrating beneficial effects of social support in old age, and may explain the incongruous results in the area. Some of the methodological and conceptual problems indicated are typical for research with older populations, but others reflect general problems in definition, operationalization, and measurement that exist in the social support field as a whole. These will be discussed below. Before doing so, however, I shall elaborate on the opportunity for therapeutic and preventive intervention provided by the social support approach.

The Opportunity for Intervention

Although the relative incidence of functional mental disorders in the elderly does not seem to exceed the rate for the population as a whole (Mechanic, this volume), the expected increase in the sheer number of old people (cf. Hauser, this volume) makes old age mental health a social concern of prime importance. While the causes of functional mental disorders in the elderly are multiple, a fair proportion of them can probably be attributed to the occurrence of stressful events and conditions which are characteristic for old age, and for which one's socialization and personal history provide no ready-made coping strategies. Among those typical stressful experiences are: retirement; death of spouses, relatives, and friends; status changes; poverty; and ill health (cf. Hooyman 1983). Their detrimental effect on mental health is well documented (e.g., Kay et al. 1964a, 1964b; Stein and Susser 1970; Richardson 1965). At the same time, old people are generally characterized by low levels of social support which, the inconsistencies in the relatively few studies of elderly populations notwithstanding, does seem to protect against mental distress and disorder. While relatively little can be done to prevent stressful events and conditions, the low support levels present a great opportunity to improve the situation of a large and increasing proportion of the population (cf. Cassel 1976). The potential benefits include also financial savings for society as a whole. O'Brien and Whitelaw (1978; quoted after Hooyman 1983) reported that low social support is associated with a greater probability of (expensive) institutionalization. Kammeyer and Bolton (1968; quoted after Hooyman 1983) showed that the use of formal service agencies tends to be higher in old people without supportive relationships. With the expected dramatic increase in the number of old people, a focussed and effective policy of creating and improving opportunities for supportive social structures and transactions would probably pay off handsomely. Unfortunately, the empirical results in the field are too inconsistent to allow the definition of precise targets for social support intervention. These empirical inconsistencies, as argued above, are rooted in theoretical and operational ones. Before intervention programs can be set up, therefore, a number of conceptual and methodological issues have to be resolved.

Current Issues in Social Support Research

These issues concern the nature of social support, the direction of causality of the reported associations, and the psychological mechanisms that mediate the beneficial effects.

What is "Social Support"?

The number of different definitions and operationalizations of social support that are offered in the literature is enormous. Among the most often cited theoretical authors on social support, Cobb (1976), for example, defines it as *information* that one belongs to a socially coherent community and that one is loved and esteemed. Kaplan et al. (1977) define it as the *state* of presence of social resources or, alternately, of satisfied basic needs, and House (1981) regards it as an interpersonal *transaction* including concern, aid, and information about oneself and the environment.

The theoretical confusion indicated here is mirrored in the multitude of different operationalizations and measures used in empirical investigations, such as "intimate relationships" (Brown and Harris 1978), social activity and number of friends of relatives available (e.g. Bell et al. 1982; Andrews et al. 1978; Williams et al. 1981), perceived supportiveness (e.g. Schaefer et al. 1981), marital status and other socioeconomic parameters (e.g., Myers et al. 1972), and a number of network characteristics (e.g., Warheit et al. 1982). It is quite unlikely that all these different operationalizations and measures capture the same thing. While there have been a number of attempts to systematize the different aspects of social support (e.g., House 1981; Kaplan et al. 1977), Thoits (1982) was quite accurate in stating that "most investigators have not attempted to formulate a precise definition of social support, and few have attempted to develop valid or reliable indicators of the concept" (p. 146), and the inconsistent results currently found in the literature bear witness to that. As I have argued elsewhere (Veiel 1985), the implicit assumption of a single commodity "social support" that is provided by a variety of social transactions and relationships is largely to blame for this confusion, and the establishment of a comprehensive and differentiated conceptual framework overdue.

The "Buffer" Controversy

The notion of social conditions as pathogenic factors was initially, i.e., in the early epidemiological studies, quite straightforward, being based on the direct association of social parameters with mental health variables. With the emergence of the social support concept in the 1970s and probably because of its narrower focus on individual rather than social parameters, the beneficial influence of the social environment seems to have been increasingly conceptualized as a *protective* one, "buffering" against psychosocial stress (Nuckolls et al. 1972; Cassel 1976; Kaplan et al. 1977). An increasing number of reports claim to have found such buffer effects, to witness recent volumes of the relevant journals, but it is still debatable whether these are real and/or substantial (cf. Thoits 1982; Gore 1981). Although the notion of social support as a kind of armor against the vicissitudes of life is appealing, there are methodological problems in empirically proving that it is so. In empirical research, the presence of statistical interactions of stress variables with support variables is generally taken as proof for a stress-buffering effect of social support. If social support measures are confounded with measures of psychosocial stress, and they usually are (death of a spouse, for example, is commonly counted as a "stressful life event," but also has obvious consequences for the social support system of the individual), spurious interaction effects arise in empirical investigations (Thoits 1982; Kessler 1983). However, the issue of buffer or no buffer effects is probably overblown in the literature. With respect to theoretical and practical implications, it is of arguably little importance whether or not social support interacts with stressful events and situations in general: given the ubiquity of psychosocial stress in life, even direct (statistical main) effects of social support could have been produced by its buffering against stress. On the other hand, if a particular social support factor could be found to buffer against a particular stressful condition and not against others, meaningful deductions could be made. Such differential effects were only rarely examined in recent investigations, however. The discussion about buffer effects shows the relatively atheoretical character of current research in the field: it is held on a methodological level, and the psychological mechanisms mediating the supposed effects of social support are rarely addressed. If more were known here, the issue of buffer or no buffer effects might well disappear in a broader theoretical perspective.

Causality Issues

The emergence of social support as an important concept in research on mental health is based on the assumption of its causal role in the etiology of mental disorder. This is but an assumption, albeit a plausible one, which is difficult to prove. Most research in the field uses cross-sectional designs that do not allow firm inferences regarding the direction of causality of observed associations, and a number of alternative causal mechanisms should be considered:

a) Mental disorders may make the social support context disintegrate. Blazer (1983) found low social support to be a *consequence* of major depressive disorder in the elderly. Henderson and Moran (1983), however, could not find such a reverse effect in a general population sample.

b) Stressful life events may make the social support system disintegrate. It stands to reason that typical social support indicators that reflect everyday social patterns involving unknown proportions of fair-weather friends is only loosely related to support in times of crisis. Dean and Lin (1977) made the more specific prediction that "life events will decrease social support in an inverse relationship to initial levels of social support" (p. 411). Few, if any, empirical investigations exist to shed light on the issue.

c) Social conditions may influence, at the same time, the amount of support individuals receive, the amount of psychosocial stress impinging on them, and also, perhaps, their mental health directly. With respect to the elderly, a likely source of confounding is age itself: it may, via separate causal mechanisms, induce social isolation, high stress levels, and poor mental health (e.g. through accumulating degenerative effects). Another such background variable may be social status. A substantial association of such third variables with both psychosocial stress and social support would leave open whether the support measured with a particular instrument, or the concomitant increase in psychosocial stress, or the third variable directly, is responsible for any observed change in the dependent variable.

d) Social support may be confounded with personality variables. Henderson (Henderson et al. 1978; Henderson, 1984) has argued that it is not so much the objective social circumstances but the attitudes and needs of the individual concerned that determine the presence or absence of supportive effects. This is reflected in the apparently paradoxical findings of Lowenthal and Haven (1968) and Kobasa et al. (1981) about the lack of detrimental effects of low support in certain categories of individuals. Generally, personality variables can be expected to influence social support on three levels: firstly by determining the size and character of the social network, i.e., of the potentially available resources (cf. Henderson et al. 1978); secondly by determining the extent to which the individual is able and willing to *use* these resources (cf. Pearlin and Schooler, 1978); and thirdly by influencing the subjective perceptions of magnitude and adequacy of available and/or received support.

It is very likely that all the above effects combine with a genuinely causal effect of social support factors on mental health to produce the associations reported in the literature. In order to determine which aspect of the social context is relevant in a given context, differentiated measures and multidimensional investigations of supportive social factors are necessary. Together with psychological models of the mechanisms by which social support affects mental health (another weak point of current research), they may eventually allow us to make sense of the present multitude of incompatible results. If such differentiated measures are to go beyond a mere separation of questionnaire items, however, a correspondingly different-tiated theoretical elaboration of the social support concept is needed. As the above discussion of the different and divergent definitions and operationalizations indicates, such a comprehensive theory is nowhere in sight.

Summary and Conclusions

While there is a large body of literature documenting the beneficial influence of supportive social structures and transactions on mental health, the evidence of such effects in the elderly is relatively sketchy. The reasons are multiple and partly due to specific problems of social support research in the elderly, partly characteristic for the field as a whole. Among the former figure the general low level of support the elderly receive and its probably reduced variance, which makes it more difficult to detects its effects statistically; the particular situation of the elderly regarding the etiology of their mental health problems and also regarding the importance of particular support indices; and the removal of the mentally ill without social support to institutions, which makes for biased survey data. For the field as a whole it can be stated that the poor development of the social support concept has led to a multitude of different operationalizations and measurement instruments which are not directly comparable, and which may well capture irrelevant aspects of the social context.

The opportunity for preventive and therapeutic intervention offered by the social support concept underscores the need for more precise empirical data than are available to date. Meaningful research will have to take account of the particular conditions of elderly populations, and to be methodologically sophisticated enough to be able to demonstrate causal effects. Since these may be, at least partly, specific to particular types of support and to particular problems, empirical efforts should be embedded in a comprehensive and differentiated conceptual framework.

References

Andrews G, Tennant C, Hewson DM, Vaillant GE (1978) Life event stress, social support, coping style, and risk of psychological impairment. J Nerv Ment Dis 166:307–316

Barnes JA (1972) Social networks. Addison-Wesley, Reading MA

Bell RA, Leroy JB, Stephenson JJ (1982) Evaluating the mediating effects of social support upon life events and depressive symptoms. J Community Psychol 10:325–340

Berkman LF, Syme SL (1979) Social networks, host resistance, and mortality: nine-year follow-up study of Alameda County residents. Am J Epidemiol 109:186–204

Billings AG, Moos RH (1981) The role of coping responses and social resources in attenuating the stress of life events. J Behav Med 4:139–157

Blau ZS (1961) Structural constraints on friendship in old age. Am Sociol Rev 26:430–440

Blazer DG (1982) Social support and mortality in an elderly community population. Am J Epidemiol 115:684–694

Blazer DG (1983) Impact of late-life depression on the social network. Am J Psychiatry 140:162–165

Bowlby J (1969) Attachment and loss, vol 1, Attachment. Basic Books, New York

Bowlby J (1973) Attachment and loss, vol 2, Separation. Hogarth, London

Broadhead WE, Kaplan BH, James SA, Wagner EH, Schoenbach VJ, Grimson R, Heyden S, Tibblin G, Gehlbach SH (1983) The epidemiologic evidence for a relationship between social support and health. Am J Epidemiol 117:521–537

Brown GW, Harris T (1978) Social origins of depression. Tavistock, London

Cassel J (1976) The contribution of the social environment to host resistance. Am J Epidemiol 104:107–123

Cobb S (1976) Social support as a moderator of life stress. Psychosom Med 38:300–315

Dean A, Lin N (1977) The stress-buffering role of social support. J Nerv Ment Dis 165:403–417

Durkheim E (1897) Le suicide. Presses Universitaires de France, Paris

Faris REL (1934) Cultural isolation and the schizophrenic personality. Am J Sociol 40:155–164

Gottlieb BH (1981) Social networks and social support in community mental health. In: Gottlieb BH (ed) Social networks and social support. Sage, London

Gore S (1981) Stress-buffering functions of social supports: An appraisal and clarification of research models. In: Dohrenwend BS, Dohrenwend BP (eds) Stressful life events and their contexts. Prodist, New York

Gurland B, Bennett R, Wilder D (1980) Planning for the elderly in New York. An assessment of depression, dementia, and isolation. Proceedings of the Research Utilization Workshop. Community Council of Greater New York, New York
Henderson S (1984) Interpreting the evidence on social support. Soc Psychiatry 19:49–52
Henderson S, Byrne DG, Duncan-Jones P, Adcock S, Scott R, Steele GP (1978) Social bonds in the epidemiology of neurosis. A preliminary communication. Br J Psychiatry 136:574–583
Henderson S, Byrne DG, Duncan-Jones P (1981) Neurosis and the social environment. Academic Press, London
Henderson S, Moran PAP (1983) Social relationships during the onset and remission of neurotic symptoms: a prospective community study. Br J Psychiatry 143:467–472
Hooyman N (1983) Social support networks in services to the elderly. In: Whittaker JK, Garbarino J (eds) Social support networks. Aldine, New York
House JS (1981) Work stress and social support. Addison-Wesley, Reading (Mass)
Jaco EG (1954) The social isolation hypothesis and schizophrenia. Am Sociol Rev 19:567–577
Kammeyer K, Bolton C (1968) Community and family factors related to the use of a family service agency. J Marriage Fam 30:488–498
Kaplan BH, Cassel JD, Gore S (1977) Social support and health. Med Care 15:47–58
Kay DWK, Beamish P, Roth M (1964a) Old age mental disorders in Newcastle upon Tyne, Part 1. Br J Psychiatry 110:146–158
Kay DWK, Beamish P, Roth M (1964b) Old age mental disorders in Newcastle upon Tyne, Part 2. Br J Psychiatry 110:668–682
Kessler RC (1983) Methodological issues in the study of psychosocial stress. In: Kaplan HB (ed) Psychosocial stress: recent developments in theory and method. Academic Press, New York
Kobasa SC, Maddi SR, Courington S (1981) Personality and constitution as mediators on the stress-illness relationship. J Health Soc Behav 22:368–378
Leighton AH (1959) My name is Legion. Vol. 1 of the Stirling County Study. New York
Lin N, Simeone RS, Ensel WM, Kuo W (1979) Social support, stressful life events and illness. J Health Soc Behav 20:108–109
Lowenthal MF (1964) Social isolation and mental illness in old age. Am Sociol Rev 29:55–70
Lowenthal MF, Haven C (1968) Interaction and adaptation: intimacy as a critical variable. Am Sociol Rev 33:20–30
Merton RK (1938) Social structure and anomie. Revisions and extensions. In: Anshen RA (ed) The family: its function and destiny. Harper, New York
Miller PM, Ingham JG (1976) Friends, confidants and symptoms. Soc Psychiatry 11:51–58
Murphy E (1983) The prognosis of depression in old age. Br J Psychiatry 142:111–119
Myers JK, Lindenthal JL, Pepper MP, Ostrander DP (1972) Life events and mental status: a longitudinal survey. J Health Soc Behav 13:398–406
Nielsen J (1962) Geronto-psychiatric period-prevalence investigation in a geographically delimited population. Acta Psychiatr Scand 38:307–330
Norbeck JS, Tilden VP (1983) Life stress, social support, and emotional disequilibrium in complications of pregnancy: a prospective, multivariate study. J Health Soc Behav 24:30–46
Nuckolls KB, Cassel J, Kaplan BH (1972) Psychosocial assets, life crisis, and the prognosis of pregnancy. Am J Epidemiol 95:431–441
O'Brien J, Whitelaw N (1978) Planning options for the elderly. Institute of Aging, Portland State University, Portland (OR)
Pearlin LI, Schooler L (1978) The structure of coping. J Health Soc Behav 19:2–21
Phillips BS (1957) A Role theory approach to adjustment in old age. Am Sociol Rev 22:212–217
Richardson IM (1965) Retirement and health. In: Psychiatric disorder in the aged. Geigy (UK), Manchester

Schaefer C, Coyne JC, Lazarus RS (1981) The health-related functions of social support. J Behav Med 4:381–406
Sosna U (1983) Soziale Isolation und psychische Erkrankung im Alter. Campus, Frankfurt.
Stein C, Susser M (1970) Bereavement as a precipitating event in mental illness. In: Hare EH, Wing JK (eds) Psychiatric epidemiology. Oxford University Press, London
Stephens RC, Blau ZS, Oser GT (1978) Aging, social support systems, and social policy. J Gerontol Soc Work 1:33–45
Thoits PA (1982) Conceptual, methodological, and theoretical problems in studying social support as a buffer against stress. J Health Soc Behav 23:145–159
Townsend P (1957) The family life of old people. Routledge and Kegan Paul, London
Tunstall J (1961) Old and alone. Routledge and Kegan Paul, London
Veiel HOF (1985) Dimensions of social support: A conceptual framework for research. Soc Psychiatry 20:156–162
Warheit G, Vega W, Shimizu D, Meinhardt K (1982) Interpersonal coping networks and mental health problems among four race-ethnic groups. Am J Community Psychol 10:312–324
Williams A, Ware JE, Donald CA (1981) A model of mental health, life events, and social supports applicable to general populations. J Health Soc Behav 22:324–336

3.4 Environmental and Behavioural Factors in Psychiatric Disorders in the Elderly: An Approach Through Risk Groups

R. C. Taylor

Introduction

It is widely assumed that some groups of elderly are particularly at risk. The WHO Expert Group on Mental Disorders in the Elderly (WHO 1977) identified seven risk groups:

1. The very old, those aged 80 and over
2. The recently widowed
3. The never married
4. Those living alone
5. Those who are socially isolated (not necessarily those living alone)
6. Those without children
7. Those in poor economic circumstances

But this WHO listing does not exhaust all possibilities. In Britain, two groups have been identified on the basis of recent changes in their circumstances (Arie 1981; Williamson 1981b):

8. Those who have recently been discharged from hospital
9. Those who have recently changed their dwelling

Finally, there is some evidence that those from working class backgrounds are disadvantaged in a number of respects (Taylor and Ford 1982):

10. Those in social class V (manual non-skilled)

This paper consists of a critical examination of the extent and nature of the risk/disadvantage experienced by each of these ten risk groups. Before proceeding with this examination it must be acknowledged that the concept of risk as applied to the elderly does not, as with younger age groups, mean susceptibility to speciefied disorders. When applied to the elderly it is more holistic, encompassing decrements in physical and social as well as mental functioning. Indeed, for the elderly the concept is ultimately defined in terms of the loss of independent functioning and the need for various forms of domiciliary or institutional care (Williamson 1981a).

Sample

The data were collected as part of the first stage of a continuing longitudinal study of coping behaviour and adjustment in later life, the target population consisting of all those aged 60 and over living in their own homes in Aberdeen, a Scottish city of 250 000 inhabitants.

The Risk Profiles

The risk profile which will be presented for each risk group has its origins in the concept of "personal resources", i.e. those reserves which individuals draw upon when coping with difficulties. For present purposes 19 key variables have been selected from our data set and arranged into six "domains".

They have all been standardised to have a mean of zero and a standard deviation of one. The score for the group on each variable is represented as a bar on a bar graph; a bar above the line represents a variable on which the average score for the group is above that of the sample as a whole, while a bar under the line represents a below average score. The bigger the bar, the more different the group from the sample as a whole. Those scores on which the departure of the group from the sample mean is statistically significant are represented in the figures by stippling.

Group Profiles

1. Those Living Alone. Accounting for about one-third of the elderly population, those living alone constitute the largest of the ten risk groups considered here. In our sample of 619, 216 or 35% lived alone. They are disproportionately old, 40.5% being aged 75 and over, cf. 29.7% in the sample as a whole ($P<0.05$), and disproportionately female, 80.3% cf. 60.7% in the sample as a whole ($P<0.05$).

For most of the measures of physical health, psychological functioning and confidence it can be seen that while the group scores slightly worse than the population as a whole, the only departure which is statistically significant occurs in the number of chronic conditions experienced (Fig. 1). It is in relation to various forms of social support that those living alone differ most. They have fewer intimates or confidantes available to them, and viewing their profile as a whole, this is the most distinctive feature. However, despite having few confidantes, the group is not characterised by low levels of psychological functioning. One reason for this may be the compensatory effect of many friends, those living alone having significantly more friends than the rest of the population. The only other significant departure from the sample mean occurs in relation to household amenities, those living alone being less likely to have such household amenities as hot water, fitted bath, etc.

Considering their profile as a whole it can only be concluded that those living alone do not stand out as being significantly disadvantaged. Of course, it is a large and heterogeneous group and entailed within it are members of other risk groups – the single, the divorced/separated and the recently widowed – whose profiles will be examined later.

2. The Childless. Those without children constitute the second largest of the ten risk groups. In the sample of 619, 123 or 20% are childless. Compared with the rest

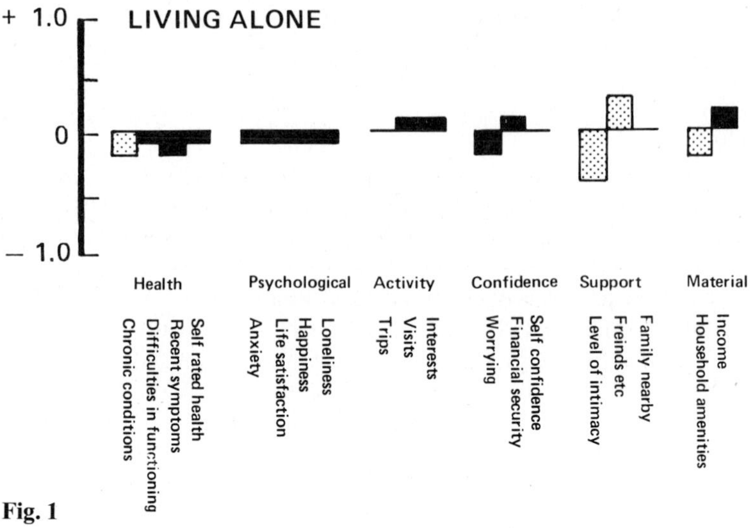

Fig. 1

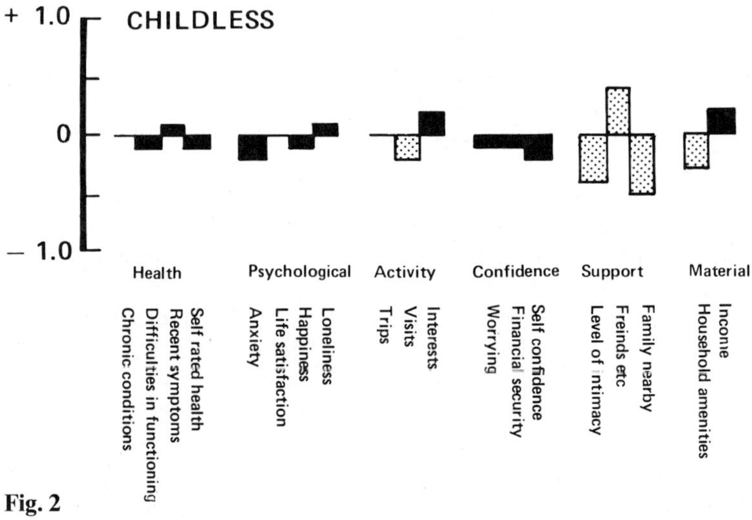

Fig. 2

of the elderly population they are indistinguishable in terms of age and sex, but they are disproportionately middle class, 55.8% cf. 35.0% in the sample as a whole ($P<0.5$).

The most distinctive feature of their profile is found in the domain of social support. They have fewer intimates or confidantes and fewer family members living nearby, but this loss is partly compensated by the comparatively large number of friends (Fig. 2).

But being childless is not associated with levels of health, psychological functioning and confidence which are significantly lower than those pertaining in the elderly population. It is possible that they are slightly more anxious and have rather less self-confidence, but they just fail to achieve statistical significance on both measures. As far as social activities are concerned, they are significantly less likely to receive visits, and this is probably a direct consequence of being childless.

The reason for their comparatively poor showing on household amenities is not immediately apparent. However, children constitute a major incentive for such home improvements as installing a bath or an inside toilet, and they also provide local authority tenants with housing points in any attempt they might make to secure better accommodation. Thus, in a city such as Aberdeen, in which over 60% of the housing stock is local authority owned, over the years the childless seem to have been left behind in the poorer inner city areas, and they have to live with the consequences in their old age.

3. The poor. Defining as poor those whose weekly income was below the Supplementary Benefit level, identified a subgroup of 93, or 15% of the sample. They are indistinguishable from the rest of the elderly population in terms of age and sex but they are disproportionately from working class backgrounds, 73.6% cf. 65.0% in the sample as a whole ($P<0.05$). Widows are also over-represented, 45.1% cf. 32.6% in the sample as a whole ($P<0.05$), and the married are under-represented, 37.3% cf. 52.2% in the sample as a whole ($P<0.05$).

By comparison with the elderly population as a whole they are clearly and massively deprived as far as income is concerned (Fig. 3), but since this is the measure on which they are defined, the observation is completely tautologous. On the related measure, household amenities, they are also significantly worse off than the sample as a whole, but this could also be seen as rather tautologous.

Apart from being financially disadvantaged, the group is also rather comprehensively disadvantaged on health grounds, scoring significantly lower than the sample on all four health measures. This is an important finding, and additional analysis (not shown here) shows that the extent of health disadvantage is even greater among the poor who are widowed and divorced/separated. Turning

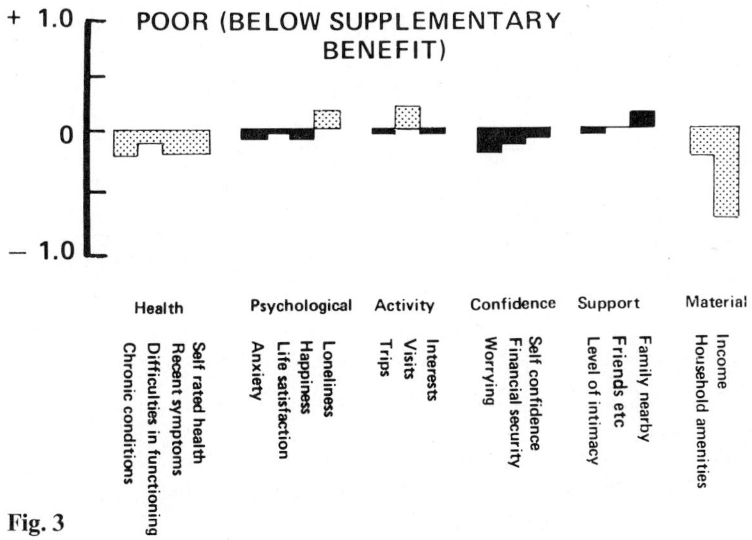

Fig. 3

attention to their mental health, evidence of risk or disadvantage is less conclusive. The group scores worse than the sample as a whole on all confidence measures, but the differences are not statistically significant; a similar situation pertains in respect of scores on anxiety, life satisfaction and happiness.

The major exception, and this is statistically significant, occurs on the measure of loneliness. As a group, the poor are not as lonely as the rest of the elderly sample and this finding is consistent with the rest of their profile. They receive significantly more visits than the sample as a whole and they tend to have more family members living locally. These departures above the sample mean are clearly related; the poor are less likely to experience loneliness because they get more visits and they probably get more visits because they tend to have more family members living locally.

On the basis of the data available it is clear that the poor are not just disadvantaged in terms of their income and housing. Compared with the rest of the elderly population they experience more illness and difficulties in functioning and have lower self-estimates of their health. However, it is important to note that this disadvantage is partially offset by their greater social contacts.

4. The Very Old. Almost 15% of the sample (86 cases) were aged 80 and over.

The group's composition is rather predictable, disproportionately female, 74.1% cf. 60.7% in the sample as a whole ($P<0.05$) and less likely to be currently married, 19.5% cf. 52.2% in the sample as a whole ($P<0.05$). They are also disproportiontely from middle class occupational backgrounds, 40.4% cf. 35.0% in the sample as a whole, but this result could have occurred by chance.

The risk profile of the very old generally confirms what is already known about their health; they have a greater number of chronic conditions and difficulties in functioning, and they tend to report more symptoms and to have lower self-ratings of their overall health (Fig. 4). As a consequence, they make fewer daily trips outside the house, but they do not seem to have fewer visits made to them.

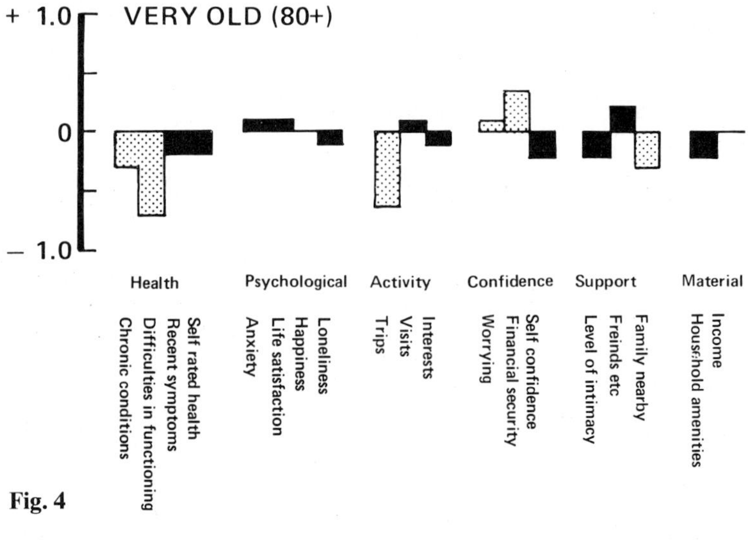

Fig. 4

On most measures of psychological functioning the very old are either indistinguishable from the rest of the elderly population, or they are significantly better off. It is clear that they worry less and feel greater financial security. This later finding is of particular interest in view of the objective evidence that over half of the very elderly (80>) have incomes below or on the margin of the State's standard of poverty. A number of factors might account for this discrepancy; for example, the very old may have fewer needs, income may have a lower salience for them than, say, health or it may be that by their own time perspective, present levels of provision seem generous.

The only other respect in which the very old are indisputably disadvantaged in relation to the rest of the elderly is the number of family members living locally. This difference is almost entirely explained in terms of differential survival. The very old are, by definition, survivors. Many of their siblings, and in some cases even their adult children, are not.

5. The Recently Moved. Contained within the sample were 85 elderly (13.7%) who had moved home within the last 2 years. They are indistinguishable in terms of age, sex and marital status but they are disproportionately from working class occupational backgrounds, 75.8% cf. 65.0% in the sample as a whole ($P<0.05$).

It is immediately apparent that most deviations from the sample mean occur below the line, so that as a group they tend to be rather comprehensively disadvantaged (Fig. 5). This disadvantage is particularly noticeable, and statistically significant, on three measures – anxiety, loneliness and worries – and containment within the psychological domain indicates the specific nature of the risks associated with residential mobility. It is worth observing that this psychological distress coincides with higher than average levels of intimacy and availability of family members.

6. The Recently Discharged. The sample contained 83 cases (13%) who had been discharged from hospital in the 2 years preceding the interview. As a group they

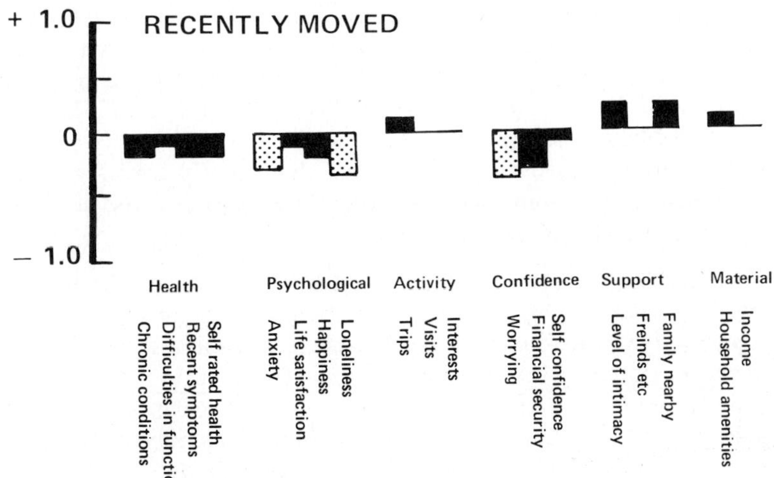

Fig. 5

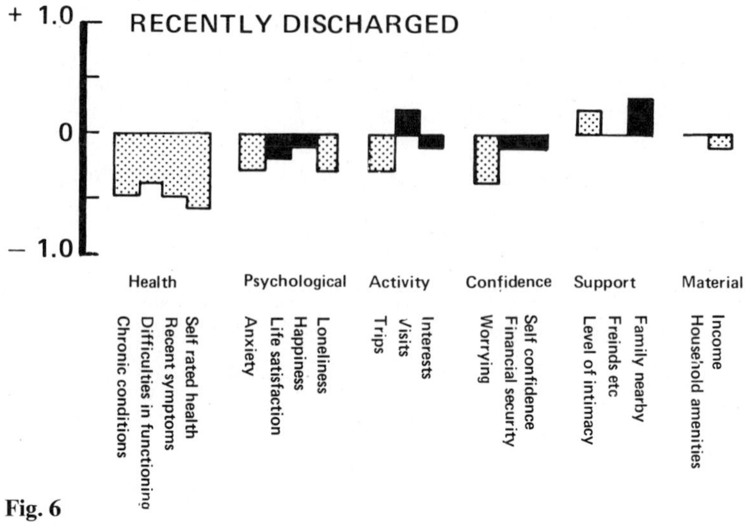

Fig. 6

are indistinguishable from the rest of the population in terms of age, sex, marital status and social class.

To define them as a risk group is partially tautological. They must all have been ill to enter hospital, and while some may have completely recovered after discharge, there will be many whose recovery is delayed, and some who never recover. But the frequency with which they are defined as a group at risk may also stem from more pragmatic considerations. Their entrances and exits from the hospital are documented, they are clearly identifiable and can (at least in theory) be routinely followed up as part of normal discharge procedure.

Their profile is dominated by poor health (Fig. 6). They score significantly worse than the rest of the sample on all measures of physical health and also on our psychological measures of anxiety, loneliness and general worrying. They also make significantly fewer trips outside the house, and have lower incomes. On the credit side, they report more confidantes and they tend to receive more visits and to have more family members living nearby. There is therefore a sense in which their physical and psychological condition mobilises higher levels of personal support than are available to the rest of the population.

Of all the risk groups we have so far examined, the recently discharged are clearly the most disadvantaged, and the profile merely underscores the need for follow-up services and support of various kinds.

7. The Never Married. The sample contained 70 cases (11.3%) who had never married, 46 spinsters and 23 batchelors. Apart from containing a greater proportion of females, 76.0% cf. 60.7% in the sample as a whole ($P<0.05$), the group is also disproportionately middle class, 49.0% cf. 35.0% ($P<0.05$).

The most pronounced feature of their profile is found in the support domain (Fig. 7). Compared with the rest of the elderly population they have fewer confidantes and fewer family members living nearby. But, as already observed for other groups, there is clear evidence of compensation through friendship.

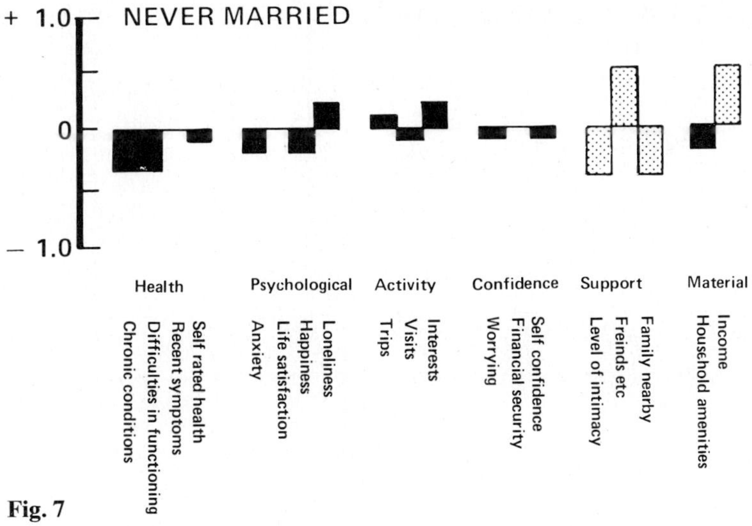

Fig. 7

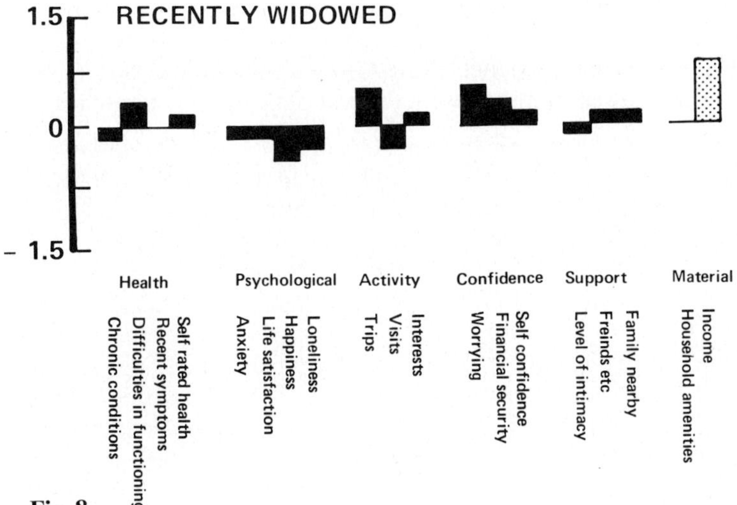

Fig. 8

8. The Recently Widowed. The sample contained 202 widows and widowers, the majority of whom had been without their spouses for many years. Studies of widowhood have suggested that its psychosocial impact begins to tail off after about 2 years. Accordingly, 37 cases bereaved in the last 2 years have been identified as a potential risk group.

Their profile reveals little conclusive evidence of comprehensive decline. Indeed, the only respect in which the group departs significantly from the sample mean is in their income (Fig. 8), and here it can be observed that the departure is in a favourable direction. While departures on other measures fail to reach statistical significancc, thcy comc closcst on happiness, trips out and worrying –

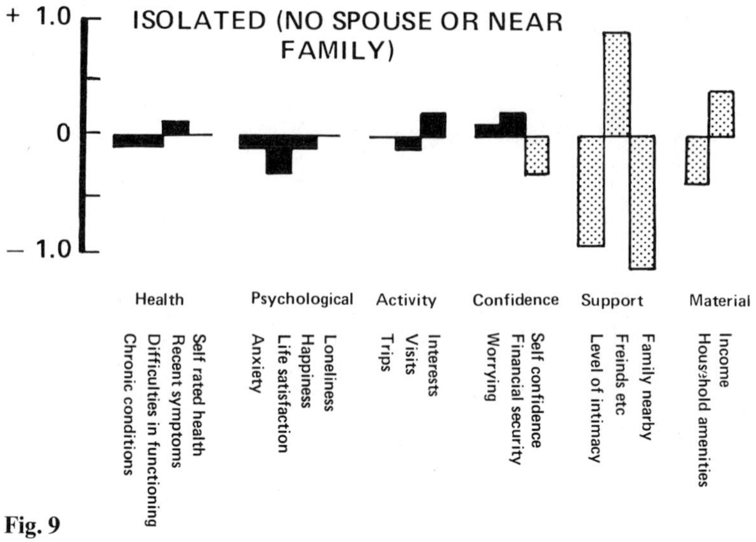

Fig. 9

all in the expected direction. But there are compensating tendencies, particularly in the confidence domain.

On the basis of the available evidence this group cannot be claimed to be significantly disadvantaged by comparison with the rest of the elderly population.

9. The Isolated. While 216 of the sample members lived alone and, by definition had no current spouse, 54 were additionally disadvantaged in having no children or siblings living locally. They have been defined as socially isolated. This group contains a higher proportion of the older cohort than the sample as a whole, 48.1% cf. 29.7% ($P<0.05$). It also contains more females, 78.1% cf. 60.7% ($P<0.05$), and more of those from middle class occupational backgrounds, 45.9% cf. 35% ($P<0.05$).

It is clear from the group's profile that the disadvantage is fairly contained. With one exception, all significant departures from the sample mean occur in the support and material domains (Fig. 9). Thus, apart from having poorer housing and better income the isolated are not significantly different from the rest of the elderly population in any respect other than those by which they have been defined.

10. Social Class V. The sample contained 51 men and women (8.2%) whose previous occupations qualified them for membership of the Registrar General's Social Class V. On other structural variables – age, sex and marital status – this group is indistinguishable from the sample as a whole.

It is clear from the group profile that social class V members are only significantly disadvantaged in terms of income (Fig. 10). On all other measures, apart from one, the group cleaves fairly close to the sample mean. The exception is the number of family members living nearby. Whatever disadvantage members of social class V may experience in health or psychological functioning, and there is not conclusive evidence in our data, the family support available to them is significantly greater than that enjoyed by the rest of the elderly population.

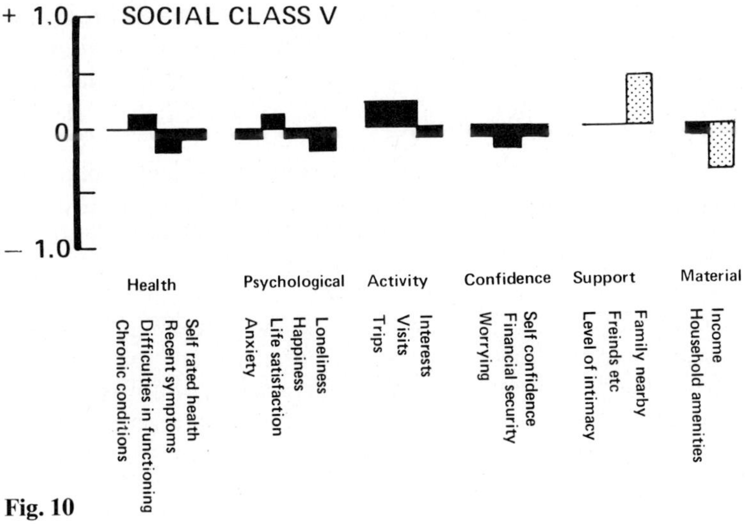

Fig. 10

Summary and Conclusions

For summary purposes, it is convenient to identify three categories of risk group.

First, there are those risk groups which are minimally disadvantaged. The Isolated, the Never Married and, to a lesser extent, the Childless, are examples of such groups. Compared with the rest of the sample they all have little social support available to them, however, and this is the most important point; their disadvantage in the domain of social support does not "spill over" into other domains. We have, for example, no evidence that their health or psychological functioning is worse than that of the sample as a whole. It is also important to note the way in which friends compensate for confidantes and family nearby.

The Recently Widowed, those Living Alone, the Poor and those from Social Class V constitute a second category. They cleave rather close to the sample mean, and are characterised by deviations both above and below. In resource terms, they have both strengths and weaknesses, an ambivalence rather clearly indicated in the resource profile of those defined as Poor.

The final category, consisting of the Recently Moved, Recently Discharged and the Very Old, is characterised by those with more deviations below than above the sample mean. Moreover, and most important, they all score worse than the sample as a whole in terms of health and/or psychological functioning. These are clearly the groups at greatest risk.

Given the crudeness of our measures these findings should be viewed as indicative rather than definitive. Nevertheless, they do pose questions for practitioners. Which, if any, of these ten risk groups are currently singled out for surveillance or case finding by the primary care team? Can a case be made for selectively screening such low risk groups as the single or those who live alone?

There are also rather more fundamental questions relating to the whole concept of risk groups. The heterogeneity of the elderly population and the tendency for poor functioning in one domain to be compensated by rather better functioning in another reduces the between-group differences. So while some of the group profiles reveal substantial risk/disadvantage, it is doubtful that they constitute a sound basis for intervention in the form of case finding or screening. In a separate paper (Ford and Taylor 1983) the efficiency of risk groups for case finding has been assessed and they have been shown to be rather inefficient. The most promising direction for future development may rest in a multi-tiered approach. The screening letter currently used in the Woodside Health Centre in Glasgow provides a good example of such an approach (Barber et al. 1980). The initial system of screening is by means of a short postal questionnaire requiring simple 'Yes' or 'No' answers. The nine questions on the screening letter are designed and phrased to cover known areas of potential risk to the patients' physical, psychological or social status. Any affirmative answer, or non-return of the questionnaire, indicates the need for a visit and a comprehensive assessment. It has been established that the screening letter identifies a higher proportion of cases than is identified by any of the pre-defined risk groups, and an attempt is currently being made to eliminate some questions (e.g. Do you live alone?) so as to reduce the proportion of the population covered without substantially reducing the proportion of "cases" identified (Taylor et al. 1984).

References

Arie T (ed) (1981) Health care of the elderly: essays in old age, Medicine, Psychiatry and Services, Croom Helm, London

Barber JH, Wallis JB, McKeating E (1980) A postal screening questionnaire in preventive geriatric care. J R Coll Gen Pract 30:49–51

Ford G, Taylor RC (1983) Risk groups and selective case finding in an elderly population. Soc Sci Med 17, No. 10:669–705

Taylor RC, Ford G (1982) Inequalities in old age: am examination of age, sex and class of differences in a sample of community elderly. Ageing Soc 3, No. 2:183–206

Taylor RC, Barber JH, Ford G (1984) Approaches to screening and case finding in elderly populations. Background Paper prepared for WHO Consultation on Assessment and Screening of the Elderly, Aberdeen, mimeo

W.H.O (1977) Expert group on mental disorders in the elderly. Copenhagen

Williamson J (1981a) The preventative approach. In: Kinnaird J, Brotherston J, Williamson J (eds) The provision of care for the elderly. Churchill Livingstone, Edinburgh

Williamson J (1981b) Screening, surveillance and case-finding. In: Arie T (ed) Health care of the elderly. Croom Helm, London

3.5 Perceptions about Old Age and Health in a Developing Country

C. A. León

Introduction

Since the process of aging in human beings is the result of a very complex interaction of physiological, psychological, and social factors, it is not surprising that the notion of old age should show a wide variability related to different modes of perception and to the diversity of sociocultural conventions. Under these circumstances the meaning of such terms as "the elderly," "old age," "advanced age," "the third age," etc., oftentimes used interchangeably, is vague and inconsistent and needs to be made more precise to be useful. Even though chronological age may not correspond to biological state in a given person, there is need for agreement on the setting of age limits for referring to a group of persons as the "elderly." Depending on various factors, the lower age limit used to define the elderly seems to vary, from 50 to 70 or 75 years of age, and even in statistical and demographic publications there is no uniformity in this regard. Predictably, in developing countries people are regarded as elderly at a rather early age. A man of 45 years may be turned down for a factory job because he is "too old" and under the newspaper caption "Old man killed by a truck," one finds that the man's age was 49.

In the present paper any reference to the elderly will apply to people 60 years of age and over.

Because of the scarcity of reliable publications and the enormous difficulties in obtaining references from other developing countries, most of the material presented will deal only with what has been observed in Colombia. I will therefore refer in succession to some aspects of demographic factors and health and psychosocial conditions related to the elderly in Colombia.

Demographic Aspects

In Colombia, as in several other countries in Latin America and the developing world, the population group of 60 years and over has represented throughout most of this century about 5% of the total population because of the stability of the demographic growth. However, during recent decades this situation has been altered by remarkable changes in the mortality and birth rates. In fact, the crude death rate has fallen from 16.5‰ in 1950–1955 to 8.3‰ in 1978–1983, and the live birth rate has been reduced from 123.3‰ in 1950–1955 to 53.3‰ in 1980–1983, (Bayona and Rico 1983). Whereas previously it took 26–30 years to double the absolute number of older people, it is now expected that doubling will take only 20 years (Fig. 1).

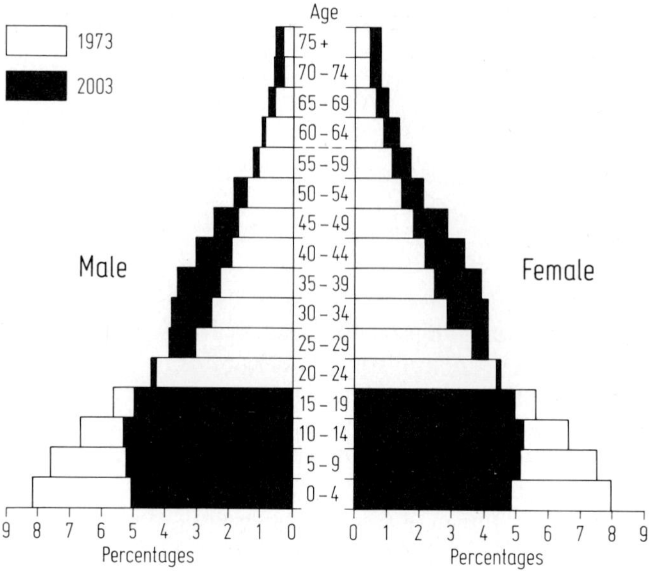

Fig. 1. Composition of population according to age groups and sex, Colombia 1973–2003 [2]

Although at present the population structure of Colombia shows the typical pyramidal shape of the developing countries, a projection for the year 2003 contemplates a significant structural change, and the expected proportion for people of 60 years and over is 6.8% of the total population[1]. The life expectancy index has increased from 44 years for people born in 1937–39 to 61 years for those born in 1978–83 and is expected to be 70 years for people born in the year 2000. At present, life expectancy for a person of 60 years is 15.7 additional years (16.6 for women, 14.9 for men). In the year 2000 the figures will be 18.6 additional years for women and 16.6 for men.

As a result of the aforementioned demographic changes, by the end of this century there will be a substantial increase in the number of persons aged 60 and over (almost double the present number).

In 1977 the death rate for people 60 years and older was about 55‰ representing 34% of all deaths. The figures for women were lower than for men in all age groups. Turning to the subject of internal migration, we find that according to the 1938 census only 30% of the population of Colombia lived in urban areas; in 1973 this figure had risen to approximately 61%, and a recent estimate places it close to 70% (Rico 1983).

Migration from rural to urban areas is occurring everywhere in the developing world. As seen in Table 1, the situation for Latin American countries and the

1 The absolute figures are: total population for Colombia in 2003: 40 327 941; people 60 years and over: 2 742 300. This last figure represents the survivors of the cohort who were 40 years and over in 1983. It is expected that about 50% of this cohort will die before 2003 [1]

Table 1. Estimated percentage of urban population in Latin America and the Caribbean

1950	1980	2000
41.4	65.3	75.4

Source: World Bank (1984) Report on World Development

Table 2. Latin American cities with population of over 10 000 000 inhabitants

1950	1975	2000
None	Mexico City 11.9	Mexico City 31
	Sao Paulo 10.7	Sao Paulo 25.8
		Rio de Janeiro 19
		Buenos Aires 12.1
		Bogotá 11.7

Source: World Bank (1984) Report on World Development

Caribbean is one of a steady increase. As a result of this it is expected that several Latin American cities will experience phenomenal growth, turning into veritable megalopoles by the end of the present century (Table 2).

Developing nations will contribute a very large share of the world population increase, and it is estimated that by the year 2000 approximately 78% of all people on earth will live in developing countries. The largest proportion living in developing countries will be in the age group under 15 (85%), but among people aged 65 and over the figure will be a sizable 54% (Table 3).

Table 3. Estimates of the world population for the year 2000 and percentage living in the less developed regions

Age groups	Population (000's)	Percent in less developed regions
<15	2 025 831	85
15–24	1 157 934	83
25–34	931 692	80
35–44	769 627	80
45–64	973 274	69
65–74	264 161	61
75–79	74 252	55
80+	57 605	46
Total	6 254 377	78

Source: Population Division, United Nations 1976

Because of selective migration practices combined with a higher reduction of the birth rate in urban areas, it is expected that there will be changes in the composition of the Colombian family. Estimates made for recent years show a trend toward a reduction in the average number of family members in urban areas, from 5.8 in 1964 to 5.4 in 1978. The proportion of families in Colombia with 6 or more members was reduced from 51.2% in 1964 to 47.7 in 1973 and 45.5 in 1978 (Rico de Alonso 1983).

Health Aspects

There is very little information about the health of the elderly in most of the developing countries. In Colombia, only in recent decades has it been possible to collect information in a systematic way. As mentioned before, one very important finding is a noticeable decrease in the general mortality.

As shown in Table 4, the ten most frequent causes of death for people of 60 yers and over in Colombia in 1981 were predominantly malignancies and degenerative diseases. Specific comparison with previous figures can only be made for the year 1973 and shows an apparent increase in the rate of malignancies, hypertensive diseases, and diseases of arteries and capillaries as causes of death in the elderly. Only six of the ten most frequent causes of death are represented among the causes of hospitalization, and only five among the causes of outpatient consultations. The rank order is quite different for the three categories (Ministerio de Salud 1984).

In a survey conducted in 1981 on a sample of 400 pensioners affiliated to Caja Nacional de Previsión Social (C.N.P.S. – a government institution for retired

Table 4. Ten most frequent causes of death and their relation to morbidity in Colombia for persons aged 60 years and over, 1981–1982

	Mortality			Morbidity, 1982	
	Rank 1981	Rate per 1000, 1981	Rank 1973	Hospital, rank	Ambulatory rank
Malignancies	1	7.80	2	5	6
Heart and circulatory diseases (other)	2	7.20	1	2	7
Ischemic heart disease	3	6.40	3		
Cerebrovascular diseases	4	5.42	4	6	
Hypertensive diseases	5	3.13	6	7	1
Diseaes of arteries, capillaries	6	1.68	9		
Acute respiratory infections	7	1.55	5	9	8
Diseases of the digestive system (other)[a]	8	1.5	8	1	5
Diabetes mellitus	9	1.47	10		
Chronic respiratory diseases	10	1.04	7		

Source for 1981, 1982: Ministerio de Salud, Colombia Encuesta Nacional de Salud; source for 1973: Bayona A, Pabón A (1982) La mortalidad en Colombia, vol II

[a] Including hernias

Table 5. Percentage of first admissions to a psychiatric hospital accounted for by persons aged 60 and over. Cali, Colombia, 1963, 1973, 1983

Year	Inpatients	Outpatients
1963	1.87	3.43
1973	2.22	3.82
1983	2.51	4.69

Source: Hospital Psiquiátrico San Isidro, Cali

public officials), the informants, urban dwellers who had an average age of 65 years, were asked if they had been ill during the previous 6 months. Sixty-nine percent replied affirmatively and identified their ailments as follows: cardiovascular 38%, musculoskeletal 24%; bronchopulmonar 10%; genitourinary 6%; eye, ear, nose and throat 6%; digestive 6%; nervous 3%; other 7% (Caja Nacional de Previsión Social 1983).

In an evaluation conducted by occupational therapists of a sample of 1000 institutionalized elderly persons in Bogota, with an age range of 57 to 99 (no average age stated), it was found that 71% could walk without help, 16.5 needed crutches, 4.4% required a walker; 2.7% needed a wheelchair, and 4.8 were bedridden. Gross coordination was preserved in 69%. Vision was normal in 52.5% and 66.3% were "mentally lucid" (Ortega and Muñoz 1983).

No study on the prevalence of mental disorders in the elderly has ever been conducted in Colombia, and the distribution of patients in mental institutions according to age is not available. An interesting fact observed at Hospital Psiquiátrico San Isidro in Cali, which for several years was the only public psychiatric institution, serving about 80% of the population, is an apparent steady increase in the demand for psychiatric services by the elderly. As seen in Table 5, elderly patients accounted for 1.87% of first psychiatric hospitalizations in 1963, 2.2% in 1973, and 2.51% in 1983. Elderly patients seen at the outpatient department increased from 3.43% of first admissions in 1963 to 3.82% in 1973 and 4.69% in 1983.

At a global level and given the fact that the rates of mental disorder are the same as those estimated for developed countries in 1975, it is expected that several disorders will show a great increase by the year 2000. Because of their population growth dynamics, the changes could be huge for developing countries (see Table 6), reaching the scale of a true "pandemic of mental disorders" (Kramer 1980). It should be noticed that senile dementia shows the highest percentage increase of all the disorders considered. The most frequent diagnoses made in Cali for elderly psychiatric patients during 1983 were, in order: senile dementia, psychosis associated with other cerebral conditions, nonpsychotic disorder associated with brain lesion, affective psychosis, schizophrenia, neurosis, and other psychoses. Alcoholic psychosis and alcoholism were conspicuously absent. A personal impression shared with colleagues in Colombia and other Latin American countries is that Alzheimer disease seems to be quite a rare disorder in this part of the world.

Table 6. Projection of the effect of population changes on selected mental disorders (based on estimated rates for 1975)

Disorder	Percentage of change, 1975 – 2000 More developed countries	Less developed countries
Serious mental disorder	20.2	72.6
Schizophrenia	15.0	83.0
Senile dementia (over 65)	54.0	123.0
Epilepsy	15.9	61.5

Source: Kramer M (1980) The rising pandemic of mental disorders and associated chronic diseases and disabilities. Acta Psychiatr Scand [Suppl 285] 62:382 – 396

In a careful study conducted in 1962 – 64 on urban mortality, Cali and Bogotá were included along with eight other Latin American cities. This study showed that the annual suicide rate for Cali was 14 per 100 000 for males aged 55 – 64 years and that there were no suicides among females in this age group. No deaths by suicide were registered during this period for either males or females in the age group 65 – 74 years. For Bogota the corresponding figures for the 55 – 64 year were 22.9 per 100 000 for males and 0 for female. In the 65 – 74 year age group the rates were 13.8 for males and 11.9 for females. In general, it was found that suicide in Cali, Guatemala City, and Mexico City tended to decline according to advancing age, while in the other seven Latin American cities it tended to increase with age but never in the same proportion as that observed in European and North American cities. The authors comment that "when Latin American cities are compared with the English speaking [sic] ones there is a close similarity in mortality rates for the age group 15 – 34 and a deep difference in older groups" (Puffer and Griffith 1968). Death by motor vehicle accidents showed a rate increasing directly in proportion with age in all Latin American cities.

One of the persistent notions, or perhaps myths, in the developing world is that in some remote and hidden region a certain group of people enjoy remarkable longevity and its members are spared from the common ailments and diseases of old age. This unusual condition is variously attributed to climatic factors, genetic stock, dietary habits, and general life-style. Most of the attempted studies to substantiate such claims seem to have been inconclusive and lacking in comparable methological frames, but nevertheless the question remains open and seems to demand a collaborative effort for its clarification. A recent report about observations made in the Amazonian region of Venezuela (Ariel et al. 1979) describes the study of a random sample of 30 aborigines of this area whose estimated age was 60 or over (19 women, 11 men). Interviews, physical examinations, and laboratory tests showed that the health of the sample was "very good, regarding degenerative illnesses but there was a high proportion of infections and nutritional deficiencies". It was also noticed that "they remain quite active and try to adapt to the possibilities of their organism".

A final point regarding the health of the elderly in Colombia concerns the number of doctors who practice geriatrics in the country. Out of a total of 18 000[1] physicians it is estimated that only about 80 specialize in geriatrics, most of them without any previous formal training. Geriatrics as a subject is not taught in medical schools and there are no postgraduate training programs for this specialty. However, there is an adequate 600 bed geriatric hospital in the city of Manizales. In a group of about 600 medical students in Cali, only one expressed interest in specializing in geriatrics.

Psychosocial Aspects

There are very few studies in Colombia dealing with characteristics of the elderly population. During 1981 and 1983 the Institute of Social Security (ISS) conducted a series of regional surveys aimed at studying the pensioners covered by the Institute. The size of this population is estimated as 103 208 (February 1984), of whom 55.5% are old age pensioners, 30.5% are survivors of deceased pensioners receiving pensions, and 14% have been disabled by accidents or professional diseases. The disparity in methods used by the different regional branches made the joint analysis of data quite difficult and it was decided to supplement the survey with uniformly designed forums with the pensioners and their relatives. The following information could be abstracted from a recently published interim report (Instituto de Seguros Sociales 1984): About 78% of the pensioners are men. Their modal age group is 60–69. Approximately 90% live in urban areas and over 60% are married. About 95% live with relatives. The main daily activities consist of house chores or repairs for the men and housekeeping for the women. Recreational activities are mostly passive, such as listening to radio, watching TV, and playing table games. Group activities are almost nonexistent. Responses to questions in the survey showed high indexes of well-being and personal satisfaction for about 80% of the respondents but under probing during the forums most of them acknowledged a predominance of feelings of depression, irritability, low self-esteem, dissatisfaction, and uselessness. In a controlled independent study conducted on a sample of 200 elderly Colombians (Dulcey and Ardila 1976) using the Tuckman-Lorge questionnaire it was found that the informants assigned to elderly people mostly negative characteristics.

It was also found that there were statistically significant differences between the elderly and a group of young controls (whose evaluation was mostly positive) and that the evaluation tended to be more negative in respondents of both groups belonging to lower economic class. In a survey conducted by C.N.P.S., 60% of the respondents had a positive image of the elderly. In this same group 12% expressed dissatisfaction with family, 19% with friends, 20% with society in general, and 30% with self (Caja Nacional de Previsión Social 1983).

During the forums with the pensioners of the I.S.S. it was learned that most of the elderly would like to continue working in an "independent way" and with a

1 The estimated figure for 1981 was a total of 17 999 doctors, which gives a ratio of 66.7 doctors per 100 000 inhabitants (10). A similar ratio for geriatrics would be 5.5 per 100 000 elderly Colombians

flexible schedule in such activities as cottage industries, small cooperatives, repairing appliances, baby sitting, and gardening. They also expressed a need for organized recreational activities: excursions and other group activities shared with relatives.

Of the pensioners in the C.N.P.S. sample, 73% admitted to having an interest in new activities – mostly of a recreational nature (63%) but also paid work (27%). In the same group the subjective experience of disability was found to change according to age group as follows: the highest proportion of those with "many disabilities" were in the 55–59 age group; most of those with "few disabilities" were in the 60–64 age group; and most of those with "no disabilities" were in the 65–69 age group. This suggests the existence of a gradual process of acceptance or tolerance of disabilities and that perception of disabilities is keenest immediately following retirement[1].

Questioned about their feelings during this period, 57% complained of feeling physically unfit; 50% reported decreased sexuality; 36% a reduction in daily activities; and 34% a lack of a "wish to live".

An important area of enquiry in the I.S.S. forums had to do with the notions, feelings, and attitudes of relatives toward the pensioners living with them. A predominant profile of the pensioner as perceived by his or her relatives was that of a person who seems to be depressed, worried, bored, irritable, withdrawn, passive, and oversensitive – at times demanding and torn between the need to go out and the fear of doing so. Yet in spite of all these characteristics there was consensus among informants that pensioners *should remain with the family*, even though facilities may be lacking. This, of course, suggests that traditional family values persist strongly despite formal structural changes in family composition. It is evident that there is a strong affective disposition to retain the pensioners within the family group in spite of limitations on care. It is common knowledge that the process of rural – urban migration and subsequent industrialization tends to undermine the family patterns of influence. However, an alternative view is presented by Carlos and Sellers (1972), who present evidence suggesting that Latin American family networks play an important role in enhancing group cohesion and adaptation.

In trying to explore some ways and means of helping to solve problems presented by pensioners, the I.S.S. forums made the following suggestions:

1. Keeping the pensioner active by assigning him or her specific tasks such as repairs around the house, looking after the children, handiwork, and participation in home industries
2. Organized social and recreational activities under the sponsorship of an agency, as well as educational activities aimed at self-improvement and retraining
3. Preparation for retirement through group meetings and discussions, also involving the relatives
4. Services for guidance to the family on how to handle the problems of the retired
5. Preferential social services to families who keep retired people with them

1 According to Colombian legislation, the lower age limit for retirement in certain occupations is 50 years, after having worked for a minimum of 20 years

6. Special subsidies to these families, especially if the pensioner is chronically ill or disabled (requiring extra care)[1]
7. Domiciliary medical services when necessary.

The number and the capacity of institutions caring for the elderly in Colombia are not known with certainty. In 1982 it was estimated that there were 270 public institutions caring for 14 623 people. Medical services were provided in 11 of them (Marroquin 1982). No information is available about the number and capacity of private nursing homes, private residences for elderly people, or other similar institutions. It can be estimated, however, that less than two per thousand of the Colombian elderly are lodged in institutions (Ministerio de Salud 1983).

General Comments

After having focused on some of the most salient problems related to the elderly in a developing country, it may be useful to try to summarize some of the implications they may have for health in general and specifically for mental health.

The increase in both the absolute and relative number of the elderly brought about by a shift in demographic factors such as a decrease in mortality and live birth rates create new problems for planning, distribution, and implementation of health services. Increased service demands for chronic and degenerative diseases represent an added and rather unexpected burden for programs aimed predominantly at dealing with sanitation and infectious, parasitic, and carential diseases. In the field of mental disorders an increase in the life span of the population will generate a higher number of cases of senile and involutional disorders. In populations with high mortality rates, the mortality of psychotics is even higher (because of higher risk), and if for any reason general mortality rates decrease, this may also bring about an increase in the prevalence of psychosis.

Migration from rural to urban areas and the process of modernization-/industrialization produce changes in adaptation, life-style, and family dynamics. In spite of the persistence of traditional values, the image of the elderly becomes negative and they may be regarded as a burden. In agricultural societies the elderly are a repository of practical knowledge, experience, and principles, all of which become useless when the setting changes abruptly and skills and knowledge of a different kind are required. Youth is worshipped and promoted ubiquitously and old age is something to be dreaded and despised. Also, pressing problems of space place a limit on the size of families and they tend more and more to become nuclear whereas previously they were extended. However, excessive feelings of rejection toward the elderly are usually not detected among relatives, and there is a disposition to keep them in the family provided that certain minimal requirements are met. The suggestions made at forums by relatives of pensioners in Colombia point to important and very realistic needs which, once fulfilled, will reinforce the role of the family as the main protecting and socializing agent for the elderly.

---

1 Paradoxically, in Colombia subsidies are paid to families who *do not* keep the retired person at home but place him or her in a nursing home or other similar institution

The whole area of training of health personnel has to be modified in accordance with the new needs created by increasing numbers of elderly people. Research activities dealing with this group need to be stimulated, especially in such fields as prevalence studies, comparison between different populations, special groups at risk, and groups with unusual characteristics. International cooperation should be seen as a crucial element for facilitating these developments.

Acknowledgment. The preparation of this paper was partially supported by the Fund *Margarita de Pacini – Fundación para la Educación Superior*.

References

Ariel A, Castillo HM, González AC (1979) Rol que desempeña el gerente en las comunidades indigenas del territorio federal del Amazonas. Publ Soc Col Geront Geriat 2:167–170

Bayona A, Rico J (1983) Socio-demografia de la tercera edad en Colombia Data estudios. Mimeographed pbulication

Caja Nacional de Previsión Social (1983) El pensionado: un potencial desconocido. Bogota

Carlos ML, Sellers L (1972) Family, kinship structure and modernization in Latin America. Lat Am Res Rev 7:95–125

Dulcey E, Ardila R (1976) Actitudes hacia los ancianos. Rev Lat Am Psychol 8:57–67

Instituto de Seguros Sociales, Oficina Nacional de Planeación (1984) Plan nacional de atención al pensionado del I.S.S.-Marco general. Bogota (Mimeographed publication)

Kramer M (1980) The rising pandemic of mental disorders and associated chronic diseases and disabilities. Acta Psychiatr Scan [Suppl 285] 62:382–397

Marroquin G (1982) El anciano en la sociedad colombiana. Publ Soc Col Geront Geriat 5:138–141

Ministerio de Salud (1983) Hacia la equidad en salud. Plan Nacional 1983–1986. Bogota

Ministerio de Salud, Organización Panamericana de la Salud, Organización Mundial de la Salud (1984) Colombia, diagnóstico de salud, politicas y estrategias. Bogota

Ortega MA, Muñoz CM (1983) Macrodiagnóstico de la situación del anciano en Bogota. Publ Soc Col Geront Geriat 6:185–191

Puffer RR, Griffith GW (1968) Caracteristicas de la mortalidad urbana. Organización Panamericana de la Salud, Washington

Rico J (1983) Tendencias futuras de la población colombiana. Universidad del Valle, Cali

Rico de Alonso A (1983) Incidencia de la urbanización y de la disminución en la fecundidad sobre el tamaño, composición y funciones de la familia colombiana. Universidad Javeriana, Bogota

3.6 Psychological and Social Aspects of Mental Health in the Elderly: A Summarizing Co-lecture

R. F. W. Diekstra, G. Stafleu

In a most remarkable novel entitled *The Devils of Loudun* the following statement is made: "Civilisation can in one of its aspects be defined as a systematic attempt to prevent the individual citizen from being exposed to situations that invite barbaric behavior." The author is the renowned Aldous Huxley and the book was first published in 1952, when most of the research in psychology on situational determinants of individual behavior had yet to be carried out. But in the 30 years to follow, Huxley was proven to have been a very keen observer of some of the major determinants of the behavior of the human species. In 1981 the outstanding social psychologists Furnham and Argyle published a book under the title *The Psychology of Social Situations* that summarized the major findings of scientific psychology in this domain. One important conclusion from their review is that when one fills out Kurt Lewin's famous formula that $B=f(S,P)$, on the basis of the available empirical evidence more than half of the variance in behavior (0.52) has to be attributed to S(ituation) and less than one-quarter (0.24) to P(ersonality). It is evident that one has to be careful in using a generalizing statement like this since its tenability is among other things dependent upon what definitions of situation and personality one uses, an issue that will not be pursued in the present context.

Nevertheless given this summary finding and paraphrasing Huxley's statement, one way to define health care is as "a complex of systematic attempts to prevent the individual from being exposed and from exposing himself to situations that provoke unhealthy or health-risk behavior." An important task for the health disciplines implied by this definition is that of devising what could be called a grammar of evil or health-risk situations. One could imagine such a grammar to be a sort of classification scheme for pathogenic situations or characteristics of pathogenic situations comparable to what WHO's International Classification of Diseases (ICD) is for (symptoms of) pathogenic somatic conditions. Actually one wonders why such an international classification of health-threatening situations has not already become available. Presumably political factors, and not so much a lack of scientific progress, are among the most powerful forces that have prevented its appearance thus far.

Let us consider a few examples of the kind of information that such a system could contain. Developmental psychologists and child psychiatrists in different parts of the world have found in longitudinal studies of children from the time they were born onwards, that the early parent – child interactions are highly consistent over time and situations and that some well-defined patterns of interaction are closely related to behavioral problems and coping styles of children in puberty and early adolescence [no longitudinal studies are at present available that have followed children for more than 14 years (ISSBD 1982)]. One of the obvious conclusions from this finding is that one should prevent children from being exposed to the harmful patterns of interaction. This could be done by training and guiding young parents with newborns or even before the birth of their child.

Another example is the well-documented relationship between the intellectual development of children and the degree of (cognitive and intellectual) stimulation the environment provides. Long-term exposure to an environment that is deprived in this respect can lead to intellectual retardation that might be very difficult to compensate for. Knowledge of what constitutes a deprived environment and prevention of exposure to it therewith become important aspects of mental health promotion (Diamond 1984).

One can easily see that the last example applies mutatis mutandis to the elderly as well. Both from the Bonn Longitudinal Study of Aging (BSLA), as Lehr points out in this volume, and from a number of similar studies (Schaie 1983), it has become evident that there is a relationship between cognitive and intellectual functioning on the one hand and situational determinants on the other. High socioeconomic status is related not only to high levels of intellectual functioning but also to the maintenance of such functioning into late life. The mechanism involved here, as the report from the Seattle Longitudinal Study puts it, "is likely to be the maintenance of varied opportunities for environmental stimulation" (Schaie 1983). According to the same report this implies that environmental and educational stimulation – for example microcomputerized brain jogging programs – holds inordinate promise for the psychological well-being of the elderly. Studies in the field of neuroanatomy, such as those by Diamond and her colleagues (1984), lend support to this claim. Experiments with "elderly" rats have shown that, given the right stimulation, the aging brain is capable of remarkable change. The implication for human life according to Diamond is "use it or lose it".

Interestingly, one common theme in the papers of Lehr, Mechanic, and Taylor in this volume is that they all provide information on situations that are supposed or proven to be detrimental to well-being in late age. Although their inventories of such situations as well as the terminology used vary somewhat, which makes them not directly comparable, there seem to be at least some striking similarities.

The Complex Relationship Between Network and Well-Being

Emphasis is often placed on the importance of supportive social networks and of "confidant" relationships for somatic and psychic well-being. However, there are exceptions to this rule, such as the elderly male bachelors in Taylor's study (this volume) a finding which is in accordance with the results of Ehrlich's study in St. Louis on the so-called SRO (single room occupant) elderly men. In this group emotional wellbeing was not related to the existence of a network of confidant relationships: "... the SRO norms of utilitarianism, freedom and privacy govern the types and frequency of social relationships permitted among them. Opportunity for forming relationships with tenants on a personal basis was restricted. Maintaining privacy went beyond staying out of each other's room; it also included not sharing one's personal affairs with one another" (Ehrlich and Ehrlich 1982, p. 76). But clearly, groups like the SRO elderly men form only a small minority of the elderly population.

Remaining Active and Well-Being

Another common observation, especially in Lehr's and Mechanic's papers (this volume), seems to be the importance of activity, of remaining active both in the physical and in the psychological sense. One wonders whether there are also exceptions to this rule. According to Schaie (1983) one could divide the elderly population into three groups in terms of their level of activity: the go-go's, the slow-go's, and the no-go's. It could well be that the level of well-being in the second group might be higher than in the other groups because such a level of activity is more appropriate to late age.

However, one can hardly say that the finding that social support and staying active are conducive to health is surprising. Its relevance would have been much greater if, for example, deprivation in these respects had been proven to be more detrimental among the elderly than among younger age groups. As far as we know it is unlikely that this is actually the case. From the available evidence one even gets the impression that the reverse might be true. Sainsbury et al. (1981), for example, found that loss of employment had a much greater impact on males between 35 and 50 years of age than on those 50 years and over. This is explainable by the fact that loss of work when one is still in the process of forming one's career and often has responsibility for a family with one or more young children, while at the same time one is at an age at which it has already become more difficult to find other employment and start a new career, is more detrimental than losing one's job at a time close to the moment one had to retire anyway. The implication of the foregoing is that our knowledge about psychological and social factors specific to mental and physical health in the elderly requires research that focuses on the differential impact of well-defined conditions at different ages or different life stages.

Attitudes Towards Aging

Another important social factor relevant to well-being in late age, which has thus far received far too little attention in quantitative research, is the influence that intergenerational differences in attitudes toward aging and corresponding behavioral patterns might have on the situation of the elderly in our society. Implicitly Mechanic (this volume) refers to the same point when he states: "Given the concerns about the growing proportions of elderly relative to the working population, it is ironic that we provide few incentives for the young elderly who retain their motivation and vitality to remain in the work force" and "The elderly population constitutes a large untapped reservoir of skill and potential productivity we have not been particularly imaginative about."

Tibitts, in his Donald P. Kent Memorial lecture in 1978, discussed the issue of negative attitudes or stereotypes towards the aged at length. The core of the old age stereotype was described by him as follows: "The elderly are seen as noncreative, very slow thinkers, and as persons that cannot continue to grow and learn and be a contributing functional being." Such a stereotype is clearly contradicted by the fact that the majority of the older population is a healthy and functioning group that contributes or is able to contribute to our society.

The stereotype is based on the 5% or less who manifest the negative characteristics. But it neglects the majority of older persons according to Tibbits, precisely because they are healthy and functioning beings and capable of and willing to contribute to our society. Atchley (1982, p. 33), in a very interesting paper entitled *Culture and Aging*, provides an explanation for this peculiar fact. According to this author attitudes and beliefs about the elderly depend a lot on the economic context of the time.

During labor shortages the value of older workers is extolled, but in times of economic recession and labor surplus age discrimination is frequently used to cut down the size of the labor force. When 65 was established as the minimum age of retirement in most western countries, by implication 65 was the age at which a person was too old to contribute. High unemployment in recent years in most of the countries in the industrialized part of the world has promoted age discrimination in employment even further, for it has made the minimum age of eligibility for retirement drop further. While at the same time the general health of the older population has improved, the attitudinal link between being an elderly person and disabled or incapacitated has become even more absurd.

This analysis shows that high unemployment or economic instability also has a strong impact on older persons, though not directly but via the social processes it sets in motion, like age discrimination and elimination of the elderly from the workforce, and via the emergence of attitudes such as the stereotypes mentioned, whose predominant function is to justify certain social measures post hoc.

In my opinion these complex processes deserve more study, both empirical and theoretical, than has thus far been devoted to them. A related topic is the attitudes the elderly themselves have toward aging. Lehr and her colleagues from the BLSA have, among others, provided evidence that there are considerable differences between older persons in this respect and that these differences are related to adjustment or well-being (Lehr, this volume). However, relatively little is known about the factors or processes that are responsible for these differences in attitudes and how they can be influenced or modified. Data from the AT&T longitudinal study (Schaie 1983) of managers suggest that quite complex processes are at work here. For example, it was found that the emotionally healthy middle-aged managers developed in a way that distinguished them from those less healthy. Over time, most men in the study lowered their expectations, became less positive (i.e., often more realistic) about the company, and reduced their drive to move ahead. However, the emotionally healthiest men changed less in this direction, as if less willing to give up their initial positive attitudes. They also increased their motivation to lead and direct others, while the less well-adjusted became less dominant over time and, what is most noteworthy, devoted more and more time to worrying. Whether this might be explained by differences in adverse social circumstances, whether it is itself the consequence of ill-health, or whether it is related to possible constitutional differences in susceptibility or sensitivity to stressors remains obscure. What has become clear is that emotional health in middle age is not related to career success, but is strongly associated with career satisfaction. It might be that the emotionally healthy men predominantly concentrate on the activities or aspects of their work and life they enjoy and on the situations and behaviors they are capable of controlling or mastering, while tending to ignore or deny that which they are unable to master or to which they do not have access. The emotionally less healthy men, on the other hand, might devote a lot of time and energy on their "impossiblities." This hypothesis is in accordance with the findings of both Vaillant and Lazarus (see Diekstra and Hawton 1986). According to these authors the ability to use the cognitive defense mechanism of denial with regard to social, psychological, and physical adversities, is closely associated with subjective emotional healthiness. Although such a hypothesis squarely contradicts the dominant idea behind the majority of psychotherapeutic approaches in psychiatry and psychology, the empirical data, especially those collected by Lazarus, unequivocally point to the negative emotional consequences of the inability to denial.

In the study by Ehrlich in St. Louis, mentioned above, it was found that one of the characteristics of the comparatively healthy SRO elderly was that they did not let health problems, identified by a like-aged group of persons, become problems for them; they seemed to disregard typical symptoms and resulting diseases and to survive the disease or conditions by sheer power of will. It seems likely that Lehr's finding (Lehr, this volume) that longevity in terms of survivorship was more closely related to subjective health than to objective health reflects the same psychological processes. Leading behavioristically oriented researchers on depression (see Diekstra and Hawton 1986) raise a point that is very relevant in this respect. The seemingly insoluble problems with regard to the classification of depression can be reduced to the false assumption that depression is a specific syndrome. Instead depression should be considered to be an affect or an affective state, which individuals generally try to avoid through specific modes of thinking, feeling, and behaving. These coping responses constitute what are called the symptoms of depression and vary according to the stage of psychological development and socio-cultural factors, which explains why symptoms of depression can be so diverse and why, for example, depressive adolescents sometimes show symptoms that are completely the opposite of the classical adult depressive reactions. One of the most ominous but typical coping responses is the helpless – hopeless reaction pattern or the inability to ignore those negative aspects of oneself or one's life situation that cannot be controlled or changed. The implication for treatment is that in general only those therapies that help to redirect attention and energy, i.e. that support denial, can be supposed to be effective in the treatment of serious depressive disorders. The relatively great effect of pharmacotherapy and of that form of psychotherapy called cognitive therapy directed at selfcontrol, especially when combined, might be considered as evidence for this point of view (Smith et al. 1980). A recent study by Engels and Diekstra (1986) which seems to indicate that compared with other psychological treatment modalities, cognitive therapy is most promising in the treatment of the depressed, appears to substantiate this point of view.

The question then arises as to which factors determine whether a person will acquire the capacity for denial to a sufficient degree or not, especially when one takes into account the fact that the installment of such capability at late life stages is more difficult and costly. Not only the classical psychoanalytic authors but also contemporary investigators in the field of developmental psychology refer to the importance of experiences in the early stages of life for the development of cognitive coping styles for later life. In their review of the literature, Troll and Bengtson (1978) found that, in general, life and coping styles show less intergenerational differences that is usually supposed. Or in other words, the previous generation, through the specific social and psychoemotional situations they provide for their offspring, play an important role in how the latter might cope with old age in their turn.

This implies that research on social and psychological factors related to mental health in the elderly should be carried out within a life span developmental frame of reference and should especially try to identify those "evil conditions" that prevent optimal well-being throughout life up to a late age. One of the first steps in this respect could and should be an internationally accepted standardized terminology for such conditions. In my opinion this is one of the most needed projects for the short-term future, in which both national working groups and WHO have an important role to play. As long as the present ICD does not have a generally accepted and widley used 'Situational' counterpart in the form I have described above, by default the medical dominance of long-term care for the elderly will continue to exist, and I wholeheartedly agree with Mechanic (this volume) when he states that: "a narrow medical approach can be a real disservice to meeting the health needs of the elderly."

References

Atchley RC (1982) Culture and aging. In: Lesnoff-Caravaglia G (ed) Aging and the human condition. Human Sciences, New York

Diamond M (1984) A love affair with the brain. Psychology Today November:62–73

Diekstra RFW, Hawton K (eds) (1986) Suicide in adolescence. Nijhoff, International Publishers: Den Haag/Boston

Ehrlich PH, Ehrlich JF (1982) SRO elderly: a distinct population in a viable housing alternative. In: Lesnoff-Caravaglia G (ed) Aging and the human condition. Human Sciences, New York

Engels G, Diekstra RFW (1986) A meta-analysis of RET outcome studies. Journal of Clinical and Consulting Psychology. (accepted)

Furnham D, Argyle M (1981) The psychology of social situations. Pergamon, London

Huxley A (1952) The Devils of Loudun. Penguin, Harmondsworth

ISSBD (1982) The relevance of developmental psychology for WHO mental health programs. WHO, Geneva

Sainsbury P, Baert AE, Jenkins J (1981) Suicide in Europe. WHO informal paper. Copenhagen, WHO/Euro

Schaie K (1983) Longitudinal studies of human development. Rhinehart and Winston, New York

Smith ML, Glass GV, Miller TI (1980) The benefits of psychotherapy. John Hopkins University Press, Baltimore

Tibbits C (1978) Can we invalidate negative stereotypes of aging? Gerontologist, 19:1

Troll LE, Bengtson VL (1978) Generations in the family. In: Burr W et al. (eds) Contemporary theories about the family. The Free Press, New York

4 Biological and Medical Aspects of Aging and Age-Specific Brain Diseases

4.1 Morphology of the Brain in Normal Aging and in Processes of Dementia: Neuropathology and CT Findings

K. Kohlmeyer

This contribution on normal brain aging and dementias will not consider the not so frequent cerebral diseases leading to dementia during the senile or presenile period of life, such as Parkinson's, Huntington's, Pick's and Creutzfeldt-Jakob's diseases, because altogether they account for at most 5% of all cases of dementia. Only the morphology of normal brain aging and the two most frequent causes of dementia in old age – senile dementia of Alzheimer's type (SDAT) and multi-infarct dementia (MID) – will be discussed.

One of the most impressive signs of normal cerebral aging macroscopically is the so-called age-dependent cerebral atrophy. This is connected with an increase in the solid compounds in contrast to the fluid parts of the brain tissue, leading to diminution of the brain mass and to a reduction in the weight of the brain. The surface of the aged brain is marked by a more pronounced outlining of the sulci and convolutions, the former being dilated and the latter narrowed. These changes result in dilatation of the inner and still more the outer cerebral spinal fluid (CSF) spaces, so-called hydrocephalus internus et externus ex vacuo.

One of the most important processes of normal brain aging causing the diminution of the brain mass as a whole is a marked decrease – up to 20%–50% – in the number of nerve cells and dendrites (Brody 1955) localized within different cerebral regions and most prominently in the upper temporal areas. However, not only the loss of brain tissue indicates the process of aging, but also some new appearances not to be seen microscopically in the brains of younger persons. Proliferation and hypertrophy with increasing formation of glial fibers replace the diffuse loss of nerve cells and dendrites. A well-known characteristic phenomenon in aging cells is the presence of a pigment called lipofuscin. The cytoplasm of large neurons of humans aged between 80 and 100 years may be completely occupied by lipofuscin. Also the two microscopic lesions first described by Alzheimer (1906/1907) in his patient with a disease later called after him – neurofibrillary tangles and neuritic plaques – are observed during the brain aging of normals to some extent.

The following list summarizes the age-dependent changes of the central nervous system (Volk 1982; Wisniewski and Terry 1976)

- *Neurofibrillary tangles
- Increase of lipofuscin
- Hirano bodies
- *Granulovacuolar degeneration
- *Neuritic plaques
- *Loss of dendrites
- *Neuroaxonal dystrophy
- Congophilic angiopathy

Turning to the neuropathology of SDAT, it is surprising that the macroscopic appearance of the sulci and convolutions on the surface of the brain of patients with SDAT does not essentially differ from that of the sulci and convolutions in a normal of the same age. Actually the mean weight of the SDAT brain is only 8% less than that of an age-matched normal. The differences are mainly at the microscopic level; these changes, however, are not different in principle, rather only the quantity of the changes is decisively greater (Terry 1963). The features marked by an asterisk in the above list indicate the changes that are predominant in SDAT (Volk 1982). The loss of nerve cells and dendrites is, on average, more than 20% higher in SDAT and this increases to 45% in respect of the large neurons only; one is also able to observe a remarkable decrease in the number of cortical synapses. Of particular significance in SDAT is the occurrence of neuritic plaques and neurofibrillary tangles. When present in small numbers they are, as mentioned, signs of a normal aging brain; already however, both plaques and tangles are present in great numbers throughout the neo- and paleocortex in patients with Alzheimer's disease in the narrow sense, i.e., presenile dementia. Many patients with SDAT have plaques only in the neocortex. It is very interesting that there is a close correlation between the numbers of tangles and/or plaques and the degree of dementia (Blessed et al. 1968). The fact that plaques are also found in the deep gray areas of diseased brains (Hirano and Zimmermann 1962), in contrast with the brains of normals, in which they mainly concern the cortex (Matsuyama et al. 1966), may explain the greater dilatation of the lateral and third ventricles in patients with SDAT than in normal aged subjects.

Arteriosclerosis is one of the common changes of the blood vessels in old age, and cerebral arteriosclerosis is the most frequent cause of occlusions of cerebral arteries and thus also the most frequent cause of cerebral infarction. Therefore it may be surprising that dementia due to cerebrovascular disorders occurs far more rarely than that due to SDAT. This group accounts for only 20% of all dementias and is called multi-infarct dementia (Tomlinson et al. 1970). Such dementias are relatively infrequent because arteriosclerosis of the larger and smaller cerebral vessels per se never leads to such a severe decrease of cerebral blood flow that a global brain atrophy comparable to that of SDAT will follow. Similarly, a single cerebral infarction per se never causes dementia. Rather, its results are focal cerebral signs like hemiplegia, aphasia, apraxia, and hemianopia. If repeated multiple brain infarcts occur, one can expect such an extensive loss of brain tissue that it will lead to cerebral atrophy and dementia. Since multiple infarcts occur independently of arteriosclerosis, for example due to cerebral emboli in patients with heart diseases, the term "multi-infarct dementia" is much more correct than the old diagnosis of "cerebral arteriosclerosis" or, to use the German term, "Zerebralsklerose."

The neuropathological appearances of cerebral infarctions are dependent on their age. There is a characteristic time course of such changes. MID and the brain atrophy are chronic processes. It takes some time for them to become obvious in a clinical sense. Therefore, while it is important to be aware of the acute and early stages of infarcts (like necrosis, resorption, and liquefaction) with regard to strokes, they are not so interesting for the neuropathology of MID. The organic basis of MID is chronic multiple glial scars and cysts localized within the cortex, the white matter, and the basal ganglia. The characteristic picture of multiple small cortical scars is that of so-called granular atrophy of the cerebral cortex (Pentschew 1934; Spatz 1939). In the deep structures of the hemispheres we see more frequently small and multiple cysts filled with CSF, situated predominantly in the basal ganglia; the term for this condition is "status lacunaris" (Marie 1901). The chronic stage of large infarcts affecting the cortical – subcortical areas or the regions of the inner capsule and the basal ganglia is marked by a huge brain tissue defect.

Finally, there is a specific, though not so frequent, type of MID called Binswanger's disease, or as originally described by Binswanger (1894), encephalopathia chronica progressiva subcorticalis. Its neuropathology is characterized by focal, confluent, or diffuse demyelinizations and cysts situated exclusively within the white matter. The cortex is spared from pathological changes. The cause of this subcortical degeneration is arteriosclerosis of the arteries supplying the white matter, and chronic very high blood pressure is present in nearly every case of Binswanger's disease. Deterioration in the permeability of the walls of arterioles and capillaries with focal edema of the white matter is also discussed as a pathogenetic factor.

Computed tomography (CT), as a morphological method for in vivo imaging of the brain and the cerebral spinal fluid (CSF) spaces, can be used to demonstrate the normal and pathological changes of the brain in old age (macroscopically only, of course).

Computed tomography was performed on 300 subjects between 60 and 98 years of age, half with and half without dementia (Kohlmeyer 1983; Kohlmeyer and Shamena 1983). The mean age of the nondemented group was 73.3 years and that of the demented group 74 years. The nondemented group was not composed of completely healthy subjects. The clinical diagnosis in this group included reactive depression, neurosis, and headache. Patients with a history of drug or alcohol abuse, epileptic seizures, head trauma, transient ischemic attacks, or strokes were excluded from the study.

The following measurements were obtained: width of the third ventricle at the level of its greatest diameter (Fig. 1); the Huckman number as the sum of the greatest and the smallest distances between the frontal horns (Fig. 2); the ventricular index, calculated as the quotient of the widest distance of the choroid plexus of the lateral ventricles and the widest distance of the frontal horns (Fig. 3); the cella media index, calculated as the quotient of the largest biparietal diameter measured from the tabula externa to the tabula externa and the greatest width of the cella media (Fig. 4); and the width of the cortical sulci, expressed as the sum of the measurements of the widest sulcus frontally, temporally, and parietally of both hemispheres. All the values mentioned were tabulated, and the mean values and standard deviations were determined for each category by age group and dementia condition. Statistical analysis was by Student's t-test.

The mean brain measurements and indices, standard deviations, and the results of statistical calculations are demonstrated in Table 1. From the measured and calculated values demonstrated, we drew the following conclusions on the size of the inner and outer CSF spaces of the brain in demented and nondemented subjects over 60 years of age.

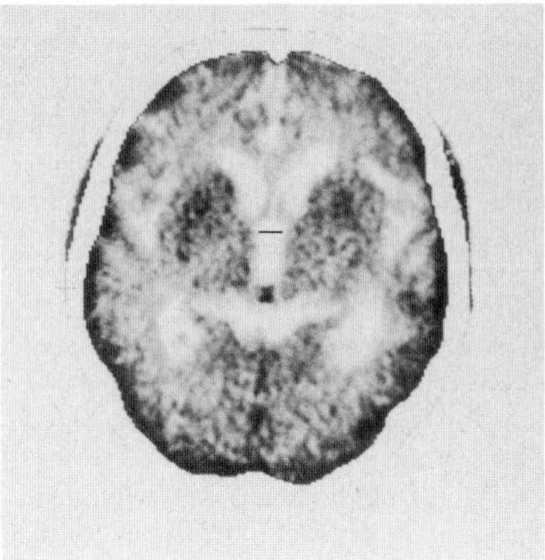

Fig. 1. Largest diameter of the third ventricle

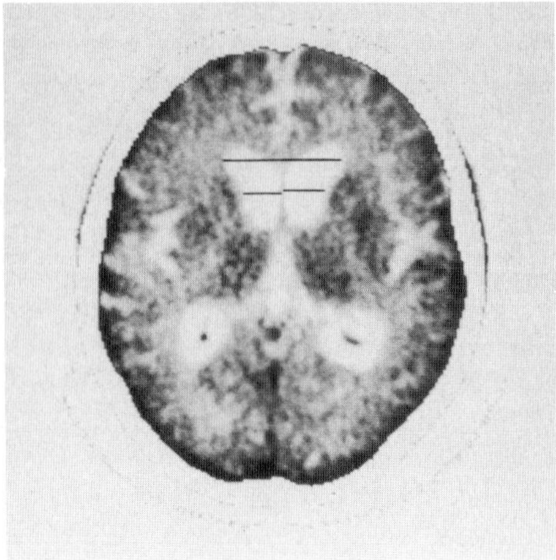

Fig. 2. Huckman number

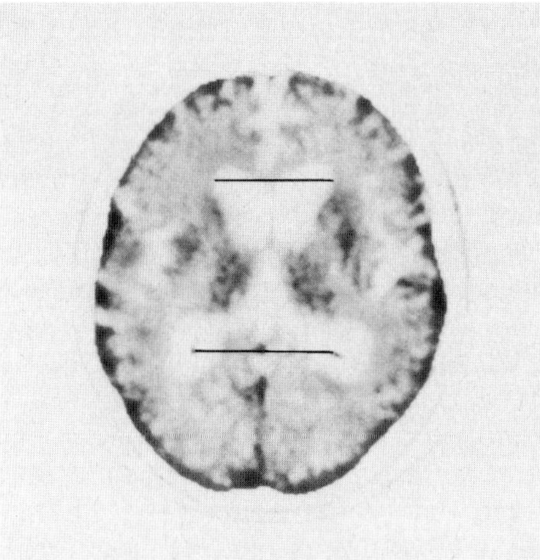

Fig. 3. Ventricle index

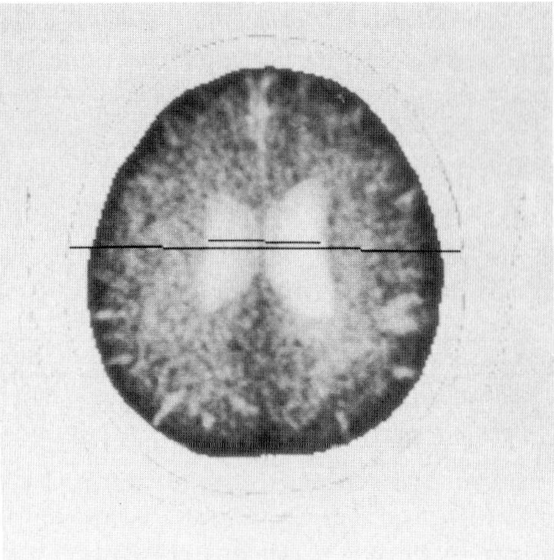

Fig. 4. Cella media index

The width of the third ventricle was increasingly age dependent in nondemented persons from 60 to over 90 years of age (Grumme 1977). But in patients with dementia in comparable age groups the third ventricle was enlarged significantly. Its width in those with dementia who were aged between 60 and 64 years exceeded the mean width in a normal group over 60 years of age.

There was a certain enlargement of the lateral ventricles in relation to age in nondemented subjects, but we never found mean values of the Huckman number, the ventricular index, and the cella media index exceeding the normal maximal values as indicated in the literature (Meese et al. 1976). On the other hand, each of

Table 1. The size of the third ventricle, the lateral ventricles, and the cortical sulci (mean values and SD) in 300 subjects aged between 60 and 100 years, iso with and iso without dementia

Age range, condition	Mean values (±SD)				
	Third ventricle <8 mm	Huckman no. 52 mm	Ventricular index >1.6	Cella media index >4.0	Cortical sulci (mm)
60–64					
Nondemented (29)	5.44 (0.58)	47.37 (3.51)	1.83 (0.12)	4.78 (0.27)	10.32 (3.3)
Demented (25)	9.5 [c](3.82)	63.83[c](4.89)	1.25[c](0.09)	3.38[c](0.28)	18.33[b](8.7)
65–69					
Nondemented (27)	6.53 (1.38)	49.56 (3.83)	1.85 (0.17)	4.78 (0.86)	14.26 (3.59)
Demented (26)	9.12[c](3.06)	64.92[c](7.2)	1.35[c](0.13)	3.76[b](0.40)	18.00[a](4.05)
70–74					
Nondemented (40)	7.91 (1.40)	49.98 (5.00)	1.81 (0.20)	5.03 (0.75)	15.28 (3.90)
Demented (39)	11.18[c](4.15)	69.62[c](8.10)	1.26[c](0.13)	3.46[c](0.33)	17.37 (3.6)
75–79					
Nondemented (35)	8.04 (1.96)	51.21 (5.10)	1.76 (0.17)	4.87 (0.90)	16.33 (3.96)
Demented (41)	11.10[c](2.98)	68.40[c](9.90)	1.26[c](0.19)	3.51[c](0.42)	17.95 (4.66)
>80					
Nondemented (19)	8.68 (2.03)	52.04 (4.04)	1.78 (0.09)	4.80 (0.07)	17.67 (4.04)
Demented (19)	11.38[a](1.81)	70.74[c](5.60)	1.22[c](0.15)	3.36[c](0.24)	18.05 (5.26)

[a] $P<0.05$; [b] $P<0.01$; [c] $P<0.001$

these values in the demented group indicated a statistically significant enlargement of the lateral ventricles compared with the nondemented groups.

Turning to the cortical sulci, there was a difference in the width between the nondemented and demented subjects from 60 to 69 years of age. This difference, however, was only of low statistical significance and no longer existed after 70 years of age. Therefore, it seems that the observation of a greater or lesser number of however dilated cortical sulci in CT studies of the brain in old people has nothing to do with dementia, but is a sign of a process of physiological involution of the cerebral cortex. By contrast, dilatations of the lateral and the third ventricles are much more suspicious of a pathological cerebral atrophy as a cause of dementia. However, it must be mentioned that this holds true only for patients aged over 50 – 60 years, while cerebral diseases leading to dilatation of the inner CSF spaces during childhood, adolescence, and early adulthood may not lead to any intellectual impairment, probably due to the greater plasticity of the brain during the earlier periods of life.

According to the clinical – neuropathological correlative studies of Tomlinson, Blessed, and Roth, SDAT is the most frequent cause of the loss of intellectual capacity in old age, while cerebrovascular diseases as a cause of dementia, so-called multi-infarct dementia (MID), are rarer. There is general agreement, with the exception of Japan, that dementia in those aged over 60 years is caused by cerebral atrophy of Alzheimer's type in about 60%, and that cerebrovascular disease is the causal process in about 20% only. The remaining 20% are either mixed cases or are of unclear etiology. The clinical differential

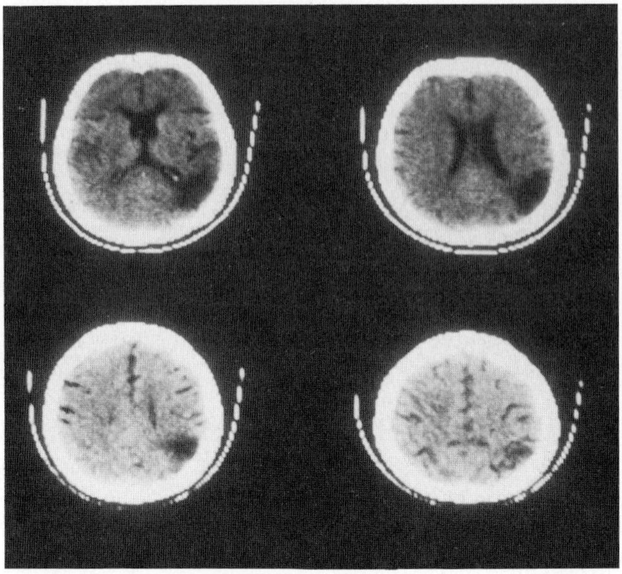

Fig. 5. Infarction in the left temporal – partietal region and cerebral atrophy

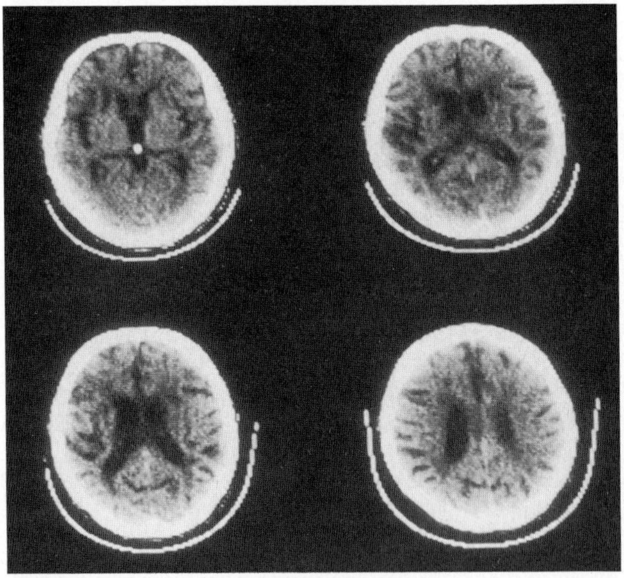

Fig. 6. Multiple small infarctions bilaterally and severe cerebral atrophy

diagnosis is a problem indeed, and is possible only in typical cases (Hachinski et al. 1974). Taking into consideration that not only the microscopic aspect of these two diseases but also their macromorphological appearances are very different, we put forward the hypothesis that CT, as a morphological method, could contribute to differential diagnosis in many cases (Kohlmeyer 1983; Kohlmeyer 1982). The

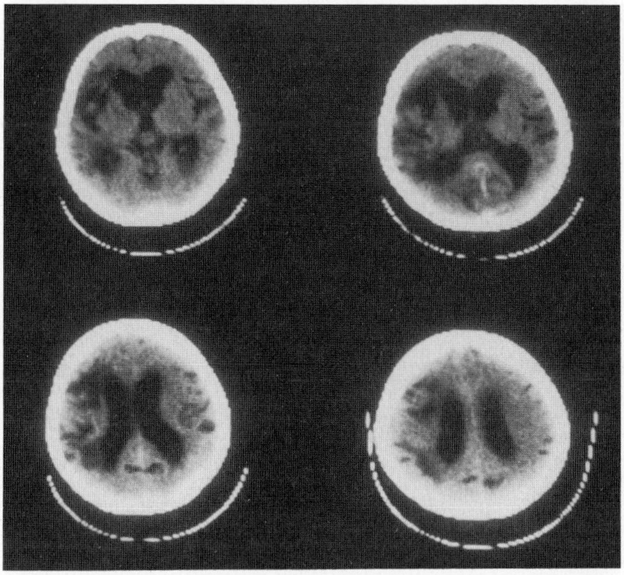

Fig. 7. Multiple large infarctions bilaterally and severe cerebral atrophy

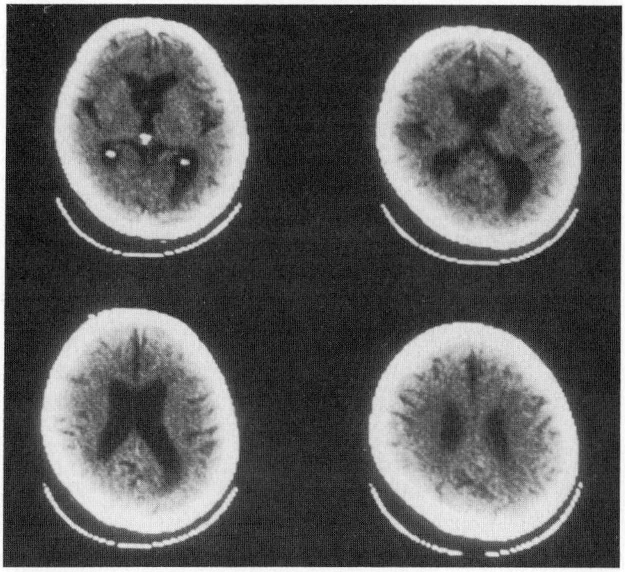

Fig. 8. Local enlargment of the left frontal horn and moderate cerebral atrophy

most prominent sign of a cerebrovascular disease in CT is the occurrence of focal hypodensities corresponding to the supply of a cerebral artery and to be interpreted as residuals of one or more cerebral infarcts, considering their localization, size, and density (Figs. 5–7). The lateral ventricles, too, can show local changes in size, e.g., a pronounced widening of one frontal horn (Fig. 8). In

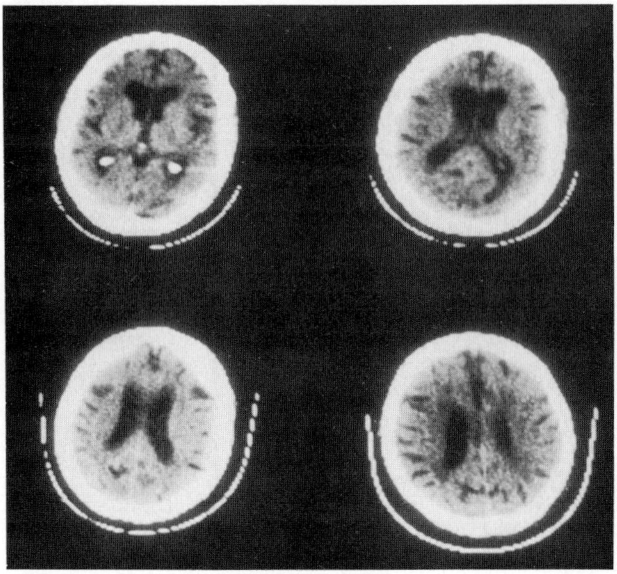

Fig. 9. Severe global cerebral atrophy without focal vascular lesions

cases of SDAT, CT reveals moderate or severe dilatation primarily of the inner CSF spaces but also of the cortical sulci (Fig. 9), even though these cases can hardly be differentiated from normal CT changes of the brain in old age.

Approaching the question of differential diagnosis, we analyzed the CT pictures of 400 consecutive patients diagnosed clinically as demented. Their mean age was 70.1 years. The clinical diagnoses and their relations with the CT findings are demonstrated by Table 2.

Clinically, 64% were classified as SDAT and 23% as MID; 13% were not classified. One of the most important findings of CT was the presence of treatable cerebral diseases (brain tumors, subdural hematomas, communicating hydrocephalus) in 26 cases (7%) of the 400 diagnosed as chronic progressive dementia by very experienced neurologists and psychiatrists. Surprisingly, CT was

Table 2. Clinical and CT diagnoses in 400 patients with dementia

	Clinically	CT			
		Atrophy with vascular signs	Atrophy without vascular signs	Tumor, subdural hematoma, hydrocephalus	Normal
SDAT	256 (64%)	36 (14%)	171 (67%)	8 (3%)	41 (16%)
MID	92 (23%)	39 (42%)	40 (44%)	8 (9%)	5 (5%)
Not classified	52 (13%)	16 (31%)	13 (24%)	10 (20%)	13 (25%)
Total	400	91 (23%)	224 (56%)	26 (7%)	59 (15%)

normal in 59 patients (15%) despite clear clinical signs of dementia. Global cerebral atrophy without signs of vascular brain lesions was found by CT in 56%, and cerebral atrophy in combination with vascular lesions of brain tissue in 23%. A comparison of the clinical classification and the CT findings shows that vascular dementia is diagnosed too often clinically, for of the 92 patients clinically classified as having MID, only 39 (42%) exhibited vascular brain lesions in CT while 40 (44%) had CT patterns that more probably corresponded to SDAT than to cerebral vascular diseases. The clinical diagnosis of SDAT was more reliable; 171 of 256 cases diagnosed clinically (67%) were also classified by CT as brain atrophy without any signs of vascular damage. The 36 patients (14%) with vascular signs in CT belonged to a special group of 61 cases with signs of demyelinization of the white matter in CT to be interpreted as Binswanger's disease, which was described as a subgroup of MID by de Reuck et al. (1980).

One problem remains: those cases with normal CT findings despite clear and severe dementia. Sophisticated methods like positron emission tomography and magnetic resonance imaging, demonstrating not only cerebral morphology but also metabolism, i.e., cerebral function, will be more reliable in diagnosing precisely such cases of dementia.

References

Alzheimer A (1906/1907) Über einen eigenartigen schweren Krankheitsprozeß der Hirnrinde. Zentralbl Nervenheilk 25:1134, 30:177–179

Binswanger O (1894) Die Abgrenzung der allgemeinen progressiven Paralyse. Berl Klin Wochenschr 49:1103–1105, 1137–1139, 1180–1186

Blessed G, Tomlinson BE, Roth M (1968) The association between quantitative measures of dementia and of senile change in the cerebral grey matter of elderly subjects. Br J Psychiatry 114:797–811

Brody H (1955) Organization of the cerebral cortex III. A study of aging in the human cerebral cortex. J Comp Neurol 102:511–556

Feigin I, Popow N (1963) Neuropathological changes late in cerebral edema: the relationship to trauma hypertensive disease and Binswanger's encephalopathy. J Neuropathol Exp Neurol 22:500–511

Grumme T (1977) Die Breite der 3. Hirnkammer vom Frühgeborenen bis ins 10. Dezennium. Fortschr Neurol Psychiatr 45:223–268

Hachinski VC, Lassen NA, Marshall J (1974) Multi-infarct-dementia – a cause of mental deterioration in the elderly. Lancet II:207–209

Hirano A, Zimmermann HM (1962) Alzheimer's neurofibrillary changes. A topographic study. Arch Neurol 7:227–242

Kohlmeyer K (1982) Computertomographischer Beitrag zur Differentialdiagnose vaskulär bedingte Demenz (Multiinfarkt-Typ) und primär degenerative Demenz (Alzheimer Typ). Z Gerontol 15:321–324

Kohlmeyer K (1983) The aging brain: normal and pathological aspects in computed tomography. In: Gispen WH, Traber J (eds) Aging of the brain. Developments in neurology, vol 7. Elsevier Science, Amsterdam New York Oxford pp 9–21

Kohlmeyer K, Shamena AR (1983) CT assessment of CSF spaces in the brain in demented and nondemented patients over 60 years of age. AJNR 4:706–707

Marie P (1901) Des foyers lacunaires de désintégration et de différents autres états cavitaires du cerveau, Rev Med (Paris) 21:281

Matsuyama H, Namiki H, Watanabe I (1966) Senile changes of the brain in the Japanese. Incidence of Alzheimer's neurofibrillary change and senile plaques. In: Lüthy F, Bischoff

A (eds) Proc 5th Internat Congr Neuropathol. Excerpta Medica Series No. 100, Amsterdam, pp 979–980

Meese W, Lanksch W, Wende S (1976) Cerebral atrophy and computerized tomography – Aspects of a qualitative and quantitative analysis. In: Lanksch W, Kazner E (eds) Cranial computerized tomography. Springer, Berlin Heidelberg New York, pp 222–232

Pentschew A (1934) Die granuläre Atrophie der Großhirnrinde. Arch Psychiatr Nervenkr 101:80–136

Reuck J de, Crevits L, Costor W de, Sieben G, Eecken H van der (1980) Pathogenesis of Binswanger chronic progressive subcortical encephalopathy. Neurology 30:920–928

Spatz H (1939) Pathologische Anatomie der Kreislaufstörungen des Gehirns. Z Neurol 167:301–351

Terry RD (1963) The fine structure of neurofibrillary tangles in Alzheimer's disease. J Neuropathol Exp Neurol 22:629–642

Tomlinson BE, Blessed G, Roth M (1970) Observations on the brains of demented old people. J Neurol Sci 11:205–242

Volk B (1982) Morphologische Aspekte der senilen Demenz. In: Fischer B, Lehrl S (eds) Differentialdiagnose Depression – beginnende chronische zerebrovaskuläre Insuffiziens. Pharmazeutische Verlagsgesellschaft, Munich, pp 69–85

Wisniewski HM, Terry RD (1976) Neuropathology of the aging brain. In: Terry RD, Gershon S (eds) Neurobiology of aging. Raven, New York, pp 265–280

4.2 Determination of Regional Cerebral Function and Structure in Normal Aging and Dementia with Positron Emission Tomography, Magnetic Resonance Imaging and X-Ray Computed Tomography [1]

A. Alavi, J. Chawluk, H. Hurtig, R. W. Dann, A. Saykin, R. Gur, M. Reivich

Dementia is a progressive clinical state characterized by the deterioration of intellect, memory, judgment, and abstract thinking (Diagnostic and Statistical Manual III 1980). The syndrome has many etiologies and is a leading cause of disability among the elderly in the U.S. and Europe. A prevalence of as high as 5% in people over 65 years has been estimated in recent surveys (Katzman 1976; Terry 1976). By far the most common cause of dementia in the world today is Alzheimer's disease, or dementia of the Alzheimer type (DAT), a primary degenerative process identifiable pathologically by its classic microscopic findings of amyloid plaques and neurofibrillary tangles (Blackwood and Corsellis 1976). DAT produces a highly variable spectrum of symptoms and it progresses at an equally variable rate. It is a clinical diagnosis of exclusion unless a brain biopsy is done, but as many as 80% of *all* demented people are probable victims of DAT (Wells 1978; Maisden and Harrison 1972). The other principal cause of dementia is atherosclerotic cerebrovascular disease, as diagnosed by *history* and X-ray computed tomography (*XCT*) *scan*, which has been labeled multi-infarct dementia (MID) by Hachinski et al. (1974).

Until recently, a vascular etiology was assigned to DAT, but Tomlinson et al. (1970) showed that the distinctive cerebral pathology of this dementia has no relationship to arteriosclerotic vascular disease. Moreover, these investigators identified similar, but less pronounced pathologic changes in the brains of nondemented old people (Tomlinson et al. 1968), thus suggesting that plaques and neurofibrillary tangles in modest numbers are normal accompaniments of aging. The quantitative correlation between the severity of dementia and intensity of brain pathology was also established by Tomlinson et al. (1968, 1970), but the mechanism for the proliferation of pathologic changes and associated clinical symptoms still remains unknown.

During the past decade, research on the central nervous system (CNS) has benefited from an unanticipated explosion in tomographic techniques. Based on principles developed by Cormack (1963), Oldendorf (1961), Kuhl and Edwards (1968), and Hounsfield (1973), tomographic scanning systems have, for the first time, allowed the detailed study of the human brain's structure and function in vivo.

XCT has become firmly established as an essential diagnostic step in the evaluation of any CNS disorder. Magnetic resonance imaging (MRI), which has been in serious preliminary clinical use only since 1980, has already demonstrated the potential for better resolution than XCT in certain neurologic conditions. Positron emission tomography (PET), through limited to major research centers in

1 Supported by NIH grants NS 14867–01 and AGO3934–01

the United States, Europe, and Japan, has nevertheless begun providing valuable insight into normal and abnormal brain function.

Rather than following a linear evolution, with each tomographic method superseding its predecessor, XCT, PET, and MRI are developing concurrently, providing complementary information in many instances. This paper reviews the applications of each of these imaging techniques in normal aging and dementia, concentrating on the newer investigative tools, PET and MRI.

Methods and Materials

In our ongoing study of regional cerebral metabolic and structural changes associated with normal brain aging and dementia, we have studied 23 cognitively impaired patients and nine elderly controls over the past year. A separate group of nine young control subjects studied under the same experimental conditions is used for comparison. Of the 23 demented patients studied, 14 had probable DAT by the criteria of the Diagnostic and Statistical Manual III (1980) and of the NINCDS-ADRDA work group (McKhann et al. 1984). A breakdown of the demographic data on the subjects included in this preliminary analysis is listed in Table 1. The normal young controls were carefully screened by a neurologist and a psychiatrist and found to be free of mental or physical disorders. The elderly subjects were evaluated by a neurologist and received an extensive battery of psychometric tests, after which they were categorized as normal or demented. Every subject was studied with both XCT and PET within a short period of time. A certain number of normal controls and patients underwent MRI. All PET studies were done under similar resting, unstimulated conditions (eyes open, ears unplugged, dimmed lights, low-level ambient machine noise).

XCT. The majority of patients were examined with GE 8800 or GE 9800 CT scanners. The brain was imaged with and without contrast enhancement.

PET. ^{18}F-labeled 2-fluorodeoxyglucose ([^{18}F]FDG) was used to determine local cerebral metabolic rates for glucose (LCMRgl) in all subjects studied. A modified version of the PETT-V system (Ter-Pogossian et al. 1968) was employed to obtain brain images of LCMRgl. This machine generates simultaneously seven cross-sectional images of the brain along the rostrocaudal axis. The

Table 1. Demographic data on demented and normal subjects studied by PET

Group	Subjects	Age ± standard deviation
	(n)	(years)
Young controls	9	28±6
Elderly controls	9	61±10
Alzheimer's disease	14	64±8
mild-moderate	8	62±9
severe	6	65±6

average of eight sections is the "whole brain" value and is used as a reference point that is relatively insensitive to slight differences in positioning.

Regional metabolic data were generated using an atlas overlay system (Dann et al. 1982), which defines approximately 50 structures covering the entire cerebral cortex, white matter, basal ganglia, and cerebellum. For each structure, the region/whole brain ratio was calculated as a measure of relative activity.

In calculating metabolic rates, the rate constants and lumped constant values used are those actually measured by our group (Reivich et al. 1984). All data are automatically entered into a data base system which allows a wide variety of subsequent statistical tests to be applied.

MRI. A developmental resistive magnet (0.12 T, 5.1 MHz), designed and built by GE, was used for this study. For brain imaging, a tightly fit head coil was used. MRI on our unit is performed with spin-warp technique, which has been described in detail (Edelstein et al. 1980). In this form of MRI, while spatial encoding is performed along the x-axis, spatial information also is phase encoded on the y-axis, and a two-dimensional (2D) Fourier transform is performed. This method of imaging is advantageous in that it is less sensitive to local magnetic field inhomogeneities. Both planar (2D) and multiplanar (3D) data collection are available. Slice thickness is 1.3 cm.

As initially configured, both saturation recovery (SR) and inversion recovery (IR) data collection schemes are available. Although SR with long repetition times has been reported as a method of obtaining proton-density-weighted scans, SR techniques with short repetition times may provide T_1-weighted information as well. IR scanning is another method commonly used to provide T_1-weighted information.

A comparison of the effectiveness of these two pulse sequences in MRI has recently been described. Edelstein et al. (1983) found that, when compared for similar imaging times, SR is superior to IR in distinguishing tissues of the same proton density but of different values of T_1. Our initial experience confirmed their findings, and as a result, T_1-weighted images on our system were typically performed with SR pulse sequences and a 0.15-s repetition rate (TR). The short TR permitted shorter scan time and increased patient acceptance of the examination procedure.

Since atrophy as demonstrated by current-generation, high-resolution XCT scanners appears to be a feature of normal aging and dementia, and since currently used PET scanners are only capable of relatively poor spatial resolution, we have also investigated the effect of cerebrospinal fluid (CSF) spaces on regional and global metabolic rate calculations, as determined by PET (Chawlule et al. 1984). We have completed a preliminary analysis of the effect that global atrophy, determined volumetrically using a technique similar to that of Gado et al. (1984), has upon calculations of global metabolic rates. Relative volumetric estimates of ventricular size, sulcal size, and residual brain tissue (intracranial cavity − [ventricle + sulci]) were obtained from the anatomical images. Global metabolic rates are then corrected for atrophy using the formula: Corrected metabolic rate = (uncorrected metabolic rate: relative brain volume) × 100.

Results

Of the nine demented patients who were not classified as DAT patients, one had probable Huntington's disease exhibited profound bilateral basal ganglia hypometabolism. Two patients had an apparent focal degenerative disorder characterized by slowly progressive aphasia, without other significant cognitive impairments. These two individuals demonstrated striking left temporoparietal hypometabolism, without other significant regional metabolic abnormalities. Neither patient demonstrated significant global atrophy on XCT or MRI or focal atrophy, which would explain the apparent regional hypometabolism. The remaining six patients suffered from MID or dementia secondary to Parkinson's disease.

Young controls, old controls, and DAT patients were compared in order to investigate changes in the pattern of regional glucose metabolism with aging and with DAT. These findings are presented in Table 2. When young normal subjects are compared with elderly normals, we note a significant relative decrease in frontal metabolism with aging, and a corresponding relative increase in posterior metabolism. In addition, the elderly normals demonstrate significantly reduced

Table 2. Significant changes in patterns of regional cerebral glucose metabolism with aging and dementia

Region	R/WB Value			
	Young controls	Old controls	Mild-moderate DAT	Severe DAT
Left anterior calcarine	123	142[a]	141[a]	169[a–c]
Right anterior calcarine	120	144[a]	144[a]	173[a–c]
Left posterior calcarine	104	123[a]	117[a]	154[a–c]
Right posterior calcarine	101	125[a]	121[a]	150[a–c]
Left inferior parietal	83	69	66[a]	48[a, b]
Right inferior parietal	89	79[a]	71[a]	66[a, h]
Left superior temporal gyrus	71	74	66	47[b]
Left sensorimotor strip	105	95[a]	108[b]	108[b]
Right sensorimotor strip	107	101	112[b]	118[b]
Left motor-premotor	109	94[a]	113[b]	112[b]
Left frontal eye field	119	101[a]	107[a]	89[a]
Right frontal eye field	125	108[a]	112[a]	99[a]
Left frontal lobe	106	92[a]	97[a]	77[a]
Right frontal lobe	110	96[a]	99[a]	84[a]
Left cortex	99	96	97	89[b, c]
Left brainstem	70	82	76	110[b, c]
Right brainstem	76	83	81	121[b, c]
Left cerebellum	100	112	112	152[b, c]
Right cerebellum	101	113	123	161[b, c]

R/WB, (regional glucose metabolic rate: global glucose metabolic rate) × 100
[a] $P<0.02$ compared with young controls
[b] $P<0.02$ compared with old controls
[c] $P<0.02$ compared with mild-moderate DAT

metabolism in the right inferior parietal region, an area of the brain which appears to be integral to attentional networks in humans (Mesulam 1981). Pre- and postrolandic metabolic activity also appeared relatively decreased in the elderly normals, perhaps reflecting known decreases in somatosensory and motor functions accompanying normal aging.

In comparing regional cerebral metabolic patterns of patients with mild to moderate DAT, as defined by mini-mental state examination (MMSE) scores of 19 or greater, with normal age-matched controls, we have demonstrated several interesting results. The first is a further decrease in right inferior parietal metabolism beyond that noted with normal aging. Primary sensorimotor metabolic function is relatively preserved in the DAT patients. When individuals with severe DAT (MMSE scores of less than 14) are compared with the patients with mild to moderate disease, the relative preservation of metabolic function in primary sensorimotor and vegetative centers is further illustrated. In addition, the severely demented patients demonstrate significant reductions in left hemispheric cortical and, specifically, perisylvian metabolism.

The brain volume by subject group and the changes in global metabolic rates after correction for cerebral atrophy are shown in Tables 3 and 4. These data show that significantly greater cerebral atrophy is present in demented patients than in age-matched controls. Furthermore, demented individuals reveal a significantly

Table 3. Brain volume by subject group

	Subjects (n)	Age ± standard deviation (years)	Brain volume ± standard deviation (%)
Elderly controls	4	61 ± 11	91.0 ± 2.3
Dementia	8	66 ± 9	82.7 ± 4.1[a]
DAT	6	64 ± 10	82.4 ± 4.8[b]
multi-infarct	1	69	83.9
parkinsonian	1	74	82.0

[a] $P \leqq 0.001$ compared with controls
[b] $P \leqq 0.005$ compared with controls

Table 4. Change in global metabolic rates after correction for cerebral atrophy

Diagnosis (n subjects)	Increase ± standard deviation (%)
Elderly controls (4)	9.9 ± 2.7
Dementia (8)	21.2 ± 6.1[a]
DAT (6)	21.8 ± 7.2[b]
multi-infarct (1)	19.1
parkinsonian (1)	20.1

[a] $P \leqq 0.001$ compared with controls
[b] $P \leqq 0.01$ compared with controls

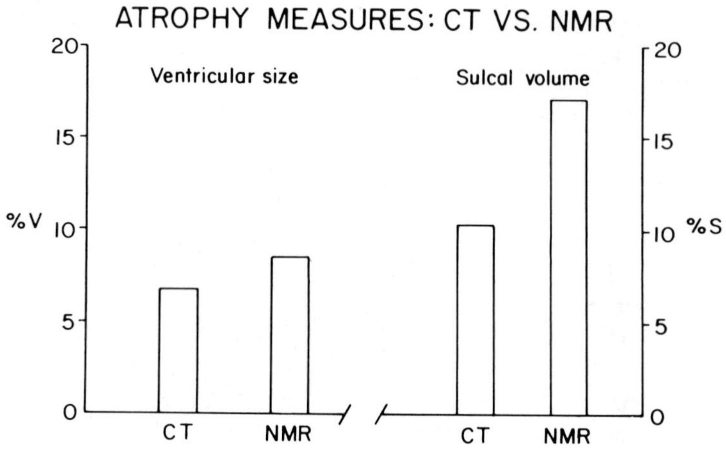

Fig. 1. Comparison of volumetric estimates from transaxial CT and NMR scans ($n=3$).

greater increase in metabolic rates after correction for atrophy than age-matched controls.

When volumetric estimates from XCT and MRI were obtained on the same patient, we noted that sulcal volumes appeared larger on the MRI scans, as illustrated in Fig. 1. Since MRI is potentially capable of demonstrating greater CSF-parenchyma contrast and is not subject to bony artifacts over the convexities, we believe that MRI may prove superior to XCT in estimating the degree of sulcal enlargement in aged and demented individuals. Our preliminary data also indicate that MRI may prove superior to XCT in diagnosing patients with multi-infarct dementia (MID). Subcortical infarcts, for example, were more clearly demonstrated with MRI than with XCT.

Discussion

The first clinical reports of XCT scanning indicated that atrophy demonstrable with pneumoencephalography was also seen on XCT images (Earnest et al. 1979). A number of groups subsequently looked at linear, planimetric (single-slice areas), or subjective (rank order) estimates of ventricular dilatation and cortical atrophy by XCT (Kasniak et al. 1979; Jacoby et al. 1980; Hughes and Gado 1981; Barron et al. 1976; Jacoby and Levy 1980). Diverse methodologies, including the manner of XCT analysis, type of cognitive tests administered, and selection of control groups, led to conflicting conclusions. These studies generally showed increasing ventricular volume with age (Earnest et al. 1979; Kasniak et al. 1979; Jacoby et al. 1980; Hughes and Gado 1981; Barron et al. 1976). Sulcal atrophy was an inferior discriminator, presumably due to convexity artifacts, arbitrary measurement techniques, and relatively poor scanner resolution (Jacoby et al. 1980, Jacoby and Levy 1980; Roberts et al. 1976).

Attempts at associating atrophic changes with cognitive impairment were even less successful. Several centers found no correlation between the degree of dementia and the extent of cerebral atrophy (Earnest et al. 1979; Claveia et al. 1977; Hughes and Gado 1981).

These initially disappointing data have been improved upon with the advent of better resolution XCT scanners and sophisticated computer programs for the analysis of CSF volumes and brain parenchyma characteristics. Yamaura et al. were the first to report relative volume estimates from XCT scans of CSF spaces, examining 228 normal subjects, 2 – 89 years old (Yamaura et al. 1980). Miller et al. found a significant increase in atrophy beginning at age 50, in agreement with previous autopsy findings (Miller et al. 1980). Ito et al. (1981), from the same center as Yamaura et al., refined its technique for volumetric analysis of CSF spaces (excluding cortical sulci, however) and applied a dementia rating scale to the study population. Their finding that atrophy correlates inversely with mental function is weakened by an associated direct correlation between atrophy and age. Gado et al., using a similar method for estimating relative ventricular and sulcal volumes, noted a highly significant separation of controls from mildly demented patients on the basis of XCT scan atrophic changes (Gado et al. 1984). Measurements of ventricular volumes in the two clinical groups did not overlap, in contrast to their previous study, which employed a linear quantification of ventricular size (Hughes and Gado 1981). A less clear-cut but still significant separation of demented patients from age-matched controls was obtained by George and co-workers, who measured only ventricular volumes, while ignoring sulcal changes (George et al. 1983). Since their correlations were still relatively weak, they further speculated that ventricular enlargement reflects the underlying pathology of DAT only partially.

Given the prominence of cortical changes seen histopathologically, one might expect to find an increase in sulcal volumes before ventricular dilatation becomes apparent in DAT. Recently Arai et al. (1983) reported a highly significant increase in cortical atrophy measured volumetrically when young patients (54 years old at onset) with mild DAT were compared with age-matched controls. The increase in ventricular volume was less dramatic until cognitive and functional disturbances became severe. Their results suggested that cortical atrophy is detectable in early (mild) disease and that ventricular dilatation is a later, perhaps secondary, occurrence (Arai et al. 1983). If their hypothesis is correct, an imaging modality capable of demonstrating sulcal enlargement more accurately would in theory prove superior to XCT in diagnosing early dementia.

Unlike XCT, proton MR scanning can image brain surfaces without interference from beam-hardening (bone) artifacts. In addition, pulse sequences can be modified to maximize the contrast between adjacent structures with different proton environment characteristics, such as CSF and gray matter. Preliminary studies by our group suggest that MRI shows greater sensitivity in detecting cortical atrophy than XCT. The validity of these measurements awaits appropriate phantom studies, the feasibility of which is being explored at our institution (G.T. Herman, personal communication; H. L. Kundel, personal communication).

Acute and chronic cerebral infarcts can be well-detected by MRI (Buonanno et al. 1983a,b; Spetzler et al. 1983; Pykett et al. 1983; Bydder et al. 1983; Brand-Zawadzki et al. 1983). In animal experiments, changes consistent with cerebral infarcts were noted as soon as 2 h after carotid artery occlusion. The infarcted hemisphere has significantly prolonged T_1 and T_2 values compared with the contralateral hemispheres (Buananno et al. 1983b; Spetzler et al. 1983). Successful application of MRI has been reported in identifying acute infarcts by several groups (Buonnano et al. 1983a; Pykett et al. 1983. Bydder et al. 1983; Brant-Zawadzki et al. 1983). These investigators have pointed out that MRI is at least as sensitive as XCT in detecting acute infarctions, and, in locations such as the posterior fossa, MRI is superior to XCT imaging in identifying structural abnormalities (Buonanno et al. 1983a; Bydder et al. 1983; Brant-Zawadzki et al. 1983).

Chronic infarcts also exhibit prolonged T_1 and T_2 relaxation times (Bydder et al. 1983; Brant-Zawadzki et al. 1983). The characteristic feature of the infarcted area is the loss of the gray-white matter contrast. Lacunar infarcts are generally circular, deep-seated, and often multiple (Bydder et al. 1983). In some patients with chronic infarcts, XCT may show no abnormality, while MRI reveals evidence of old infarction with the above-mentioned prolonged relaxation times and loss of gray-white contrast.

These preliminary data indicate that MRI may be the study of choice in the examination of patients with old infarcts. Small infarcts are readily detected by the MRI technique. These lesions are especially well visualized in coronal sections.

Using PET, Lammertsma et al. (1981) found a diminution of gray matter oxygen metabolism with increasing age, but only up to the fifth decade. Samples of older persons showed no further average changes. Kuhl at al. determined LCMRgl in 40 normal volunteers aged 18 – 78 years using the [^{18}F]FDG technique (Kuhl et al. 1982). At age 78, mean LCMRgl was, on the average, 26% less than at age 18. This alteration is of the same order as the variance among subjects at any age. Glucose consumption was symmetrical in the hemispheres. The mean glucose metabolic rate in cortex, caudate, and thalamus was equal in each age group by decade. The slopes of decline of metabolic rates with advancing age were similar for cerebral cortex (frontal, temporal, parietal, occipital, and visual), centrum semiovale, caudate, and putamen. However, the metabolic rate ratio of superior frontal cortex to superior parietal cortex declined with aging, possibly due to the selective degeneration of the superior frontal cortex or to a difference between younger and older age groups in the sensory and cognitive responses to the study. Several investigators report no age-related changes in glucose utilization (Alavi et al. 1980; Ferris et al. 1981, 1983; de Leon et al. 1983; Rapoport et al. 1983; de Leon et al. 1984).

Several studies, including our own, reported diminished metabolic activity in the brain of DAT patients. In our first study (Alavi et al. 1980; Ferris et al. 1981, 1983; Alavi et al. 1982; Farkas et al. 1982), we studied seven DAT patients (aged 72.7±4.9 years) and three normal subjects (aged 63.0±6.6 years). Our results indicated substantial regional diminutions of the metabolic rate for glucose that ranged between 33% and 37%. We also demonstrated significant correlation ($P < 0.05$) between the magnitude of the regional metabolic rates and measures of cognitive performance.

Frackowiak et al. (1981) used the $^{15}0_2$ steady-state technique to study CBF and cerebral 0_2 metabolism in 22 dementia patients (aged 66±9 years) and 14 normal controls (aged 61 ± 8 years). Of the dementia patients, 13 were classified as having degenerative dementia (probably DAT) and nine as suffering from vascular dementia. The results of this study indicated that, compared with controls, the DAT group had diminished CBF and diminished metabolic rates for 0_2. The brain regions at the basal ganglia level showed metabolic rate diminutions ranging from 19% to 29%. It was also reported that the more severe dementia cases had the greatest reductions in metabolic rates. In addition, these authors demonstrated a regional coupling of the CBF to cerebral 0_2 metabolism in both degenerative and vascular dementia. This result suggests the use of CBF as an estimate of brain metabolism. Furthermore, in both the degenerative and vascular groups, there was no change in the 0_2 extraction ratio across different severity levels of DAT, a result which supports the view that the brain changes found in DAT are not a consequence of chronic ischemia.

In a larger series of 24 DAT patients (aged 73.4 ± 6.9 years) and 22 elderly normal controls (aged 66.6 ± 7.6 years) significant decreases in glucose metabolic rates were found in the DAT patients (Ferris et al. 1983; de Leon et al. 1983). For regions of interest at the basal ganglia level of the brain, the range of diminution was 17% – 23% while at the centrum semiovale level, the range of diminution was 18% – 24%. In this large study, significant correlations were noted between measures of cognitive impairment and the metabolic rate. Specifically, the mental status evaluations were correlated with the regional metabolic rates in the range of $r = 0.5 - 0.6$ ($P < 0.01$). The extent to which decreased glucose utilization in DAT may be of diagnostic value was examined. A series of discriminant function classification analyses were carried out to determine the accuracy with which individual subjects can be classified as DAT patients or controls, based only on regional glucose utilization values. For predictions based on single PET regions of interest, the overall classification accuracy ranged from 70% – 80%.

Foster et al. studied 13 right-handed patients with DAT using the [^{18}F]FDG technique (Foster et al. 1983). For this project, three subjects with predominant language deficits, four with disproportionate failure of visuoconstructive function, and six others who suffered primarily from memory loss were selected. The group with language deficits showed marked reduction in LCMRgl in the left frontal, temporal, and parietal regions. Those with predominately visuoconstructive dysfunction demonstrated focal hypometabolism in the right parietal cortex. Patients with memory loss had no significant asymmetry of metabolic activity in cortical regions. In all subjects, a good correlation between verbal competence and left frontotemporal metabolic activity was noted, while visuoconstructive test performance was linked to glucose utilization in the right parietal lobe. In the studies by Friedland et al. (1983) left-right asymmetries were *not* found in DAT patients, although significant bilateral temporoparietal decrements in glucose metabolism were seen.

XCT and isotope clearance blood flow studies have in general proven disappointing in differentiating DAT from MID. PET studies to date have met with somewhat better success. Benson et al. (1983), Kuhl et al. (1983) and Frackowiak et al. (1981) and collaborators have reported small series including both DAT and MID patients. Patients with DAT appeared to have more symmetrical and global pattern of reduced metabolism compared with the focal and asymmetrical reductions associated with MID. XCT was nondiagnostic in Benson's three cases of MID, all of whom had focal abnormalities of glucose metabolism. Kuhl et al. (1983) demonstrated that patients with DAT had a global decline of LCMRgl of 33% as contrasted with a 17% reduction in MID, when both groups were compared with age-matched controls. Patients with MID showed a pattern of multiple focal defects compared with a DAT group which consistently revealed metabolic depressions in the parietal and occipital regions. These results show some promise of distinguishing DAT from MID by using metabolic imaging. In their six patients with MID, 39 lesions were found with either XCT or [^{18}F]FDG scans. The 24 lesions not seen by XCT had an average decrease in LCMRgl of 17%, compared with a 48% decline in lesions seen on both XCT and [^{18}F]FDG scan. However, five lesions seen on XCT were not visualized on [^{18}F]FDG scans. These lesions were small white-matter lacunar infarcts which are not readily identified with metabolic examinations. Moreover, Foster et al. (1983). have suggested that DAT itself may produce focal and asymmetric regions of depressed metabolism that correspond to neuropsychological deficits. In summary, the above results show that further investigation is needed before a true delineation of these two major diagnostic subtypes can be established with any degree of certainty.

Our own preliminary data indicate that, with aging, a significant relative decrease in frontal metabolic rate occurs. In contrast, metabolic rates in the posterior structures are preserved. Similarly, some decline in right inferior parietal area, an area of the brain associated with attentional tasks, accompanies aging. In patients with a probable diagnosis of DAT, a further decline of relative metabolic rate compared with that noted in normally aged control subjects is noted in the inferior parietal lobe area. Primary sensorimotor metabolic rate is relatively preserved in patients with DAT. This observation fits with the standard clinical impression that, in contrast to higher integrative cognitive functions which are affected early on, crude sensory and motor functions in this disorder are preserved until late in the course of the disease. Patients with severe dementia undergo significant reduction in left hemisphere cortical metabolism, which is especially pronounced in the perisylvian area. This may correspond to the language function disturbance that occurs late in the course of DAT.

Our data also demonstrate that both XCT and MRI are excellent techniques for detecting structural changes secondary to normal aging and dementia, although the degree of cortical atrophy can be better estimated by MRI than by XCT scan. Both techniques are useful in delineating ventricular dilatation. Small subcortical infarcts in patients with MID are seen more distinctly with MRI. PET techniques, on the other hand, offer the unique opportunity of visualizing regional functional abnormalities and of quantifying regional function and metabolism.

References

Alavi A, Ferris S, Wolf A, Reivich M, Farkas T, Dann R, Christman D, Fowler J (1980) Determination of cerebral metabolism in senile dementia using F-18-deoxyglucose and positron emission tomography. J Nuclear Med 21:21

Alavi A, Ferris S, Wolf A, Christman D, Fowler J, MacGregor R, Farkas T, Greenberg J, Dann R, Reivich M (1982) Determination of regional cerebral metabolism in dementia using F−18 deoxyglucose and positron emission tomography. Hoyer S(1982) The aging brain. Springer, Berlin Heidelberg New York (Experimental brain research supplement, vol 5)

Arai H, Kogayashi K, Ikeda K, Nagao Y, Ogihara R, Kosaka K (1983) A computed tomography study of Alzheimer's disease. J Neurol 229:69−77

Barron SA, Jacobs L, Kinkel WR (1976) Changes in size of normal lateral ventricles during aging determined by computerized tomography. Neurology 26:1011−1013

Benson DF, Kuhl DE, Hawkins RA et al. (1983) The fluorodeoxyglucose 18F scan in Alzheimer's Disease and multi-infarct dementia. Arch Neurol 40:711−714

Blackwood W, Corsellis J (eds) (1976) Greenfield's textbook of neuropathology. Chicago, pp 796−849

Buonanno FS, Pykett IL, Brady TJ, Pohost GM (1983a) Clinical applications of nuclear magnetic resonance (NMR). DM 29 (8):1−81

Buonanno FS, Pykett K, Brady TJ, et al. (1983b) Proton NMR imaging in experimental ischemic infarction. Stroke 14:178−184

Brant-Zawadzki M, Davis PL, Brooks LE, et al. (1983) NMR demonstration of cerebral abnormalities: comparison with CT. AJR 140:847−854

Bydder GM, Steiner RE, Young IR, et al. (1983) Clinical NMR imaging of the brain: 140 cases. AJR 139:215−236

Chawluk J, Alavi A, Dann R, Kushner MJ, Hurtig H, Zimmerman RA, Reivich M (1984) PET measurements of cerebral metabolism corrected for CSF contributions. J Nuclear Med 25 (5):P56

Claveria LE, Moseley IF, Stevenson JF (1977) The clinical significance of "cerebral atrophy" as shown by C.A.T. In: du Boulay GH, Moseley IF (eds) The first european seminar on computerized axial tomography in clinical practice. Springer, Berlin Heidelberg New York, pp 213−217

Cormack AM (1963) Representation of a function by its line integrals, with some radiological applications. J Appl Phys 34:2722

Dann R, Muehllehner G, Rosenquist A (1982) Computer-aided data analysis of ECT data. J Nucleic Med 24:P82

de Leon MJ, Ferris SH, George AE, et al. (1983) Positron emission tomographic studies of aging and Alzheimer disease. Am J Neuroradiol 4:568−571

de Leon MJ, George AE, Ferris SH (1984) Positron emission tomography and computerized tomography of the aging brain. J Comput Assist Tomogr 8:88−94

Diagnostic and Statistical Manual III (1980) American Psychiatric Association, Washington, D.C.

Earnest MP, Heaton RK, Wilkinson WE, Manke WF (1979) Cortical atrophy, ventricular enlargement and intellectual impairment in the aged. Neurology 29:1138−1143

Edelstein WA, Hutchison JMS, Johnson G, Redpath T (1980) Spin warp NMR imaging and applications to whole-body imaging. Phys Med Biol 25:751−756

Edelstein WA, Bottomley PA, Hart HR, Smith LS (1983) Signal, noise and contrast in nuclear magnetic resonance (NMR) imaging. J Comput Assist Tomogr 7:391−401

Farkas T, Ferris SH, Wolf AP, de Leon MJ, Christman DR, Reisberg B, Alavi A, Fowler JS, George AE, Reivich M (1982) 18-F-2-deoxy-2-fluoro-D-glucose as a tracer in the positron emission tomographic study of senile dementia. Am J Psychiatry 139:352−353

Ferris SH, de Leon MS, Wolf AP, Farkas T, Christman DR, Reisberg B, Fowler JS, MacGregor R, Goldman A, George AE and Rampal S (1981) Positron emission tomography in the study of aging and senile dementia. Neurobio Aging 1:127−131

Ferris SH, de Leon MJ, Wolf AP, et al. (1983) Positron emission tomography in dementia. In: Mayeux R, Rosen WG (eds) The dementias. Raven, New York, pp 123−129

Foster NL, Chase TN, Fedio P, et al. (1983) Alzheimer's disease: Focal cortical changes shown by PET. Neurology 33:961−965

Frackowiak RSJ, et al. (1981) Regional cerebral oxygen supply and utilization in dementia. Brain 104:753−778

Friedland RP, Budinger TF, Ganz E, et al. (1983) Regional cerebral metabolic alterations in dementia of the Alzheimer type: positron emission tomography with [18F] fluorodeoxyglucose. J Comput Assist Tomogr 7:590–598

Gado M, Hughes CP, Danziger W, Chi D, Jost G, Berg L (1984) Volumetric measurements of the cerebrospinal fluid spaces in demented subjects and controls. Radiology 144:535–538

George AE, de Leon MJ, Rosenbloom S, Ferris SH, Gentes C, Emmerich M, Kricheff II (1983) Ventricular volume and cognitive deficit: a computed tomographic study. Radiology 149:494–498

Hachinski JC, Lassen NA, Marshall J (1974) Multi-infarct dementia. Lancet 2:207–210

Hounsfield GN (1973) Computerized transverse axial scanning (tomography). I. Description of system. Br J Radiol 46:1016–1022

Hughes CP, Gado M (1981) Computed tomography and aging of the brain. Radiology 139:391–396

Ito M, Hatazawa J, Yamaura H, Matsuzawa T (1981) Age-related brain atrophy and mental deterioration – a study with computed tomography. Br J Radiol 54:384–390

Jacoby RJ, Levy R (1980) Computed tomography in the elderly 2. Senile dementia: diagnosis and functional impairment. Br J Psychiatry 136:256–269

Jacoby RJ, Levy R, Dawson JM (1980) Computed tomography in the elderly: I. the normal population. Br J Psychiatry 136:249–255

Kasniak AW, Garron DC, Fox JH, Bergen I, Huckman M (1979) Cerebral atrophy, EEG slowing, age, education and cognitive functioning in suspected dementia. Neurology 29:1273–1279

Katzman R (1976) Prevalence and malignancy of Alzheimer's disease. Arch Neurol 33:217–218

Kuhl DE, Edwards RQ (1968) Reorganizing data from the transverse section scans of the brain using digital processing. Radiology 91:975–983

Kuhl DE, Metter EJ, Riege WH, Phelps ME (1982) Effects of human aging on patterns of local cerebral glucose utilization determined by the [^{18}F] fluorodeoxyglucose method. J Cereb Blood Flow Metab 2:163–171

Kuhl DE, Metter EJ, Riege WH, et al. (1983) Local cerebral glucose utilization in elderly patients with depression, multiple infarct dementia, and Alzheimer's disease. J Cereb Blood Flow Metab 3 [Suppl 1]:5494–5495

Lammertsma AA, Frackowiak RSJ, Lenzi GL, et al. (1981) Accuracy of the oxygen-15 steady state technique for measuring rCBF and $rCMRO_2$: Tracer modeling, statistics and spatial sampling. J Cereb Blood Metabol 1 [Suppl 1]:53–54

Marsden CD, Harrison MJG (1972) Outcome of investigation of patients with presenile dementia. Br Med J 1:249–252

McKhann G, Drachman D, Folstein M, et al. (1984) Clinical diagnosis of Alzheimer's disease. Neurology 34:939–944

Mesulam M-M (1981) A cortical network for directed attention and unilateral neglect. Ann Neurol 10:309–325

Miller AKH, Alston RL, Corsellis JAN (1980) Variation with age in the volumes of grey and white matter in the cerebral hemispheres of man: measurements with an image analyser. Neuropathol Appl Neurol 6:119–132

Oldendorf WH (1961) Isolated flying-spot detection of radiodensity discontinuities; displaying the internal structural pattern of a complex object. IRE-Trans Bio-Med Elect BME 8:68–72

Pykett IL, Buonanno FS, Brady TJ, Kistler JP (1983) True three-dimensional nuclear magnetic resonance neuro-imaging in ischemic stroke: correlation of NMR, X-ray CT, and pathology. Stroke 14:173–177

Rapoport SI, Duara R, Horasitz B, et al. (1983) Brain aging in 40 healthy men: rCMRglu and correlated functional activity in various brain regions in the resting state. J Cereb Blood Flow Metab 3 [Suppl 1]:5484–5485

Reivich M, Alavi A, Wolf A, Fowler J, Arnett C, Ferrieri R, Atkins H, Dann R, Greenberg J (1984) The evaluation of the lumped constant for deoxyglucose and fluorodeoxyglucose in man. (to be published)

Roberts MA, Caird FI, Grossart KW, Steven JL (1976) Computerized tomography in the diagnosis of cerebral atrophy. J Neurol Neurosurg Psychiatry 39:909–915
Spetzler RF, Zabramski JM, Kaufman B, Yeung HN (1983) Acute NMR changes during MCA occlusion: a preliminary study in primates. Stroke 14:185–191
Ter-Pogossian M, Mullani N, Hood J (1968) Design considerations for a positron emission tomograph (PETT V) for imaging of the brain. J Comput Assist Tomogr 2:539–544
Terry RD (1976) Dementia, a selective review. Arch Neurol 33:1–3
Tomlinson BE, Blessed G, Roth M (1968) Observations on the brains of non-demented old people. J Neurol Sci 7:331–356
Tomlinson BE, Blessed G, Roth M (1970) Observations on the brains of demented old people. J Neurol Sci 11:205–292
Wells CE (1978) Chronic brain disease: an overview. Am J Psychiatry 135:1–12
Yamaura H, Ito M, Kubota K, Matsuzawa T (1980) Brain atrophy during aging: a quantitative study with computed tomography. J Gerontol 35:492–498

4.3 Regional Cerebral Blood Flow and Glucose Metabolism in Old Age and in Dementia Evaluated by PET

W.-D. Heiss, G. Pawlik, K. Herholz, K. Wienhard

Introduction

Function of neural tissue is closely linked to glucose consumption as the most important energy-supplying metabolic process. Therefore, regional disturbances as well as changes in functional activity can be detected with this metabolic variable. At the time being, only positron emission tomography (PET) affords regional and three-dimensional quantitation of glucose metabolism in the human brain, using measurements of the concentration of an injected radiolabeled glucose analogue in small volumes of tissue, and computer reconstruction of tomographic images showing the spatial tracer distribution. On those sections the individual anatomical structures of the brain are represented according to their metabolic activity.

Principles of Positron Emission Tomography

When positron emitting radionuclides decay, a positively charged particle of the mass of an electron is released. Over a distance of 1 – 5 mm this particle is decelerated to such a degree that it must combine with an electron. When those positively and negatively charged particles collide, their mass is annihilated and two gamma quanta with an energy of 511 keV each are emitted in opposite directions (angle of 180°). Without further collimation the two photons can be registered by electronically connected coincidence detectors assigning the decay event to the straight line between the two detectors. This electronic collimation permits construction of highly efficient detector systems, in which detectors that are arranged in circles or polygons are connected with each other in a fan-like fashion via coincidence counters. Cross-sections of the activity distribution in the examined structure are reconstructed from the many individual events that have been recorded in various directions, employing algorithms that ressemble those used in X-ray computerized tomography. Those tomographic images represent an object thickness of about 10 – 15 mm at an in-plane resolution of 7 – 10 mm. The necessary attenuation and scatter corrections can be made with great accuracy because of the high and identical energy of the gamma quanta. State-of-the-art machines containing numerous detector rings permit simultaneous scanning of up to nine brain slices during a single examination. A number of tracer compounds which serve the examination of different physiological processes can be labeled with the cyclotron-produced short-lived positron emitting radionuclides ^{15}O, ^{11}C, and ^{18}F (reviews in Phelps et al. 1982; Heiss and Phelps 1983). As measurements with ^{18}FDG (half-life of $^{18}F = 110$ min) of local glucose metabolism and with ^{15}O

(half-life = 2 min) of oxygen consumption and blood flow are widely used in functional studies on normal volunteers as well as in clinical examinations of various cerebral disorders, a description of these methods follows.

Determination of Local Glucose Metabolism by PET

The measurement of local glucose metabolism with ^{18}F-2-fluoro-2-deoxy-D-glucose (FDG) (Reivich et al. 1979) is derived from the ^{14}C-deoxyglucose autoradiographic technique devised by Sokoloff et al. (1977). The technique developed by Sokoloff can be applied directly as FDG labeled in position 2 behaves like deoxyglucose. FDG is transported into the cells by the same carrier system as glucose. Inside the cell, it is phosphorylated by hexokinase to ^{18}F-deoxyglucose-6-phosphate. Deoxyglucose-6-phosphate, however, cannot be metabolized to fructose-6-phosphate; rather it accumulates in the cell because the phosphatase reaction yielding deoxyglucose again takes place with much slower kinetics, and deoxyglucose-6-phosphate can penetrate the cell membrane in small amounts only. The kinetics of the accumulation of deoxyglucose-6-phosphate are described in terms of the transport and enzyme constants of a three-compartment model. The local cerebral metabolic rate for glucose (LCMRGl) is then calculated employing the corresponding model equation which, in its original form, is rather complex, but can be simplified for measurement purposes as follows:

$$\text{LCMRGl:}\ \frac{(\text{Gl})}{\text{LC}} \times \frac{\text{C}(^{18}\text{F}) - \text{C}(\text{FDG})}{\text{A}_\text{b}}$$

C(^{18}F) corresponds to the entire radioactivity in the tissue and is determined directly by PET. C(FDG) represents the concentration of free FDG in the tissue, estimated on the basis of the plasma concentration at a given time T. The difference between the two values indicates the local tissue concentration of FDG-6-phosphate. A_b stands for the total amount of FDG taken up by the tissue; it can be computed on the basis of the area under the FDG concentration curve from time 0 to time T, taking into account the measured FDG values in plasma and appropriate model constants. The second ratio to the right of the equal sign represents the phosphorylation rate of FDG. Multiplication with plasma glucose concentration (Gl) would yield the rate of glucose phosphorylation if the behavior of glucose and FDG were the same. However, as the arteriovenous extraction rate of glucose does not equal that of FDG, the value has to be corrected by an experimentally determined constant (LC = lumped constant). In measuring cerebral glucose utilization after intravenous injection of 3–6 mCi ^{18}FDG, the plasma concentration curve of FDG must be determined from the time of injection to the point of measurement. Likewise, the glucose concentration in plasma and the local ^{18}F activity in the brain must be determined after an equilibrium of FDG between blood and tissue has been reached.

Determination of Regional Cerebral Blood Flow (rCBF) and Oxygen Metabolism (rCMRO) by ^{15}0-PET

Water labeled with ^{15}0 is a freely diffusible tracer which can be used for measurements of rCBF. It is administered continuously by inhalation of ^{15}0-carbon dioxide, which is converted to $H_2{}^{15}0$ by the carbonic anhydrase in the lung, using a steady state model (Jones et al. 1976; Frackowiak et al. 1980). During inhalation of $0^{15}0$ in a second run the local brain activity measured by PET mainly represents $H_2{}^{15}0$ produced by aerobic metabolism in the tissue, also being freely diffusible. Since the distribution of water between tissue and blood is known from the first run, the production rate of $H_2{}^{15}0$, and hence the rCMRO, may be calculated. Correction for the amount of unmetabolized oxygen bound to hemoglobin is possible by measurement of local cerebral blood volume using ^{11}CO or $C^{15}0$ as a hemoglobin marker (Lammertsma and Jones 1983). The relation between rCMRO and rCBF gives the regional oxygen extraction rate (rOER).

Studies in Normal Human Subjects

In normal volunteers an average cerebral glucose utilization of 29 – 32 μmol/100 g/min (Mazziotta et al. 1981) has been found by means of FDG and PET. Under control conditions (darkened laboratory and low noise background during the examination), the anatomy of the brain is reflected in the metabolic activity of the transaxial cross-sections. Individual metabolic rates can be estimated by direct comparison with the shades of gray or with the corresponding colors on the reference scale: The highest values are found in the visual cortex (45 – 50 μmol/100 g/min) and in the striatum (42 – 46 μmol/100 g/min). Values in other areas of the cortex, in the basal ganglia (35 – 42 μmol/100 g/min), and in the gray matter structures of the posterior fossa (25 – 30 μmol/100 g/min) are much lower. The lowest LCMRGl is found in white matter (15 – 22 μmol/100 g/min).

Studies of oxygen consumption and regional blood flow have demonstrated comparable differences between gray and white matter: The mean value of $CMRO_2$ was determined as 5.9 ml/100 g × min for gray and 1.8 ml/100 g × min for white matter; the mean rCBF values were 65.3 and 21.4 ml/100 g × min, respectively (Frackowiak et al. 1980). Regional oxygen extraction rate was 0.48 – 0.49 for both compartments. Differences between various gray structures, as described for CMRGl, were not observed with the ^{15}0-method, but this might be due to its low spatial resolution.

Decreases of glucose metabolism and oxygen consumption with age observed in preliminary studies (Frackowiak et al. 1980; Kuhl et al. 1982) were not confirmed in recent investigations on larger groups of volunteers: in 40 selected healthy men neither CMRGl of the whole hemispheres nor of individual brain regions was correlated with age (Rapoport et al. 1983). Similar results were reported by Metter et al. (1983) and Leon et al. (1983), but interregional correlations of older volunteers differed from those observed in younger men (Metter et al. 1983). The previously observed age-dependent changes in oxygen consumption were also not found in recent study (Frackowiak et al. 1981).

Functional Activation During Sensory Stimulation

A number of studies (Greenberg et al. 1981, Phelps et al. 1982) have demonstrated that local glucose metabolism is increased during functional activation of the corresponding brain structures: With visual stimulations, glucose metabolic rates rise in the primary visual cortex; this increase is dependent on stimulus intensity. Upon presenting a complex scene, the increase is about 50% and spreads to the visual association cortex. With auditory stimulation, different patterns are observed depending on the modality of stimulation.

With elimination of sensory stimuli by either blindfolding the eyes or stuffing the ears, the cerebral metabolic rate for glucose decreases. The lowest rates are observed in complete sensory deprivation, which further results in an asymmetry with higher activity of the right hemisphere. By blocking sensory input from the outside and reducing brain activity, in sleep a decrease in metabolic rates between 10% and 20% as compared with wakefulness is found in all cortical and basal gray matter structures (Heiss et al. 1983).

Metabolic Disturbances in Dementia

Over the past few years PET has contributed much to the understanding of neurological disorders (for reviews see Phelps et al. 1982; Heiss and Phelps 1983). Especially in cases of focal lesions metabolic disturbances have been shown to extend far beyond the site of the primary lesions, and to include morphologically intact brain structures far away from the anatomical lesion. Decreased metabolism is particularly striking in patients with small infarctions that often cannot be detected by CT but are associated with extensive decreases in metabolic rate. Those remote metabolic effects may explain the impairments which cannot be directly ascribed to the focal lesion. They underlie the psycho-organic syndrome in stroke patients and influence the outcome of rehabilitation after a stroke.

In diseases with global impairment of brain function, such as dementia, which are often combined with unspecific findings in computed tomography, the decrease in metabolic rate is generally also diffuse and depends on the severity of the psycho-organic syndrome. However, these metabolic disturbances usually are characteristic of each disease and its typical pattern of spread. In degenerative dementia of the Alzheimer type, cerebral glucose consumption is severely impaired even in the early stages after onset, before cerebral atrophy can be documented by CT. Corresponding metabolic changes are particularly pronounced in the parictotemporal cortex (Foster et al. 1983; Kuhl et al. 1983). In senile dementia the impaired glucose metabolism was pronounced in the frontal cortex (Alavi et al. 1982). With multi-infarct dementias glucose uptake is reduced more or less in proportion to the severity of clinical symptoms and in accordance with the multifocal destruction of cortical tissue as demonstrated by CT; energy metabolism is affected mainly in the small old infarcts.

In most patients suffering from dementia CBF is decreased, but typical patterns for the various types of dementia could not be established. The primary disturbance of flow in multi-infarct dementia (MID) and the primary affection of metabolism in degenerative dementias postulated by Hoyer et al. (1975) could not be confirmed in PET studies (Frackowiak et al. 1981): In 9 MID patients and in 13 Alzheimer cases regional flow and oxygen consumption were affected similarly, and, as a consequence, oxygen extraction rate was not changed. Decreases of flow and metabolism were related only to the duration and the severity of the mental impairment, not to the type of dementia. An increase of the oxygen extraction rate was never observed, and, therefore, a "chronic ischemic syndrome" could be ruled out. Regional differences of oxygen consumption were observed in both groups. In the vascular groups disturbances were most prominent in the parietal lobe, but the pattern was highly influenced by the focal ischemic lesions. In case with moderate degenerative dementia focal abnormalities were most frequent in the parietal and temporal lobe; in severe cases disturbances were found especially in frontal regions, while the occipital lobe was least affected.

In Huntington's disease the most conspicous metabolic changes are found in the basal ganglia, particularly in the caudate nucleus and putamen (Kuhl et al. 1982), reflecting the severity of the clinical manifestations; even mild cases showing no characteristic atrophy of the head of the caudate nucleus on CT, exhibit definite metabolic abnormalities. The typical reduction of glucose uptake in the striatum of Huntington patients' family members may even allow detection of the disorder before any clinical symptoms become apparent.

Disturbances of metabolism in dementia are related to the impairment of mental function. That may be the cause, but also the consequence of the altered functional activity of the brain. In contrast to oxygen consumption and glucose metabolism the synthesis of proteins, which can be determined with ^{11}C-methyl-methionine (Bustany et al. 1983), is not directly coupled to the function in the nervous system. The decrease of protein synthesis to 60% in moderate and to 38% in severe cases of Alzheimer dementia, which again is predominant in parietal and frontal regions, could, therefore, be of pathogenetic importance.

These few examples of the application of PET to studies of local cerebral metabolism give only a vague idea of the vast potential of the method. Basically, a large number of organic compounds can be labeled with positron emitters, e.g., ^{11}C, ^{13}N, and ^{18}F, to allow quantitative imaging of such processes as the metabolism of various substrates, protein synthesis, function and distribution of receptors, tumor growth, and the distribution of drugs. With ^{15}O, produced directly in a cyclotron, local oxygen utilization can be measured. With simple compounds containing either ^{15}O or other radionuclides (^{11}C or ^{18}F), regional blood flow and blood volume can be determined quantitatively and three-dimensionally. All these applications of PET as a complex but noninvasive method grant insight into the functional anatomy, physiology, and pathology of the human brain unmatched by any other currently known technology.

References

Alavi A, Reivich M, Ferris S et al. (1982) Regional cerebral glucose metabolism in aging and senile dementia as determined by 18F-deoxy-glucose and positron emission tomography. In: Hoyer S (ed) The aging brain. Springer, Berlin Heidelberg New York

Bustany P, Henry JF, Sargent T, Zarifian E, Cabanis E, Collard P, Comar D (1983) Local brain protein metabolism in dementia and schizophrenia: in vivo studies with ^{11}C-L-methionine and positron emission tomography. In: Heiss W-D, Phelps ME (eds)

Positron emission tomography of the brain. Springer, Berlin Heidelberg New York, pp 208–211

Foster NL, Chase TN, Fedio P, Patronas NJ, Brooks RA, DiChiro G (1983) Alzheimer's disease: Focal cortical changes shown by positron emission tomography. Neurology 33:961–965

Frackowiak RSJ, Lenzi G-L, Jones T, Heather JD (1980) Quantitative measurement of regional cerebral blood flow and oxygen metabolism in man using ^{15}0 and positron emission tomography: Theory, procedure, and normal values. J Comput Assist Tomogr 4:727–736

Frackowiak RSJ, Pozzilli C, Legg NJ, DuBoulay GH, Marshall J, Lenzi GL, Jones T (1981) Regional cerebral oxygen supply and utilization in dementia. A clinical and physiological study with oxygen-15 and positron tomography. Brain 104:753–778

Greenberg JH, Reivich M, Alavi A, Hand P, Rosenquist A, Rintelmann W, Stein A, Tusa R, Dann R, Christman D, Fowler J, McGregor B, Wolf A (1981) Metabolic mapping of functional activity in human subjects with the (^{18}F) fluorodeoxyglucose technique. Science 212:678–680

Heiss W-D, Pawlik G, Herholz K, Wagner R, Wienhard K (1985) Determination of regional glucose metabolism in the brain by FDG and PET. In: Hartmann A, Hoyer S (eds) Measurement of cerebral blood flow and cerebral metabolism in man. Springer, Berlin Heidelberg New York Tokyo, pp 391–402

Heiss W-D, Phelps ME (1983) Positron emission tomography of the brain. Springer, Berlin Heidelberg New York

Hoyer S, Oesterreich K, Weinhardt F, Krüger G (1975) Veränderungen von Durchblutung und oxydativem Stoffwechsel des Gehirns bei Patienten mit einer Demenz. J Neurol 210:227–237

Jones T, Chesler DA, Ter-Pogossian MM (1976) The continuous inhalation of oxygen-15 for assessing regional oxygen extraction in the brain of man. Br J Radiol 49:339–343

Kuhl DE, Metter EJ, Riege WH, Hawkins RA, Mazziotta JC, Phelps ME, Kling AS (1983) Local cerebral glucose utilization in elderly patients with depression, multiple infarct dementia, and Alzheimer's disease. J Cereb Blood Flow Metab 3 [Suppl. 1]:S494–S495

Kuhl DE, Phelps ME, Markham CH, Metter EJ, Riege WH, Winter J (1982) Cerebral metabolism and atrophy in Huntington's disease determined by ^{18}FDG and computed tomographic scan. Ann Neurol 12:425–434

Lammertsma AA, Jones T (1983) Correction for the presence of intravascular oxygen-15 in the steady-state technique for measuring regional oxygen extraction ratio in the brain: 1. Description of the method. J Cereb Blood Flow Metabol 3:416–424

Leon MJ de, Ferris SH, George AE, Reisberg B, Christman DR, Kricheff II, Wolf AP (1983) Computed tomography and positron emission transaxial tomography evaluations of normal aging and Alzheimer's disease. J Cereb Blood Flow Metab 3:391–394

Mazziotta JC, Phelps ME, Miller J, Kuhl DE (1981) Tomographic mapping of human cerebral metabolism: Normal unstimulated state. Neurology 31:503–516

Metter EJ, Riege WH, Kuhl DE, Phelps ME (1983) Differences in regional glucose metabolic intercorrelations with aging. J Cereb Blood Flow Metab 3 [Suppl 1]: S482–S483

Phelps ME, Mazziotta JC, Huang S-C (1982) Study of cerebral function with positron computed tomography. J Cereb Blood Flow Metab 2:113–162

Reivich M, Kuhl D, Wolf A, Greenberg J, Phelps M, Ido T, Casella V, Fowler J, Hoffman E, Alavi A, Som P, Sokoloff L (1979) The (^{18}F) fluorodeoxyglucose method for the measurement of local cerebral glucose utilization in man. Circ Res 44:127–137

Rapoport SI, Duara R, Horwitz B, Kessler RM, Sokoloff L, Ingvar DH, Grady C, Cutler N (1983) Brain aging in 40 healthy men: rCMRglc and correlated functional activity in various brain regions in the resting state. J Cereb Blood Flow Metab 3 [Suppl. 1]: S484–S485

Sokoloff L, Reivich M, Kennedy D, DesRosiers M-H, Patlak CS, Pettigrew KD, Sakurada 0, Shinohara M (1977) The ^{14}C-deoxyglucose method for the measurement of local cerebral glucose utilization: Theory, procedure, and normal values in the conscious and anesthetized albino rat. J Neurochem 28:897–916

4.4 The Significance of Regional Cerebral Blood Flow and Metabolism for Processes of Aging and Dementia

R. S. J. Frackowiak

Introduction

Historically a number of important questions have dominated the field of dementia research in the last decades. Is aging a pathological process? Is dementia accelerated aging? What role does vascular insufficiency play in the process of senility? The clinical physiologists have attempted to answer some of these questions by measurement of cerebral blood flow and most recently concurrent measurement of cerebral energy metabolism. The main advances, however, have come from the neuropathologists, who have demonstrated the quantitative and qualitative differences between normally aging brains and those of demented patients. They have also pointed out that the vast majority of the dementias are due to Alzheimer's disease, a degenerative process of unknown cause, rather than cerebrovascular disease.

The physiological data have been confusing over the years. Controversy still exists whether normal aging is accompanied by a gradual progressive decline in cerebral blood flow (and by implication function) (Kety 1956; Sokoloff 1966). During the period when CBF was the only variable practically measurable in man, controversy raged over the primary or secondary nature of the frequently measured low CBF in demented patients. The concept of chronic cerebrovascular insufficiency has been the basis for numerous pharmaceutical treatments of dementia in the past. This concept arose out of the notion that the low CBF was the primary event, resulting in a kind of slow strangulation of the brain and chronic anoxic cell death.

The advent of positron emission tomography has largely clarified many of these matters. The reasons are clear. PET gives accurate regional and tomographic information allowing delineation of grey and white structures. It permits the concurrent measurement of CBF and metabolism. This is crucial, as it is the relationship between them that defines ischaemia and permits definitive statements to be made about the relationship between energy supply and demand in the cerebral tissues.

Positron Tomography

Studies of aging and dementia have been performed by a number of groups using PET. Detailed and quantitative information is available concerning oxygen metabolism and extraction, glucose metabolism and cerebral blood flow. Preliminary results are also now emerging in relation to protein metabolism and amino acid turnover. A brief résumé of these techniques is given as background.

Oxygen metabolism and extraction ($CMRO_2$ and OER) have been measured using oxygen 15-labelled CO_2 and O_2. This method also gives a measurement of CBF, and the variable OER is an expression of the relationship between CBF (i.e. oxygen supply) and $CMRO_2$ (i.e. its utilisation). The product of OER and the stable arterial oxygen content is the arterio-venous oxygen difference. The OER therefore expresses the fractional extraction of oxygen, whereas the $A-VO_2$ expresses the absolute oxygen extration in ml O_2 per ml blood. The most commonly used and carefully validated technique is the steady-state method (Frackowiak et al. 1980; Lammertsma et al. 1981, 1982, 1983; Lammertsma and Jones 1983) and all the studies of oxygen metabolism reported in aging and dementia have been done in this way.

Glucose metabolism has been measured in aging and semiquantitative studies have been published in dementia using variations of Sokoloff's deoxyglucose technique (Sokoloff 1981; Phelps et al. 1979). This is an analogue method which depends greatly on an adequate description of the relationship between the handling of the natural and analogue substrates by the tissue. If this description is readily quantified (the lumped constant), use of the analogue (e.g. ^{18}FDG) will result in an accurate measure of the consumption of the natural substrate (i.e. glucose). This is not always easy.

Protein metabolism in dementia has been studied and reported in preliminary form using ^{11}C-labelled methionine (Bustany et al. 1983). The kinetic modelling using this tracer has not been worked out completely as yet. The description of the fate of the injected tracer is possible in terms of three compartments and this, potentially, allows measurement of the free methionine pool, the permeability of the BBB to methionine and the incorporation rate into proteins.

Aging

Measurement of CBF in aging suggests that in grey matter a steady, if small, progressive decline in perfusion occurs following the third decade of life. This was also the conclusion of Kety when he summarised the findings of various authors studying this problem in whole brain with the nitrous oxide technique. There appears to be no decline of note in the white matter of the centrum semiovale (Frackowiak 1982). A significant criticism of these regional findings is that the normal human brain tends to lose weight (and volume) beyond the sixth decade. The measurements of CBF are made per volume of brain tissue. If the volume of interest contains less grey matter, then the corresponding flow value will be underestimated. The main reason for thinking that this is not a sufficient explanation of the finding is that measurements of oxygen consumption do not follow a similar pattern.

Oxygen consumption shows a tendency to decline with age between the third and eighth decades. However, this barely reaches significance and there seems to be a definite difference between the rates of decline of CBF and $CMRO_2$. This implies a gradual alteration in the relationship between supply and demand and a tendency for the fractional oxygen extraction to rise. Kennedy and Sokoloff (1957) showed, using the N_20 technique, that children had considerably higher

CBF than adults in the third decade. Oxygen consumption was, however, much more comparable with adult values. The AVO_2 was 30% lower than in adults and as the oxygen contents were similar, the fractional oxygen extraction was similarly lower than in adults. There seems, therefore, to be a trend throughout life for the fractional oxygen extraction to increase. This means that the range of normal OER varies from about 25% in childhood to 35% – 40% in adulthood and 40% – 45% in old age. It is clear that there remains a considerable oxygen reserve in the perfusing blood available for any sudden changes in flow or demand and in no sense does this represent cerebrovascular insufficiency. In an elderly person with an OER of 45%, the reserve would be capable of supporting a twofold increase in $CMRO_2$ even if no further increase in CBF were possible.

What is the structural or morphological basis for this small but apparently definite trend towards a decrease in the haemodynamic reserve with age? The answer to this is not clear but it is possible there is a decrease in the capillary density with age. In normal aging the cerebral vessels are functionally normal and capable of appropriate vasodilation and constriction. Cerebral autoregulation is maintained, as is CO_2 reactivity. There is therefore no evidence that the aging brain is chronically anoxic or somehow limited in its function by an inadequate nutrient supply.

A final question, which is in the process of investigation, relates to a methodological problem. The measurement of OER is influenced by the blood volume in the region of brain from which the measurement is made (Lammertsma and Jones 1983). A measured correction can be applied (Lammertsma et al. 1983). It is theoretically possible that the trend towards an elevation of OER is explicable in terms of an increasing CBV with age. No such increase has been demonstrated in the small number of patients studied thus far.

The studies with deoxyglucose have been less clear. This is largely because of problems of technique and possibly subject selection. Kuhl and his colleagues (Kuhl et al. 1982) have reported a fall in glucose consumption with age which was in excess of that reported independently for oxygen. This would imply consumption by the aging brain of substrates other than glucose for energy. Arteriovenous difference measurements in the past have on occasion suggested ketones may be a more significant source of energy in the elderly but these reports have not been consistently confirmed. A study measuring oxygen and glucose consumption concurrently in the same subjects would be needed to answer this point.

Rapoport and his colleagues at NIH (Duara et al. 1984) have reported no decline in glucose consumption with age. Their study seems to be consistent with the 1960s NIH study with A–V difference techniques (Dastur et al. 1963). The latter study was at variance with most other workers at the time and the discrepancy was attributed to the highly rigorous selection criteria for normality used by the NIH group. Similar criteria have been used for the PET study. The results, however, do exhibit a lot of scatter and it seems that the last word in this controversy has not yet been said. Whether the "supernormal" and "normal" aged have different cerebral physiology is one question, the significance of this is another.

In terms of regional information, there is clarification of the distributions of blood flow and energy metabolism in different cerebral structures. The hyperfrontal pattern described by Ingvar (Ingvar 1979) in the awake, alert, normal individual is much less clearly seen than with the intracarotid ^{133}Xe technique. The reason for this is most probably methodological and relates to siting of detectors and distribution of the ^{133}Xe after intracarotid injection. It appears that most cortical regions have a similar perfusion and the major difference lies between grey and white matter. The small differences registered by PET between different cortical areas are probably all explicable in terms of the resolution of the PET cameras. The cortical strip with a width averaging 3 – 4 mm is being examined by instruments with a transaxial resolution averaging 10 – 20 mm^2.

Mention should also be made of experiments investigating alterations of the normal pattern of distribution of energy metabolism by specific physiological stimuli. The Los Angeles group (Mazziotta et al. 1981, 1982a, b; Phelps et al. 1981) has demonstrated focal increases in metabolism in cortical regions in response to visual, auditory, alerting stimuli and during the performance of memory and auditory discrimination tasks. This disturbance of the resting state pattern in the normal, when fully quantified, gives the opportunity for working out intracerebral connections subserving the various functions of the brain. This is an exciting prospect both for the field of normal and diseased neuropsychology. Of particular importance to the study of aging will be the comparison between the young and elderly of the focal patterns and the capacity to augment cerebral function locally in response to a given stimulus.

Dementia

Many studies have demonstrated in dements a decline of CBF in excess of that seen in the normal population. The decline has been correlated with severity of dementia. Many of the original studies were performed at a time when arteriosclerosis and chronic cerebrovascular insufficiency were common concepts and this coloured the interpretation of these results. The controversy between the primary and secondary nature of the decline in CBF was still alive in 1981 (Plum 1981) despite the seminal work of the Newcastle group in 1969–1970 (Tomlinson et al. 1970)

PET was used to resolve this controversy definitively by a study of both CBF and $CMRO_2$ in demented patients of different aetiology (vascular and degenerative) and severity (Frackowiak et al. 1981). Furthermore, both global and regional measurements were reported in case the relationship between flow and metabolism was regionally rather than globally disturbed. Care was taken to study patients who were free of intercurrent illness and who had not suffered a recent *acute* cerebrovascular event. The results are unequivocal. In neither degenerative nor vascular dementia was any evidence of an imbalance between CBF and $CMRO_2$ in the direction of ischaemia observed. This related to mild (and therefore early phases) as well as severe dements.

The pattern of physiological disturbance was different in the two groups. The Alzheimer patients showed an initial severe decline in temporoparietal metabolism (and flow) and as the dementia became more severe so frontal metabolism fell progressively, eventually falling to the lowest values in the severest dements.

The further decline in temporoparietal metabolism was much less pronounced. Primary motor and sensory areas as well as deep grey structures were relatively spared though some decline in function also occurred. White matter metabolism fell proportionately, reflecting decreased axonal traffic and/or a loss of axons concomitant with loss of neurones. This pattern of sequential and selective functional loss has now also been reported by groups using ^{18}FDG (Benson 1982; Chase et al. 1984). Some correlation between loss of clinically measurable functions and fall in metabolism in certain appropriate cerebral areas has also been reported, though further analysis of such structure – function relationships awaits finer resolution tomographs. The implications for the neuropathologist attempting to define the anatomical and structural correlates of these changes and hence the early pathology of this illness are considerable. It is clear that any neurotransmitter-based theory of aetiology must take into account the regional distribution of dysfunction described with the PET studies.

The pattern of dysfunction in the chronic vascular dement is much more focal, with randomly distributed lesions in grey and white matter predominating in middle cerebral artery territory. These lesions, in the chronic phase, are also perfectly matched in those with early or late dementia. The distribution of lesions to some extent is appropriate to the pattern of functional deficits determined clinically. Studies of patients with acute cerebrovascular events (strokes) have clarified the formation of these lesions (Lenzi et al. 1982; Wise et al. 1983; Frackowiak and Wise 1983). When a cerebral vessel becomes occluded, the tissue distally becomes ischaemic and oxygen extraction rises precipitously to approach 100%. Depending on the depth and duration of ischaemia tissue dies, unable to maintain a level of energy metabolism sufficient to maintain structural and functional integrity. When reperfusion occurs, this is initially usually through a damaged and dysautoregulated vasculature. The CBF is thus in great excess of residual tissue metabolic need and so the OER falls to values close to 10%. The recoupling of flow to metabolism then occurs over a number of weeks as reparative processes complete their task and a focal area of low flow and metabolism results. In massive infarcts where all the nervous tissue is destroyed, the OER may remain low and recoupling does not occur. It is interesting that though this is common following massive infarcts due to major vessel occlusion, it is very rare in the demented population. This implies that the dement suffers from repeated acute minor ischaemic events sufficient to result in partial infarction of tissue manifesting as minor clinical events until the accumulation of damage results in a permanent syndrome of dementia.

Studies with patients suffering from multiple large vessel occlusion have in rare cases demonstrated areas of the brain with a chronically raised OER. The values usually lie in the range 50% – 70% and therefore the brain is not ischaemic. However, the oxygen reserve is greatly diminished and it is reasonable to suspect that such patients may be at a greater than normal risk of suffering further infarcts if haemodynamic failure occurs. Measurement of CBV and CBF has demonstrated that a further homeostatic mechanism protects the brain from infarction in the face of a falling perfusion pressure. This is the haemodynamic reserve, which is dependent on vasodilation causing decreased peripheral resistance and thus maintenance of flow. A proportionally greater number of patients with major vessel stenoses or occlusions show a diminished haemodynamic reserve as opposed to an elevated OER and a diminished oxygen carriage reserve (Gibbs et al. 1984). It seems that these protective mechanisms act in series. Initially the cerebral vasculature vasodilates, resulting in an increase in cerebral transit time but maintenance of flow (and hence $CMRO_2$). Then when vasodilation becomes maximal, the oxygen reserve is called upon and oxygen extraction rises as flow begins to fall; thus $CMRO_2$ continues to be maintained. Finally, flow falls to levels such that even with maximal oxygen extraction there is not enough oxygen delivered to maintain consumption and this also then declines with resulting clinical features. It is therefore clear that if haemodynamic and oxygen carriage reserves can be quantified, then the risk of clinical deterioration should be measurable. The haemodynamic reserve can be quantified by measuring CBF and CBV, which gives transit time measurements. The oxygen carriage reserve is quantified with the OER. Thus, potentially rational decisions, based on an adequate physiological description of the cerebral tissue, can be made concerning preventative therapy. It is clear that vasodilation in itself cannot be useful as in the first phase this is appropriate anyway and in the second phase of haemodynamic failure, maximal dilation has already been achieved.

It should be pointed out that haemodynamic failure seems to be a rare cause of infarction and hence vascular dementia. Much commoner treatable predisposing factors remain hypertension, atrial fibrillation and atheroembolism.

The studies of protein metabolism, though as yet very preliminary (Bustany et al. 1983), show a very similar distribution of disturbances of amino acid incorporation into protein as the studies with oxygen and glucose metabolism. There appears to be no change in the permeability of the BBB to methionine, the amino acid used in these studies, but the turnover of the free amino acid pool is greatly decreased, especially in frontal and temporoparietal areas.

Conclusion

This review highlights the main areas in which understanding of the physiology of aging and dementia has progressed in the last few years since the advent of PET into clinical research. It attempts to show how this improved understanding provides a more rational basis for classification, treatment and prevention of dementia and points to areas where PET seems to hold out most promise for future advances in the research of aging and dementia.

References

Benson DF (1982) The use of positron emission scanning in the diagnosis of Alzheimer's disease. Aging 19:79

Bustany P, Henry JF, Sargent T et al. (1983) Local brain protein metabolism in dementia and schizophrenia: in vivo studies with ^{11}C-L-methionine and positron emission tomography. In: Heiss WD, Phelps ME (eds) Positron emission tomography of the brain. Springer, New York, pp 208–211

Chase TN, Foster LN, Fedio P, Brooks R, Mansi L, DiChiro G (1984) Regional cortical dysfunction in Alzheimer's disease as determined by positron emission tomography. Ann Neurol 15 [Suppl] S170–S174

Dastur DK, Lane MH, Hansen DB et al. (1963) Effects of ageing on cerebral circulation and metabolism in man. In: Barren JE, Butler RN, Greenhouse SW et al. (eds) Human ageing. US Public Health Service Publication No. 985:59–76

Duara R, Margolin RA, Robertson-Tchabo EA et al. (1984) Resting cerebral glucose utilisation as measured with positron emission tomography in 21 healthy men between the ages of 21 and 83 years. Brain 107:761–775

Frackowiak RSJ (1982) Human regional cerebral blood flow and oxygen metabolism studied with oxygen-15 and positron emission tomography. MD thesis, University of Cambridge, pp 1–209

Frackowiak RSJ, Lenzi GL, Jones T, Heather JD (1980) Quantitative measurement of regional cerebral blood flow and oxygen metabolism in man using $^{15}0$ and positron emission tomography: theory, procedure and normal values. J Comput Assist Tomogr 4:727–736

Frackowiak RSJ, Pozzilli C, Legg NJ, DuBoulay GH, Marshall J, Lenzi GL, Jones T (1981) Regional cerebral oxygen supply and utilisation in dementia: a clinical and physiological study with oxygen-15 and positron tomography. Brain 104:753–778

Frackowiak RSJ, Wise RJS (1983) Positron tomography in ischaemic cerebrovascular disease. Neurol Clin 1(1):183–201

Gibbs TM, Wise RJS, Leenders KL, Jones T (1984) Evaluation of cerebral perfusion reserve in patients with carotid artery occlusions. Lancet I:310–314

Ingvar DH (1979) Hyperfrontal distribution of the cerebral grey matter flow in resting wakefulness: on the functional anatomy of the conscious state. Acta Neurol Scand 60:12–25

Kennedy C, Sokoloff L (1957) An adaptation of the nitrous oxide method to the study of the cerebral circulation in children: normal values for cerebral blood flow and cerebral metabolic rate in childhood. J Clin Invest 36:1130–1137

Kety SS (1956) Human cerebral blood flow and oxygen consumption as related to aging. Res Publ Assoc Res Nerv Ment Dis 35:31–45

Kuhl DE, Metter EJ, Riege WH, Phelps ME (1982) Effects of human aging on patterns of local cerebral glucose utilisation determined by the (^{18}F) fluorodeoxyglucose method. J Cereb Blood Flow Metab 2:163–171

Lammertsma AA, Jones T (1983) The correction for the presence of intravascular oxygen-15 in the steady state technique for measuring regional oxygen extraction in the brain: 1. Description of the method. J Cereb Blood Flow Metab 3:416–424

Lammertsma AA, Jones T, Frackowiak RSJ, Lenzi GL, Pozzilli C (1981) A theoretical study of the steady state model for measuring regional cerebral blood flow and oxygen utilisation using oxygen-15. J Comput Assist Tomogr 5:544–555

Lammertsma AA, Heather JD, Jones T, Frackowiak RSJ, Lenzi GL (1982) A statistical study of the steady state model for measuring regional cerebral blood flow and oxygen utilisation using oxygen-15. J Comput Assist Tomogr 5:566–573

Lammertsma AA, Wise RJS, Heather JD, Gibbs JM, Leenders KL, Frackowiak RSJ, Rhodes CG, Jones T (1983) The correction for the presence of intravascular oxygen-15 in the steady state technique for measuring regional oxygen extraction ratio in the brain: 2. Results in normal subjects and brain tumour and stroke patients. J Cereb Blood Flow Metab 3:425–431

Lenzi GL, Frackowiak RSJ, Jones T (1982) Cerebral oxygen metabolism and blood flow in human cerebral ischaemic infarction. J Cereb Blood Flow Metab 2:321–335

Mazziotta JC, Phelps ME, Miller J, Kuhl DE (1981) Tomographic mapping of human cerebral metabolism: normal unstimulated state. Neurology 31:503–516

Mazziotta JC, Phelps ME, Carson RE, Kuhl DE (1982a) Tomographic mapping of human cerebral metabolism: sensory deprivation. Ann Neurol 12:435–444

Mazziotta JC, Phelps ME, Carson RE, Kuhl DE (1982b) Tomogrphic mapping of human cerebral metabolism: auditory stimulation. Neurology 12:435–444

Phelps ME, Huang S-C, Hoffman EJ, Selin EJ, Sokoloff L, Kuhl DE (1979) Tomograhic measurement of local cerebral glucose metabolic rate in humans with (F-18) 2-fluro-2-deoxy-D-glucose: Validation of method. Ann Neurol 6:371–388

Phelps ME, Mazziotta JC, Kuhl DE, Nuwer M, Packwood J, Metter J, Engel J Jr (1984) Tomographic mapping of human cerebral metabolism: visual stimulation and deprivation. Neurology 31:517–529

Plum F (moderator) (1981) Guidelines for vasoactive drug studies in chronic cerebrovascular disease and stroke. In: Drugs and methods in CVD. ed, SIR. Pergamon, New York, pp 467–490

Sokoloff L (1966) Cerebral circulatory and metabolic changes associated with aging. Res Publ Assoc Res Nerv Ment Dis 41:237–251

Sokoloff L (1981) Localisation of functional activity in the cerebral nervous system by measurement of glucose utilisation with radioactive deoxyglucose. J Cereb Blood Flow Metab 1:7–36

Tomlinson BE, Blessed G, Roth M (1970) Observations on the brains of demented old people. J Neurol Sci 11:205–242

Wise RJS, Bernardi S, Frackowiak RSJ, Legg NJ, Jones T (1983) Serial observations on the pathophysiology of acute stroke: the transition from ischaemia to infarction as reflected in regional oxygen extraction. Brain 106:197–222

4.5 Neurotransmitters in Old Age and Dementia

A. Carlsson

The changes occurring in the aging brain are complex and not well understood. Degeneration of neurons obviously constitutes an important feature. This process is inevitably progressive, since lost nerve cells cannot be replaced.

Insufficient perfusion of the brain tissue, owing to arteriosclerosis and other vascular changes, sometimes in combination with extracerebral factors such as decrease in blood pressure, may be the cause of tissue damage. However, in many cases the primary change is believed to reside in the brain tissue itself. This is true of Alzheimer's disease (AD. a form of presenile dementia) and senile dementia of Alzheimer type (SDAT).

There seems to be no distinct borderline between normal and pathological aging. Presumably degenerative changes can go on for a considerable time in the brain tissue before a functional failure becomes manifest. Initially the failure may be transient and show up as a delirious state. Stressful conditions, such as trauma, infection, certain drugs, or major environmental changes, may elicit the failure. In more advanced stages persistent functional losses occur, ultimately leading to overt dementia.

Given the insidious onset of degenerative changes in old age, the examination of the brains of aged people is likely to reveal mild or moderate changes characteristic of dementia in some individuals who do not yet show any clear signs of the disorder. With increasing age this number may become considerable. It should be recalled that dementia of severe degree has been found to increase rapidly above the age of 75 and may occur in almost 50% of people aged 90 – 100 years (Adolfsson et al. 1981; Gottfries et al. 1985). We are thus facing a dilemma when trying to collect proper control material. When investigating dementia and other age-related disorders it may prove useful not to rely entirely on an age-matched control group but also to compare with a group of younger controls.

Neuronal degeneration, initially perhaps limited to a reduction in cell mass and number of processes but ultimately resulting in total loss of the neuron, will inevitably lead to a reduction in the level of neurotransmitters and in the enzymes involved in their synthesis. The age dependence of different neuronal types is not uniform. For example, catecholamine-producing neurons, especially those manufacturing dopamine, appear to be more age sensitive than, for example, GABAergic or serotonergic neurons (McGeer 1978; Carlsson 1981a), as evidenced by a more rapid decline of transmitter levels and synthetizing enzymes. This phenomenon also shows up as a decrease in cell count in substantia nigra and locus ceruleus, whose cell bodies are dopaminergic and noradrenergic, respectively; this is in contrast to several other brainstem nuclei, where the cell count is not clearly age dependent (Brody 1975; McGeer 1978).

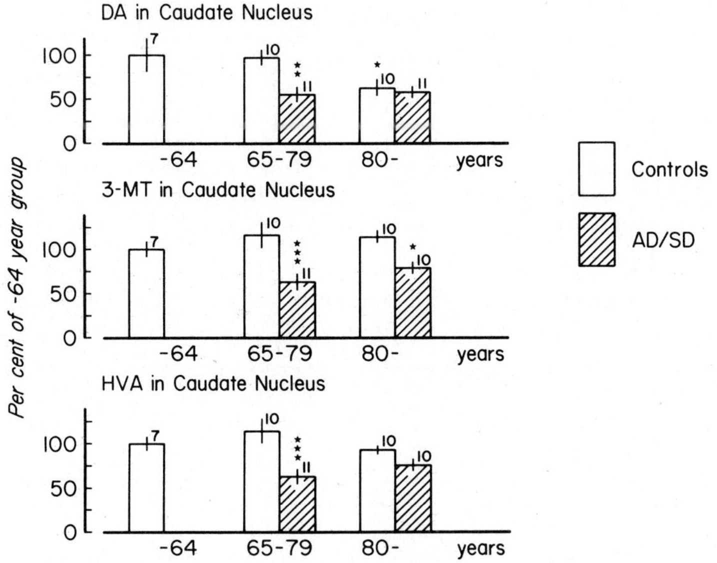

Fig. 1. Dopamine (*DA*) and its metabolites 3-methoxytyramine (*3-MT*) and homovanillic acid (*HVA*) in the caudate nucleus of different age groups of controls and of cases with dementia of Alzheimer type (AD/SDAT). Shown are the means and SEM (*n*). $^{*}P<0.05$, $^{**}P<0.01$, $^{***}P<0.001$, vs. age-matched controls or, in the case of controls, vs. – 64-year-old group

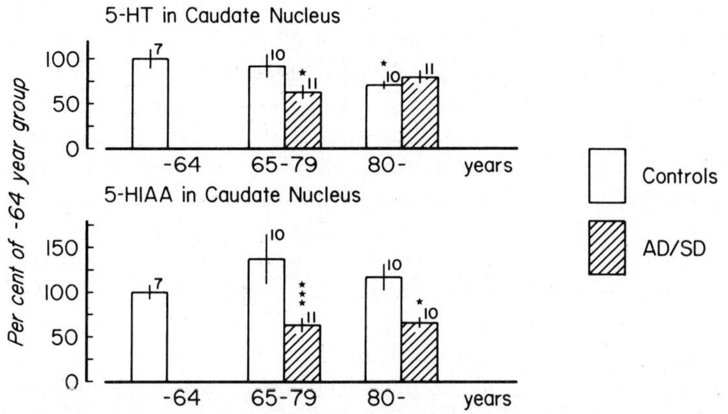

Fig. 2. Serotonin (5-HT) and its metabolite 5-hydroxyindoleacetic acid (5-HIAA) in the caudate nucleus of the same age groups as in Fig. 1

Neurons appear to possess a considerable reserve capacity. In the event of increased demand they may increase their firing rates and utilize more of their enzymatic synthetizing activity. This may explain why a decrease in neuronal number and mass is not necessarily accompanied by any detectable functional loss. In fact, in postmortem analyses of the brains of neuropsychiatrically normal aged people we have found decreases in transmitter levels, as compared with

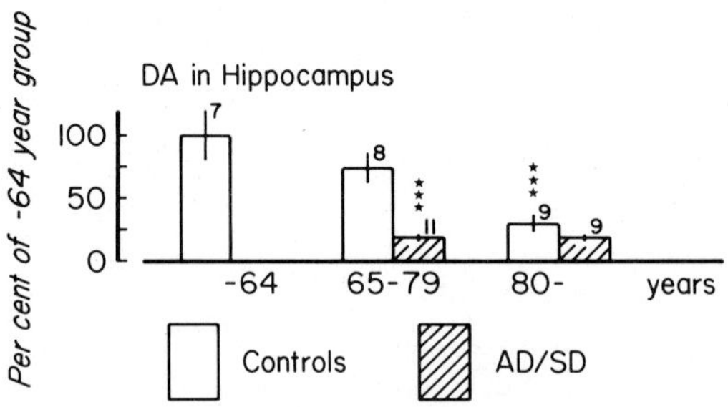

Fig. 3. Dopamine (*DA*) in the hippocampus of the same groups as in the previous figures

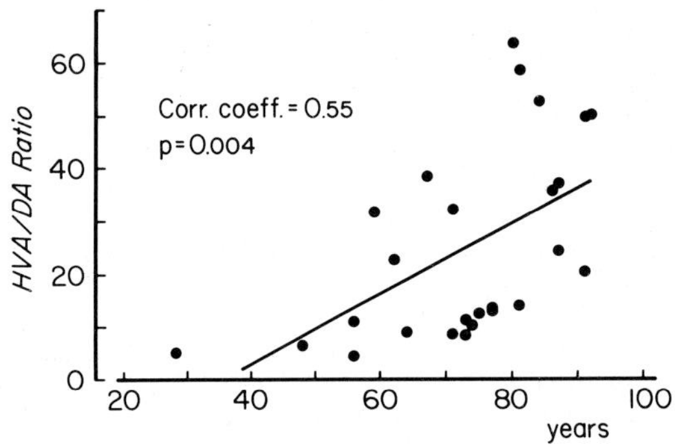

Fig. 4. Ratio of homovanillic acid (*HVA*) to dopamine (*DA*) in the hippocampus of controls, plotted versus age

younger individuals, whithout a concomitant decrease in the corresponding transmitter metabolites. Thus, in an ongoing postmortem study we confirm earlier observations (Carlsson and Winblad 1976; Carlsson 1981a) that the level of dopamine in the basal ganglia decreases in old age (C.-G. Gottfries, A. Carlsson, S.-A. Eckernäs, L. Svennerholm, and B. Winblad, unpublished data). However, there is no corresponding decrease in its metabolites 3-methoxytyramine, 3, 4-dihydroxyphenylacetic acid (DOPAC), or homovanillic acid (HVA; see Fig. 1). Similarly, serotonin (5-HT) decreases with age without any concomitant decrease in its metabolite 5-hydroxyindoleacetic acid (5-HIAA; see Fig. 2). Dopamine and homovanillic acid show a similar pattern in the hippocampus, although the age dependence is even more striking in this region (Fig. 3). Consequently there is a significant increase in the ratio of metabolites to transmitter, as illustrated in Fig. 4. The most likely explanation of this phenomenon is that the age-related loss of neurons is compensated by an increased activity of the remaining neurons, probably as a result of feedback stimulation. This stimulation causes an increased release, which in turn will lead to a further depletion of transmitter and counteract the decrease in metabolite levels. A similar phenomenon has been observed in Parkinson's disease, where the reduction of dopamine in the basal ganglia is more severe than the decrease in metabolite levels (Hornykiewicz 1966).

Increased receptor sensitivity could theoretically also compensate for neuronal losses and is likely to occur. However, in the case of dopamine in the basal ganglia the receptor density, as judged by in vitro binding, is not increased; in fact it shows a significant decrease with age in the caudate nucleus (Severson et al. 1982). The interpretation of this finding is complicated by the fact that postsynaptic dopamine receptors are believed to occur on at least three types of neuron in the striatum. Whether the age dependence of dopamine receptors refers to all these neurons, or perhaps only to one type, is not known.

When brain function finally deteriorates, this could be due to failure of the compensatory mechanisms. In fact, in our ongoing study we find that in a group of high-age dementia (age > 80 years) the most conspicuous deviation from age-matched controls is a decrease in transmitter metabolites (see Fig. 1 – 3). The decrease in transmitter levels is less striking. But here we have to take into account that the transmitter levels were reduced also in the control group, when compared with a younger control group. Reduced levels of their metabolites have been found not only in postmortem studies of brains from individuals who had suffered from dementia of the Alzheimer type, but also in clinical examinations of cerebrospinal fluid from such patients (see Gottfries 1985).

As mentioned, the "normal" age dependence of the catecholamines has been particularly well documented. In general, the cholinergic system appears to be less sensitive to the normal aging process. In contrast, the cholinergic system is clearly affected in dementia, as evidenced by a decrease in the activity of choline acetyltransferase (CAT), at least in the important subgroups belonging to the Alzheimer type (AD/SDAT). In fact, several workers have felt that these types of dementia are essentially due to failure of the cholinergic system. Although a decrease in the cholinergic system is generally recognized as an important feature of AD/SDAT, others have felt that Alzheimer dementias involve many different neurons (for a review of the different arguments, see Reisberg 1983). Evidence in favor of the latter contention has been quoted above. Table 1, with data from our ongoing study, may serve to clarify the matter somewhat further. As is evident from this table, the transmitter changes occurring in the brains of AD/SDAT cases are not uniform. Even though the changes appear to be widespread, regional differences are evident, with, for example, the hippocampus and the caudate nucleus being more affected than the putamen. A difference between the hippocampus and the caudate nucleus is evident both from the table and comparison between Figs. 1 and 3. The decrease in 5-HIAA is pronounced in all brain regions and more uniform than, for example, the decrease in CAT. Marked reductions of 5-HT, dopamine, and dopamine metabolites are also seen in certain regions.

The fact that the caudate nucleus is more affected than the putamen in dementia is in agreement with earlier observations in normal aging (see Carlsson 1981b). However, in Parkinson's disease the dopamine and HVA levels are clearly more severely reduced in the latter nucleus. As pointed out by Hassler (1980), the two nuclei appear to have different functions, judging from their neuronal connections. The putamen seems to be largely involved in motor functions, with strong connections to the motor cortex. On the other hand, the caudate nucleus communicates more intimately with the frontal cortex and may thus be more involved in mental activity. Of interest in this context is the recent finding that homologous grafting of adrenal medulla into the caudate nucleus of two

Table 1. Biogenic amines and metabolites in various brain regions of patients with Alzheimer's disease/senile dementia of Alzheimer type. Preliminary, previously unpublished data of a joint Swedish investigation (C.-G. Gottfries, A. Carlsson, S.-Å. Eckernäs, L. Svennerholm, and B. Wimblad). Values are means ± sem in percent of age-matched controls. $n=20$

	Caudate	Left putamen	Right putamen	Hippo-campus	Cort. gyr. temp.
Dopamine	71 ± 7[a]	88 ± 13	79 ± 10	36 ± 4[c]	101 ± 27
3-Methoxy-tyramine	62 ± 5[c]	68 ± 6	68 ± 7[b]	–	–
DOPAC	78 ± 8	86 ± 14	88 ± 13	66 ± 5[b]	71 ± 7
HVA	67 ± 5[b]	78 ± 7	85 ± 9	77 ± 7[a]	91 ± 10
5 HT	87 ± 7	93 ± 11	87 ± 8	59 ± 7[b]	52 ± 12[b]
5-HIAA	51 ± 4[c]	53 ± 5[c]	62 ± 6[c]	51 ± 5[c]	58 ± 5[c]
Noradren.	77 ± 15	84 ± 16	91 ± 14	86 ± 8	–
CAT	48 ± 5[c]	73 ± 10	67 ± 10	50 ± 10[b]	37 ± 8[c]

[a] $P<0.05$; [b] $P<0.01$; [c] $P<0.01$ vs. control

Parkinsonian patients did not result in more than marginal and transient improvement of motor functions, whereas one of the patients suffered from paranoid symptoms when L-DOPA therapy was reintroduced after the surgery; these symptoms disappeared after reduction of the L-DOPA dosage (L. Olson, personal communication).

The changes observed in the caudate nucleus of demented patients may thus be relevant for certain aspects of the complex symptomatology in dementia, even though the role of other brain regions such as the hippocampus may be even more important.

In addition to biogenic amines, certain peptides (somatostatin and substance P) appear to be involved (Davies et al. 1980, 1982).

Needless to say, our knowledge of brain neurotransmitters is fragmentary, and this is certainly true of their role in aging and dementia. There are two or three dozens of neurotransmitters in the brain, belonging to different chemical groups. i.e., the biogenic amines, amino acids, and peptides. To further complicate the issue, one and the same neuron may utilize more than one compound as transmitter. Up till now the discussion of the role of neurotransmitters in aging and dementia has dealt mainly with the biogenic amines, partly because they have been most extensively investigated so far. The deterioration of brain function in aging and dementia is very complex and evidently extends far beyond the memory deficit. It is thus by no means surprising that many different types of neuron and many different brain regions show changes in normal aging as well as dementia.

Even though postmortem brain studies have yielded interesting information, a detailed mapping of the various neurotransmitters in normal and pathological aging will probably have to await the advent of more sophisticted in vivo methods of investigation, such as the powerful modern imaging techniques now underway. However, the full utilization of these techniques will require a considerable methodological effort, and thus we will probably have to be patient for at least a decade or two until anything approaching a reasonably complete mapping materializes.

When investigating the neurotransmitters in normal and pathological aging, we have to realize that not all changes are necessarily the immediate consequence of neuronal degeneration. The importance of feedback mechanisms has already been alluded to. Moreover, the primary cause of a change observed may reside outside the neuron under study: it may even reside in nonneuronal elements. For example, recently the role of white matter lesions in dementia has been emphasized. In line with this contention, my colleagues in Gothenburg have observed decreases in various lipid constituents of the white matter of the brain (Gottfries et al. 1985), probably due to demyelinization. Possibly the primary lesion in such cases resides in oligodendroglia cells, and this lesion may in turn be induced by vascular lesions and circulatory disturbances. Histological observations seem to favor this interpretation (Brun 1983). However, the possibility that neuronal degeneration is the primary cause of the lesion cannot be excluded.

Another remarkable observation in aging and dementia is the increase in monoamine oxidase B with little or no concomitant change in monoamine oxidase A. Possibly this is due to glial proliferation, induced by neuronal degeneration (see Gottfries et al. 1983).

Most studies of transmitter disturbances in dementia have so far concentrated on AD and SDAT. At present there is a trend to lump these two conditions together to form "AD/S-DAT." The chief basis for this is that microscopic changes observed in Alzheimer's disease (plaques, tangles, etc.) are also seen in senile dementia with later onset. However, these lesions are probably unspecific. The biochemical profiles of the two conditions appear to differ somewhat. In the presenile form there are reductions in the levels of catecholamines and 5-HT and in the cholinergic marker choline acetyltransferase (CAT). In the senile form the levels of the monoamines are about the same as in the presenile form, but in view of the "normal" decreases seen in old age they are not strikingly different from the levels seen in age-matched controls. On the other hand, as already pointed out, the levels of monoamine metabolites are clearly reduced in comparison with age-matched controls, suggesting a failure of compensatory mechanisms, and the concentrations of various lipid constituents in white matter are reduced in the senile form; especially the last-mentioned change appears to be mild or absent in patients with dementia of early onset. At present it would thus seem appropriate to keep the two conditions apart, even though a cholinergic deficiency appears to exist in both forms.

"Multi-infarct dementia" has attracted much less attention than the two previously discussed forms of dementia. In our ongoing postmortem study we have added a group of demented individuals in whom autopsy revealed one or more infarctions in the brain. Our investigation has not yet been completed, but our impression is that the transmitter changes in this group are similar to those of demented people free of brain infarctions (as briefly described in this paper), although they tend to be less marked. The interpretation of this finding must await a more careful analysis.

What can the neurotransmitter research strategy offer in terms of future therapy and prevention? First of all, the possibility of substitution therapy, in line with the use of L-DOPA in Parkinson's disease, is opened up. Attempts in this direction, aiming at improving cholinergic and catecholaminergic transmission, have not been encouraging (for reviews. see Reisberg 1983). However, it must be realized that we are dealing with a multiple neurotransmitter deficiency. Thus the substitution of only one transmitter may not be sufficient. Moreover, there seem to be considerable differences in deficiency profile. It may therefore prove necessary to determine the deficiency profile in the individual patient and to tailor the substitution accordingly. To achieve this we have to await the development of highly sophisticated diagnostic procedures and of an arsenal of receptor agonists suitable for substitution therapy.

The marked decrease in 5-HIAA observed in the demented patients (see above) is remarkable. Therapy aiming to improve serotonergic transmission may thus prove worthwhile. For example, the specific 5-HT-uptake inhibitors now underway certainly deserve to be tried in dementia. They differ from conventional antidepressants in, among other ways, being essentially devoid of anticholinergic side-effects, which of course are especially bothersome in dementia owing to the already existent cholinergic deficiency in this disorder. Also tryptophan provides an interesting alternative and has indeed been tried in open studies with some success. Insufficient absorption of tryptophan may contribute to serotonergic failure in certain cases (Lehmann et al. 1981). The combination of tryptophan with a monoamine oxidase inhibitor may also prove useful.

More futuristic is the prospect of substitution therapy by grafting. Despite promising observations in animal experiments (Björklund 1984), this strategy will probably remain experimental for a considerable time, at least in multifactorial conditions such as dementia. In Parkinson's disease this approach would seem more promising (Olson et al. 1984).

Another fascinating aspect is the possibility of prevention. To achieve this it will prove necessary to clarify the mechanisms underlying neuronal degeneration, focussing on neuronal types showing the greatest susceptibility. In this context the special vulnerability of catecholamine neurons may provide an important clue. As is well known, these neurons, especially the dopamine neurons, in addition to being age sensitive, are uniquely sensitive to a number of noxious influences, e.g., to virus, manganese, and certain neurotoxins, especially the recently discovered NMPTP (for data and references, see Chieuh et al. 1984). The reason for this vulnerability is not well understood. However, the fact that catecholamines possess cytotoxic properties, mediated by their autoxidation quinoid products, is intriguing (see Moldéus et al. 1983). The reason why catecholamines are not overtly cytotoxic is the occurrence of highly efficient antioxidants in tissues. Partial failure of this protective system may possibly explain the special vulnerability and age dependence of catecholamine neurons. If this hypothesis proves correct, prevention may prove possible by supporting the protective system.

References

Adolfsson R, Gottfries C-G, Nyström L, Winblad B (1981) Prevalence of dementia in institutionalized Swedish old people. Acta Psychiatr Scand 63:225–244

Björklund A, Stenevi U, Schmidt RH, Dunnett SB, Gage FH (1983) Intracerebral grafting of neuronal cell suspensions. I. Introduction and general methods of preparation. Acta Physiol Scand [Suppl] 522:1–8

Brody H (1975) Cell counts in cerebral cortex and brainstem. In: Katzman R, Terry RD, Bick KL (eds) Alzheimer's disease: senile dementia and related disorders. Aging vol 7. Raven, New York, pp 345–352

Brun A (1983) An overview of light and electron microscopic changes. In: Reisberg B (ed) Alzheimer's disease. The Free Press, New York London, pp 37–47

Carlsson A (1981a) Aging and brain neurotransmitters. In: Platt D (ed) Funktionsstörungen des Gehirns im Alter. Schattauer, Stuttgart New York, pp 67–81

Carlsson A (1981b) Aging and brain neurotransmitters. In: Crook T, Gershon S (eds) Strategies for the development of an effective treatment for senile dementia. Mark Powley Association, New Canaan, pp 98–106

Carlsson A, Winblad B (1976) Influences of age and time interval between death and autopsy on dopamine and 3-methoxytyramine levels in human basal ganglia. J Neural Transm 38:271–276

Chieuh CC, Markey SP, Burns RS, Johannessen JN, Jacobowitz DM, Kopin IJ (1984) Selective neurotoxic effects of *N*-methyl-4-phenyl-1,2,3,6-tetrahydropyridine (MPTP) in subhuman primates and man: a new animal model of Parkinson's disease. Psychopharmacol Bull 20:548–553

Davies P, Katzman R, Terry RD (1980) Reduced somatostatin-like immunoreactivity in cerebral cortex from cases of Alzheimer disease and Alzheimer senile dementia. Nature 288:279–280

Davies P, Katz DA, Crystal HA (1982) Choline acetyltransferase, somatostatin and substance P in selected cases of Alzheimer's disease. In: Corkin S, Davis KL, Growdon JH, Usdin E, Wurtman RJ (eds) Aging vol 19. Alzheimer's disease. A report of progress in research. Raven, New York, pp 9–14

Gottfries C-G (1985) Senile dementia of Alzheimer's type: clinical, genetic, pathogenetic and treatment aspects. In Sorensen AB, Weinert FE, Sherrod LR (eds) Human development: interdisciplinary perspectives. (in press)

Gottfries C-G, Adolfsson R, Aquilonius S-M, Carlsson A, Eckernäs S-A, Nordberg A, Oreland L, Svennerholm L, Wiberg A, Winblad B (1983) Biochemical changes in dementia disorders of Alzheimer type (AD/SDAT). Neurobiol Aging 4:261–271

Gottfries C-G, Karlsson I, Svennerholm L (1985) Senile dementia – a white matter disease. In: Gottfries C-G (ed) Normal Aging Alzheimer's Disease and Senile Dementia. Aspects on Etiology, Pathogenesis, Diagnosis, and Treatment. Editions de l'Université de Bruxelles

Hassler R (1980) Discussion remark. In: Rinne UK, Klingler M, Stamm G (eds) Parkinson's disease. Current progress, problems, and management. Elsevier, Amsterdam, pp 213–214

Hornykiewicz O (1966) Metabolism of brain dopamine in human Parkinsonism: Neurochemical and clinical aspects. In: Costa E, Coté LJ, Yahr MD (eds) Biochemistry and pharmacology of the basal ganglia. Raven, New York, pp 171–181

Lehmann J, Persson S, Wålinder J, Wallin L (1981) Tryptophan malabsorption in dementia. Improvement in certain cases after tryptophan therapy as by mental behaviour and blood analysis. Acta Psychiatr Scand 64:123–131

McGeer EG (1978) Aging and neurotransmitter metabolism in the human brain. In: Katzman R, Terry RD, Bick KL (eds) Alzheimer's disease: senile dementia and related disorders. Raven, New York, pp 427–440

Moldéus P, Nordenskjöld M, Bolcsfoldi G, Eiche A, Haglund U, Lambert B (1983) Genetic toxicity of dopamine. Mutat Res 124:9–24

Olson L, Backlund EO, Sedvall G, Herrera-Marschitz M, Ungerstedt U, Strömberg I, Hoffer B, Seiger A (1984) Intrastriatal chromaffin grafts in experimental and clinical Parkinsonism: first impressions. In: Usdin E, Carlsson A, Daheström A, Engel J (eds) Catecholamines: neuropharmacology and central nervous system – therapeutic aspects. Alan Liss, New York, pp 195–201

Reisberg B (ed) (1983) Alzheimer's disease. The Free Press. New York London, pp 1–475

Severson JA, Marcusson J, Winblad B, Finch CE (1982) Age-correlated loss of dopaminergic binding sites in human basal ganglia. J Neurochem 39:1623–1631

4.6 The Value of Collaborative Research in Aging

B. O. Osuntokun

Cross-cultural and inter-cultural population-based studies often contribute to knowledge of the aetiology and prognosis of diseases, clear-cut examples being hypertension, ischaemic heart disease and stroke. Such cultural studies have shown, for example, that in some 30 or more isolated communities in developing countries where blood pressures do not rise with age, the major determinants of this normal phenomenon are life-style and quantity of salt intake. In the last two decades the World Health Organisation (WHO) has taken the initiative in promoting such studies in respect of a number of diseases, including the three named above, as well as the epidemiology of depression, psychoneuropharmacology and schizophrenia. Over the last 5 years the Neurological Disorders Programme, Division of Mental Health, WHO, Geneva, has also catalysed the development of research in neuro-epidemiology in developing countries. The results of this WHO-sponsored collaborative research have been very fruitful. They have contributed to our knowledge of the epidemiology, the risk factors, the prognosis and the natural history of these diseases and indicated possible means of prevention. Citing a few specific examples, age-specific incidence rates for stroke in a developing country such as Nigeria are now similar to those in developed countries and the commonest risk factors are also similar – hypertension, diabetes mellitus and heart disease – except that atherosclerosis (including coronary heart disease) is rare whilst it is common in developed countries (Osuntokun et al. 1979). The prognosis of schizophrenia is better in developing countries such as Nigeria, Colombia and India than in European countries (WHO 1979). The neuro-epidemiological research is currently being conducted in a number of developing countries – Nigeria, Senegal and Kenya in Africa; Ecuador, Venezuela, Chile, Columbia and Mexico in Latin America; India and China. The same research protocol is being used, with well defined criteria for diagnostic decisions. Preliminary results have shown that in some developing countries there is an unusually high prevalence of epilepsy, of the order of 2% – 5% (about 5 – 10 times the prevalence in developed countries), and that migraine surprisingly is as common in rural communities as in the sophisticated ones of the developed countries (Osuntokun et al. 1982; Cruz et al. 1984; Gerritts 1983; Gousmit and Van der Waals 1983).

Collaborative research into the neurobiology of aging may be rewarding. I want to use as an example dementia and specifically Alzheimer's disease.

Until the last 2 decades, Alzheimer's disease (first described by Alois Alzheimer 1906) as a nosological and diagnostic entity was a neurological curiosity. Most cases of idiopathic dementia were labelled primary degenerative dementia, senile or presenile, and were often ascribed to arteriosclerosis or just senility. In 1968, it was shown that in 50% of elderly persons with dementia, the classical neuropathological features described by Alzheimer were present (Blessed et al. 1968). Since then it appears that an "epidemic" of Alzheimer's disease (AZD) has afflicted the elderly in developed countries. AZD is now the fourth most common cause of death in those above 65 in the United States and some developed countries (US Department of Health and Human Services 1984). AZD reduces life expectancy by about 50%. In addition, the economic costs of dementia are staggering. AZD is of considerable public health importance to developing and developed countries, yet little is known about AZD in different races, in urban as against rural communities and in nations outside the developed countries of the North. It is estimated that the 400 million people in the world currently over the age of 65 will have increased to 600 million by 2000 A.D. and that two-thirds of them will live in the developed countries. If the current demographic pattern in developed countries is maintained, the proportion over 65 will double within the next 40 years, and the result will be an increasing incidence of AZD.

In AZD, recent studies have shown deficits predominantly in the brain cholinergic pathway (with severe loss of cholinergic neurons in the basal nucleus of Meynert) as well as in the noradrenergic, serotonergic, dopaminergic and GABA-ergic systems that innervate the telencephalon. Somatostatin concentration in the brain cortex is also reduced. Some specific discrete lesion in the hippocampus may be the initial pathological substrate.

The cause of AZD is unknown. Current theories include auto-immunity, aluminium and other environmental toxicity, infection by slow virus, genetically determined susceptibility and the presence of "free radicals". (These are a highly reactive class of molecule fragments that combine readily with other pieces of molecules and are probably involved in aging, causing chemical reactions that lead to damage to and plugging of vessels and cells throughout the body: free radicals are also linked to the formation of amyloid, which forms the core of neuritic plaques, characteristic of AZD). It is likely that epidemiological studies of AZD would contribute to our knowledge of the causation of the disease.

Currently, in developed countries AZD afflicts about 10% of those above the age of 65 and 30% of those aged 85 years or more. However, it is striking that AZD appears to be uncommon or rare in developing countries, especially in Africa. A Med-line bibliographic search carried out in August 1984 showed no publication on the disease in Africans. In a recent neuro-epidemiological study involving a sample of 19 000 Nigerians, 5% and 12% of whom were over the age of 65 and 50 years respectively, no patient with dementia was seen (Osuntokun et al. 1985). Yet black Americans (who are of African descent) do not differ from American whites in the incidence and prevalence of the disease (Schoenberg et al. 1984). In a recent study in Israel, the prevalence of presenile dementia of Alzheimer's type in Jews was much higher in those who emigrated from Europe and North America than in those who emigrated from elsewhere (Horcyn, personal communication, 1984).

The rarity of AZD in Africans could, however, be apparent rather than real. The manifestation of the disease in the elderly may be regarded as a sign of benign senility and thus be ignored by relatives so that the cases do not come to medical attention. The proportion of the elderly in the population of developing countries is much lower than in that of the developed countries; however, this alone would not explain the rarity of AZD in developing countries in Africa. For example, in the neuro-epidemiological study in Nigeria referred to earlier, of the 850 people above the age of 65, about 80 would be expected to suffer from AZD if the prevalence of the disease was similar to the 10% reported in whites, yet not a single patient was identifiable. Elderly Africans are not rare, but they may be different from elderly whites and American blacks. For example, 7% of Kung African bushmen are over 65 years of age, but were all slim (Truswell 1979). It is not, however, being suggested that excessive weight is causally related to AZD; in fact, one recent study suggests that at least among the Dutch, in men in the 65 – to 74-year group, the lower the weight the shorter the rest of their life (Deeg and van Sonneverld 1984).

What is likely is that people (genetic) and environment (climate including solar radiation, soil, pollutants, minerals, life-style, diet and infections) differ.

Epidemiologists are confounded by the variety of diseases in which the neurofibrillary tangles of AZD may be found: postencephalitic Parkinson's disease (which is of viral aetiology), Down's syndrome (which is genetic) and the punch-drunk syndrome (dementia pugilistica, related to trauma). Why do neurofibrillary tangles occur in AZD?

Africans in Africa rarely suffer from auto-immune disease whereas American blacks (of African descent) have an unusually high frequency of auto-immune disease, especially systemic lupus erythematosus. As pointed out earlier, AZD could possibly be an auto-immune disease.

Epidemiologists know that it is valuable to study a disease not only in communities where it is common but also in those where it is rare. It is necessary to establish whether the rarity of AZD among Africans (in Africa) is real or not. This can be done through autopsy survey of an adequate sample, looking for histological evidence of AZD, and through community studies using a structured questionnaire of adequate sensitivity, specificity and predictive value followed by thorough neuropsychiatric evaluation of positive respondents.

If AZD is truly rare among Africans it would be equally important to establish the reasons. Such research may indicate the aetiological factor(s) responsible for the disease. It would best be conducted through collaboration between centres in developing and developed countries, employing a standardised and relevant research protocol. There is urgency about such studies, as changes take place rapidly in the developing countries, and such changes may be associated with a remarkable alteration of diseases in accordance with the well-known phenomenon of epidemiological transition: With the control of infections, nutritional and other deficiency diseases, more people in the community would survive to old age, and the increased life expectancy would be associated with increased prevalence of degenerative diseases. Perhaps there are communities where senescence does not take place or not at the same rate as in others, just as there are communities where blood pressure does not rise with age. [A community with a high proportion of centenarians is said to exist in Ecuador (M. Cruz, personal communication).] A collaborative multicentric, cross-cultural and inter-cultural study on AZD could have enormous relevance to the neurobiology of aging.

References

Blessed G, Tomlinson BE, Roth M (1968) The association between quantitative measures of dementia and of senile changes in the cerebral grey matter in elderly subjects. Br J Psychiatry 114:797–811

Cruz ME, Barberis P, Schoenberg BS, Bolis L (1984) Prevalence of neurological disorders in an area of endemic goitre. Abstract No.-402. 10th Scientific Meeting, International Epidemiological Association, 10–25 August 1984. Vancouver, British Coumbia, Canada

Deeg D, van Sonneverld RJ (1984) Predicting longevity. Abstract 166. 10th Scientific Meeting, International Epidemiological Association, 19–25 August 1984. Vancouver, British Columbia, Canada

Gerritts C (1983) A West African epilepsy focus. Lancet I:358

Gousmit J, Van der Waals FW (1983) Endemic epilepsy in an isolated region of Liberia. Lancet I:528–529

Osuntokun BO, Bademosi O, Oyediran ABO, Akinkugbe OO, Carlisle RC (1979) Incidence of stroke in an African city. Stroke 10:205–208

Osuntokun BO, Schoenberg BS, Adeuja AOG et al. (1982) Research protocol for measuring the prevalence of neurologic disorders in developing countries: results of a pilot study in Nigeria. Neuroepidemiology 1:143–149

Osuntokun BO, Adeuja AOG, Schoenberg BS et al. Community diagnosis of neurological disorders in a Nigerian town: results of door to door screening of 19 000 subjects. In: 13th world congress of Neurology. 1–7 September. Hamburg, F.R.G. Abstracts. Elsevier: Amsterdam, 1985

Schoenberg BS, Anderson DW, Kokman E, Haerer AF (1984) Multi-infarct dementia: incidence and prevalence. Abstract No. 385. 10th Scientific Meeting, International Epidemiological Association, August 19–25 1984. Vancouver, British Columbia, Canada

Truswell AS (1979) Historical and geographical perspectives. In: Davidson S,Passmore R, Brock JP, Truswell AS (eds) Human nutrition and dietetics, 7th ed. Livingstone, Edinburgh, pp 1–5

US Department of Health and Human Services (1984) Task Force on Alzheimer's Disease. Alzheimer's Disease, Neurology (w.y.) 34 (1984) 939–944

WHO (1979) Schizophrenia. WHO study shows that patients fare better in developing countries. WHO Chron 33:428

4.7 Issues in Geriatric Psychopharmacology

D. M. Loew

Introduction

In this paper I shall address the question "Can the cerebral changes associated with aging be modified by pharmacotherapy?" in the context of the biological and medical aspects of aging, related to brain disease specific to or frequent in aged patients. For the purposes of this presentation I propose the following definition of psychogeriatric drugs:

a) those intended to treat any cognitive, emotional, or behavioral deficit alleged to be caused by "normal aging" and
b) those intended as a treatment of a disease or condition (or some epiphenomena of a disease or condition) that is found solely, or at least more frequently, among the elderly (Leber 1983).

The present state of geriatric psychopharmacology is characterized by the variety of drugs in therapeutic use. In addition to psychotropic drugs which have primarily been developed for younger patients, psychogeriatric drugs are available which have pharmacologic effects considered to be predictive of specific therapeutic effects in senile dementia and milder forms of cognitive dysfunction in the elderly. In terms of chemical structure and pharmacologic activity, they constitute a heterogeneous class of compounds. Typically, vasodilation, effects on brain metabolism, or actions on synaptic transmission are given as their principal mode of action (Hoffmeister and Stille 1983; Hyams 1980). In contrast to classic psychotropic agents, their therapeutic indications are less well defined and there is considerable controversy on efficacy criteria (Reisberg et al. 1981a). Indeed, as examplified by two recent reviews by European authors, opinions on their clinical role change from "no therapeutic indication can be derived from the available evidence" (Spagnoli and Tognoni 1983) to the detailed discussion of indications for individual agents (Coper and Kanowski 1983).

Let us consider the reasons for the controversies about psychogeriatric drugs. From the viewpoint of a regulator, Leber (1983) cites the following points: Problems in subject selection, lack of agreement on the rules for diagnosis, lack of a "benchmark drug" for the treatment of dementia, the fact that differences between treatment and placebo groups are small (though statistically significant), and an inadequate consensus on methods of assessment. Additional reasons may be found in the variety of pathogenetic mechanisms underlying the diagnosis of an organic brain syndrome or a dementing syndrome. Coper and Kanowski (1983) suggest that this syndrome may consist of a number of subsets, owing to partially interrelated impairments in energy, protein and transmitter metabolism affecting neuronal and vascular regulation. They suggest that, independent of pathogenesis, a common final pathway may exist, e.g. disturbance of vigilance. Their reasoning goes on to conclude that, with a particular drug, the efficacy criterion of a global improvement will only partially be met, as it will influence only a subset of alterations. Therefore, therapeutic efficacy will be seen in only a subset of patients. The theoretical consequences for the assessment of efficacy of psychogeriatric agents are clear: They concern patient characterization and outcome measures.

Patient Characterization

To characterize the patients, clear operational criteria are needed to define symptoms, syndromes, and disease entities, e.g., the definitions provided recently by the American Psychiatric Association's *Diagnostic and Statistical Manual of Mental Disorders* [DSM – III; Spitzer et al. (1980)]. It has to be kept in mind that the diagnosis of primary degenerative dementia remains a diagnosis of exclusion and that the prognosis and long-term course are largely unknown. As yet, no clinical indictor exists to predict the clinical course in an individual patient, and the variability among patients is a major source of errors, particularly in long-term drug trials. In addition, severity needs to be assessed by a standardized mental status examination [such as the Mini-Mental State of Folstein et al. (1975)]. As in other areas of psychopharmacology, target symptoms should be identified and assessed beforehand. They serve to define drug actions targeted at symptoms of cognitive impairment, confusion, or emotional dysfunction. Baselines for physiologic, psychometric, and behavioral measures of drug efficacy are required which duly control procedural responses, learning effects, and diurnal variations.

Outcome Measures

A considerable choice of methods is available to *assess drug efficacy* in geriatric psychopharmacology (Crook et al. 1983; Israel et al. 1984; Raskin and Jarvik 1979). Broadly, these techniques can be classified into rating systems, psychological performance tests, and measures of physiologic function. The decision as to which techniques are appropriate in a particular drug trial will be influenced by a number of factors, including the type of drug under investigation and the hypothesized drug effects, the subject sample in which the drug is being studied and the population to which drug effects are to be generalized, the setting in which the study is being conducted, and the phase of development of the drug under investigation. It is important to emphasize, however, that only in rare cases is a single method of evaluation appropriate. In most cases, the appropriate strategy is a multimodal assessment in which information from different sources is combined to a comprehensive assessment of the subject.

Rating Scales

The principal tools for the assessment of behavioral changes are rating scales. Psychiatric rating scales (Kochansky 1979) have the most widespread use and the best acceptance. Less frequently self-rating scales (McNair 1979) and ward behavior scales (Honigfeld 1983) are used. Experience is scarce with drug sensitive rating systems which collect information on geriatric outpatients by using lay informants and significant others, and only recently has such a rating system been described (Schwartz 1983).

It is important to note that rating scales are standardized instruments to collect a behavioral sample of general psychopathology. They are most suitable in delineating overall differences between a placebo and a drug-treated patient group. However, they are of limited value when the aim is to find specific differences between two different types of drug, or between responses of two different patient subgroups. In addition, the item content may bias measures of outcome. Take, for instance, the cognitive items in the Sandoz Clinical Assessment Geriatric Scale (SCAG) (Shader et al. 1974; Venn 1983) as compared to the Inventory of Psychological and Somatic Complaints in the Elderly (IPSC-E) (Reisberg et al. 1981b). Four out of 19 items in the SCAG, compared with 19 out of 80 items in the IPSC-E, are used to assess cognitive impairment.

The importance of assessing social functioning emerges from a review by Wittenborn (1981). This author summarized 31 published drug studies on age-related behavioral deficiencies and defined ten behavioral criteria which would consistently discriminate drug-induced changes. Four of them reflect an impairment of social functioning. This is an area where specific studies in geriatric psychopharmacology are yet to be carried out.

Psychological Performance Tests

Psychological performance tests or psychometric tests clearly occupy a more important role in geriatric drug studies than in other areas of psychopharmacology, because they provide objective and sensitive means of assessing memory and other cognitive variables which decline in senile dementia. Scores on selected psychological tests may also correspond closely to performance outside the clinic and provide sensitive indexes of drug effects. For example, the Nuremberg Gerontopsychological Inventory of Oswald and Fleischman (1981, 1983) contains six psychological performance tests and a set of rating scales consisting of a personality rating, a gerontological attitude scale, a rating of activities of daily living, and a self-rating scale. This test system has been standardized and validated in a sample of over 1000 nursing home residents between the ages of 55 and 95 years. A factor analysis of test performance identified speed and power factors. The speed component was found to be age-dependent and correlated with activities of daily living, such as maintaining personal appearance and helping with financial affairs, as well as with items such as activity and communication on the personality rating. This speed component was also shown to be sensitive to the effects of psychogeriatric agents.

Physiologic Measures

In geriatric psychopharmacology a number of physiologic measures are available. For instance, regional brain metabolism or cerebral blood flow could be suitable indicators in the study of metabolic activators. Changes in neurotransmitter metabolites and in some neuroendocrinological parameters may be used to assess effects on neurotransmitter function. Drugs increasing attention or signal processing speed could be investigated by using a combination of psychometric performance measures and evoked brain potential recording.

It is true that, at present, none of these techniques has found wide general acceptance, and that most of them lack high face validity. Thus, they are not likely to replace standardized clinical observation and behavioral assessment. On the other hand, it is obvious that the rapid increase in the understanding of the biological basis of senile mental decline is leading to new drugs which originate from pharmacologic experiments dealing with a specific mechanism possibly involved in senile dementia. If we are to assess the therapeutic potential of these new, specific drugs, evidence of their actions on biological measures in humans is required.

With regard to physiologic measures, it is important to observe the distinction emphasized by Herrmann et al. (1981) between assessing "efficacy" and "effects" of gerontopsychiatric agents. At present, physiological measures can only be taken as indicators of a drug-induced change in partial aspects of a disease, but do not constitute the disease itself. In the assessment of treatment-induced change in arterial hypertension, blood pressure is such an indicator. In Parkinson's disease, tremor, rigor, and akinesia are indicators of change. Similarly, changes in cerebral blood flow or in the electroencephalogram can be used to study changes in the dementias. As we can learn from the recent history of antihypertensive treatment, the availability of an objective, commonly accepted and readily identifiable indicator for drug action provides a powerful tool in the promotion of drug research in a defined disease area.

The Use of Indicators of Drug Action

The following examples illustrate how, as part of controlled clinical trials, physiologic and psychological measures can be used to further elucidate the biologic basis of drug action. The drug of reference is co-dergocrine mesylate, (Loew and Weil 1982; McDonald 1982), an ergot derivative which has been shown, in animals, to affect monoaminergic synaptic function and to induce behavioral stimulation (Copeland et al. 1981; Loew et al. 1979; Olpe and Steinmann 1982; Poschel and Ninteman 1981).

In a recent study, Samorajski et al. 1982 have chosen *serum prolactin assessment* as an indicator of dopaminergic function in senile dementia. These authors report that in the demented patients, serum prolactin levels were higher than in age-matched controls. In addition, the patient group treated with co-dergocrine mesylate showed a decline in prolactin levels after a daily dose of 6 mg over 6 and 12 weeks. A significant correlation was found, at week 12, between an improvement in clinical ratings and reduction in plasma prolactin levels, in particular for the factor "apathy," the overall impression, and the average of all items of the SCAG. These results demonstrate how plasma prolactin levels can be used to indicate drug effects on altered dopaminergic function in dementia.

The second example is taken from a pilot study where the effects of co-dergocrine mesylate on neuronal functioning were directly assessed by an evaluation of an *event-related brain potential*, the rebound function of contigent negative variation (CNV) (Tecce et al. 1981, 1983) CNV rebound occurs when a short-term memory task is omitted during the interstimulus interval of a warned reaction time task. In patients with mild to moderate degrees of dementia, CNV rebound is attenuated. Under treatment with co-dergocrine mesylate (6 mg/day over 10 – 11 weeks) this attenuation was reduced. At the same time, response speed was increased in the simple reaction time and the continuous performance tests. Previously, Matejcek and co-workers (Matejcek 1980; Matejcek et al. 1979) had shown correlations of quantified EEG and drug-induced behavioral changes. In contrast to the resting EEG, the importance of event-related potentials lies in their use as physiologic indicators of drug actions on impaired information processing and decision making.

The third example illustrates how *psychometric performance tests* can serve to reveal drug-induced changes in performance, relevant for behavioral effects. Oswald et al. 1982 used the Nuremberg Gerontopsychological Inventory to compare co-dergocrine mesylate (6 mg/day) with a daily dose of 2.4 g piracetam, over a 6-week treatment period, and found that improvements in the "speed" component of the psychometric assessment correlated with reduced need of care and improved subjective well-being, as rated by a nurse's rating scale and a self-evaluation. This procedure illustrates how drug-induced changes in psychometric performance can be validated by relating them to changes in activities of daily living and subjective improvement.

Conclusions and Outlook

Let me return to the remarks of Dr. Leber 1983 quoted in the introduction to this presentation. The present state of geriatric psychopharmacology is characterized by the availability of a number of drugs which provide symptomatic amelioration. Controlled studies show a significant superiority of these drugs over placebo; however, the data available do not allow us to predict which subset of patients will respond to a particular agent. It is likely that this is due to the limited knowledge regarding the selection of suitable patients both for drug trials and for treatment. In addition, from the variety of methods of outcome assessment, no particular tool has yet emerged to study a particular type of agent.

What, then, are the most urgent needs for research in geriatric psychopharmacology? An immediate necessity is to focus on improving the selection of patients for treatment by accurate diagnostic assessment and suitable outcome measures, in order to enhance the usefulness of the presently available psychotropic and psychogeriatric agents. Beyond this immediate action, basic and clinical research needs to be encouraged, to exploit fully our increase in basic knowledge on the dementing conditions.

At this very point in time we are witnessing an increasing public awareness that psychogeriatric disorders, and in particular the dementias, are accessible to and deserve medical treatment. Although the causes of the dementias are still largely unknown, a number of hypotheses have emerged which provide new bases for drug development. Early results from British laboratories indicated deficiences in brain acetylcholine synthesis. More recently, Scandinavian scientists have shown alterations of the brain metabolism of other neurotransmitters such as dopamine, noradrenaline, and serotonin, and alterations in neuropeptides have been described.

At the same time, public funding for basic and clinical research in the dementias is rising, e.g., in the United States from less than $ 4 million in 1976 to over $ 37 million in 1984. A variety of new experimental drugs are being investigated, both in laboratories and in clinical research units. These drugs are designed to compensate for deficiencies in brain metabolism, in particular for neurotransmitter deficiencies alleged to be involved in the dementias.

It appears to me that geriatric psychopharmacology has only just passed the stage of "ignorance and prejudice" which was so charaacteristic of the field of hypertension in the early 1940s (Page 1981). It is my hope that in the near future, our field will develop as fast as the pharmacotherapy of hypertension has progressed during the last 30 years. Most of the basic medicinal chemistry and technical development will have to come from the pharmaceutical industry. In addition, clinical investigators experienced in diagnostic evaluation and therapeutic assessment will have to devote considerable effort to the development and testing of suitable assessment techniques, giving due account to the biological basis of senile mental deterioration.

References

Copeland RL, Bhattacharyya AK, Aulakh CS, Pradhan SN (1981) Behavioral and neurochemical effects of Hydergine in rats. Arch Int Pharmacodyn 252:113–123

Coper H, Kanowski S (1983) Nootropika: Grundlagen und Therapie L. In: Langer G, Heimann H (eds) Psychopharmaka: Grundlagen und Therapie. Springer, Vienna, pp 409–433

Crook T, Ferris S, Bartus R (1983) Assessment in geriatric psychpharmocology. Mark Powley Associates, New Canaan, Conn.

Folstein MF, Folstein SE, McHugh PR (1975) "Mini-mental state"; a practical method for grading the cognitive state of patients for the clinician. J Psychiatr Res 12:189–198

Herrman WM, Schuster J, Stille G (1981) Gedanken zur Phase-III-Prüfung zum Nachweis der therapeutischen Wirksamkeit von Gerontopharmaka. In: Oswald WD, Fleischmann UW (eds) Experimentelle Gerontopsychologie. Beltz, Weinheim Basel, pp 23–35

Hoffmeister F, Stille G (eds) (1983) Psychotropic agents. Part II: Anxiolytics, gerontopsychopharmacological agents, and psychomotor stimulants. Springer, Berlin Heidelberg New York (Handbook of experimental pharmacology, vol 55/II)

Honigfeld G (1983) Psychopathology rating scales for use by nursing personnel. In: Crook T, Ferris S, Bartus R (eds) Assessment in geriatric psychopharmacology. Mark Powley Associates, New Canaan, Conn., pp 81–96

Hyams DE (1980) Cerebral activating drugs. In: Denham MJ (ed) The treatment of medical problems in the elderly. University Park Press, Baltimore, pp 295–331

Israel L, Kozarevic D, Sartorius N (1984) Source book of geriatric assessment. Karger, Basel

Kochansky GE (1979) Psychiatric rating scales for assessing psychopathology in the elderly: a critical review. In: Raskin A, Jarvik LF (eds) Psychiatric symptoms and cognitive loss in the elderly. Evaluation and assessment techniques. Wiley, New York, pp 125–156

Leber P (1983) Establishing the efficacy of drugs with psychogeriatric indications. In: Crook T, Ferris S, Bartus R (eds) Assessment in geriatric psychopharmacology. Mark Powley Associates, New Canaan, Conn., pp 1–12

Loew DM, Weil C (1982) Hydergine in senile mental impairment. Gerontology 28:54–74

Loew DM, Vigouret JM, Jaton AL (1979) Ergot derivatives and the central nervous system: effects of co-dergocrine mesylate (Hydergine) on cerebral synaptic transmission. In: Nandy K (ed) Geriatric psychopharmacology. Elsevier/North Holland, Amsterdam, pp 173–193 (Developments in Neurology, vol 3)

Matejcek M (1980) Clinical correlates of vigilance regulation and their use in evaluating the effects of treatment. In: Goldstein M, Calne DB, Lieberman A, Thorner MO (eds) Ergot compounds and brain function. Neuroendocrine and neuropsychiatric aspects. Raven, New York, pp 339–348

Matejcek M, Knor K, Piquet PV, Weil C (1979) Electroencephalographic and clinical changes as correlated in geriatric patients treated three months with an ergot alkaloid preparation. J Am Geriatr Soc 27:198–202

McDonald RJ (1982) Drug treatment of senile dementia. In: Wheatley D (ed) Psychopharmacology of old age. Oxford University Press, London, pp 113–138

McNair DM (1979) Self-rating scales for assessing psychopathology in the elderly. In: Raskin A, Jarvik LF (eds) Psychiatric symptoms and cognitive loss in the elderly. Evaluation and assessment techniques. Wiley, New York, pp 157–168

Olpe H-R, Steinmann MW (1982) The effect of vincamine, Hydergine and piracetam on the firing rate of locus coeruleus neurons. J Neural Transm 55:101–109

Oswald WD, Fleischmann UM (1980) The Nuremberg Gerontopsychological Inventory. Test instructions, test material, standard scores. Version 08/81. Nuremberg, August 1981

Oswald WD, Fleischmann UM (1983) The Nuremberg Gerontopsychological Inventory as a psychometric assessment in aging brain. In: Agnoli A, Crepaldi G, Spano PF, Trabucchi M (eds) Aging brain and ergot alkaloids. Aging vol 23. Raven, New York, pp 121–129

Oswald WD, Matejcek M, Lukaschek K, Dennler HJ, Oswald B (1982) Über die Relevanz psychometrisch operationalisierter Therapie-Effekte bei der Behandlung altersbedingter Insuffizienzerscheinungen des Gehirns am Beispiel des Nürnberger-Alters-Inventars NAI. Arzneimittelforsch 32 I:584–590

Page IH (1981) Antihypertensive drugs: our debt to industrial chemists. N Engl J Med 304:615–618

Poschel BPH, Ninteman FW (1981) Excitatory effects of Hydergine on intracranial self-stimulation. Drug Dev Res 1:163–166

Raskin A, Jarvik LF (1979) Psychiatric symptoms and cognitive loss in the elderly. Evaluation and assessment techniques. Wiley, New York

Reisberg B, Ferris SH, Gershon S (1981a) An overview of pharmacologic treatment of cognitive decline in the aged. Am J Psychiatry 138:593–600

Reisberg B, Ferris SH, Schneck MK, deLeon M, Crook T, Gershon S (1981b) Relationships between psychiatric assessments and cognitive test measures in mild to moderate senile dementia of the Alzheimer's type. Psychopharmacol Bull 17:99–101

Samorajski T, Ho BT, Kralik PM, Hartford JT (1982) Serum prolactin changes with age, senile dementia, and dihydroergotoxine mesylate treatment. In Giacobini E, Filogamo G, Giacobini G, Vernadakis A (eds) Cellular and molecular mechanisms of aging in the nervous system. Aging, vol 20. Raven, New York, pp 259–269

Schwartz GE (1983) Development and validation of the Geriatric Evaluation by Relatives Rating Instrument. Psychol Rep 53:479–488

Shader RI, Harmatz JS, Salzman C (1974) A new scale for clinical assessment in geriatric populations: Sandoz Clinical Assessment – Geriatric (SCAG). J Am Geriatr Soc 12:107–113

Spagnoli A, Tognoni G (1983) Cerebroactive drugs. Clinical pharmacology and therapeutic role in cerebrovascular disorders. Drugs 26:44–69

Spitzer RL, Williams JBW, Skodol AE (1980) DSM-III: The major achievements and an overview. Am J Psychiatry 137:151–164

Tecce JJ, Boehner MB, Cattanach L, Branconnier R, Cole JO (1981) Hydergine treatment and brain functioning (CNV rebound) in Alzheimer's patients: preliminary findings. Psychopharmacol Bull 17:202–206

Tecce JJ, Cattanach L, Boehner-Davis MB, Branconnier RJ, Cole JO (1983) Etude neuropsychologique de la baisse de l'attention et traitement médicamenteux chez les malades atteints de maladie d'Alzheimer. Presse Méd 12:3155–3162

Venn RD (1983) The Sandoz Clinical Assessment-Geriatric (SCAG) Scale. A general-purpose psychogeriatric rating scale. Gerontology 29:185–198

Wittenborn JR (1981) Pharmacotherapy for age-related behavioral deficiencies. J Nerv Ment Dis 169:139–156

4.8 Dementia in Later Life: Research and Action

D. M. Macfadyen, J. Henderson

Introduction

Dementia is the acquired global impairment of higher cortical function including memory, the capacity to solve the problems of day-to-day living, the performance of learned perceptuo-motor skills, the correct use of social skills, all aspects of language and communication and control of emotional reactions, in the absence of gross clouding of consciousness. The condition is often progressive though not necessarily irreversible (College Committee on Geriatrics 1981).

The Dementias of Old Age

The most common causes of failure of brain function in elderly people are senile dementia of Alzheimer type (SDAT) and multi-infarct dementia (MID), disorders which currently are classified in the International Classification of Diseases, Ninth Revision (ICD 9) within code 290. The histological features characterizing the former include neurofibrillary tangles, plaques and loss of neurons in the cortex, in the basal nucleus of Meynert and in the basal forebrain. The two last-mentioned cell losses result in diminished cholinergic activity, particularly in regard to reduction in levels of choline acetyltransfererase and acetylcholine. The causes of these histopathological and neurochemical changes have not yet been elucidated.

Public Health Consequences of Dementia

The importance of dementia as a public health problem is no longer in dispute. It is a principal cause of disability and dependence in old age. Epidemiological studies consistently show a high prevalence of this group of disorders: some 5% – 8% of persons aged 65 and above are estimated to manifest dementia of severe degree. [The generic term dementia includes dementia attributed to neuropathological Alzheimer change (SDAT), cerebral infarction (MID), dementia secondary to known disease plus others of unknown origin.]

Despite the recent huge increase in the number of mentally infirm old people admitted to long-term stay facilities, there is ample evidence that institutionalized old people represent only the tip of the iceberg. Epidemiological studies indicate, at least in Europe, that only one-fifth of elders with severe forms of mental disorder are placed in institutional care.

The yearly cost of caring for 2 million sufferers in the United States of America is estimated at 26 billion (10^9) dollars. Research expenditure on the condition amounts to US$ 22 millions.

In most countries, the upsurge of public concern on dementia is not reflected by a reordering of priorities, either in medical service provision or in scientific research. This delay in responding to a problem of increasing urgency has implications for the rate of progress in scientific knowledge. A claim to high priority in terms of public effort, financial investment and scientific endeavour can be justified with respect to the five outstanding tasks specified below. An international strategy is required to correlate the different areas of research, to finance the more promising endeavours and to work co-operatively towards reducing the risk of senile dementia as populations age, especially in developing countries (WHO 1984). The present report presents such a strategy.

Elements of Proposed Research Programme

Problems of Diagnosis and Classification

In view of the need for rigorous assessment of present and future drug treatment, an immediate task is to develop screening procedures and instruments for early diagnosis together with an agreed staging of the dementia process. Also required are measures that differentiate SDAT from other types of dementia, and that differentiate between dementia and the pseudodementia associated with treatable mental disorders.

An urgent recommendation to WHO is to convene a group that would develop agreed "core" clinical criteria and nomenclature for the diagnosis of dementia in older persons and to incorporate operational criteria for grading severity. Such a group would be charged with developing an internationally reliable and valid mental state examination instrument together with a structured clinical interview – both being linked with the Tenth Revision of the International Classification of Diseases (ICD 10). The group would also help to field test instruments for differential diagnosis at the primary health care level.

A promising area for research in administering and developing instruments is the use of portable microcomputers.

Introduction of non-invasive methods for investigating the brain, such as computerized axial tomography, positron emission tomography and nuclear magnetic resonance, may help in the development of more precise clinical differentiation, although such studies must be limited to centres with sophisticated technology.

Epidemiological Research

Clinical epidemiological studies of the natural evolution of the dementias in different cultures should be supported by WHO in advance of developments in pharmacological intervention. One way of doing this inexpensively would be to develop methods of analysing diaries kept by family members of SDAT victims.

For aetiological purposes estimates of incidence are considerably more valuable than prevalence. Such studies of incidence require longitudinal investigations and long-term funding of teams of investigators.

It would be prudent for WHO to support the few teams of investigators involved in longitudinal studies to help them co-ordinate their methodology and to achieve standard screening and case-finding instruments that would be applicable in different settings. This could be done by establishing a task force to promote the development of prospective longitudinal studies in several centres. The World Health Organization could also help this development by promoting the exchange of younger epidemiological researchers between different centres as the studies get under way.

Only two epidemiological risk factors of SDAT are known namely, family history and advancing age. The method of the case-control study offers promise of providing immediate clues as to aetiology and what is needed are hypotheses of possible risk factors, for example the hypothesis that cases do not differ from controls in terms of their nutrient intake.

Aetiology, with Particular Reference to Neurobiology[1]

In the field of neurobiological research, it is increasingly emerging that the commonest form of dementia, senile dementia of Alzheimer type, is a disease which differs from the normal process of aging within the central nervous system. Research in neurobiology is exciting great interest because of the prospect raised of yielding strategies for preventing or (as in the case of Parkinsonism) stemming the disease manifestation. However, an etiology has to be elucidated and the progress of knowledge in this domain has accelerated by the investigation of neuropathology and neurochemistry of the brain post mortem, and the correlation of these findings with clinical investigations undertaken during life.

Neuropathology and Neurochemistry

The quest for the cause of SDAT, using the most advanced biological technology, is being pursued in laboratories in several countries. While much is known about the anatomical changes in the brain of Alzheimer victims, much more is yet to be found: the chemical nature of the classical lesions is not yet completely known and our understanding of the paired helical filaments, which are the main component of the characteristic tangle, is still elusive. As stated earlier, there is a widespread loss of cholinergic activity. Evidence has also emerged on the loss of nuclei in the locus ceruleus and related reductions in noradrenergic activity. Which of these structural and chemical changes is primary is unknown, but combined chemical and immunocytochemical research may help to answer this question.

Immunology

Further work in immunology is unquestionably warranted. Immunological changes seem to be mainly non-specific. They involve an anti-brain antibody, as well as some evaluation of serum immunoglobulins. Recent work has shown elevation of an antibody against pituitary prolactin cells.

Transmissable Agents

Further investigation of possible infectious agents is necessary. The unconventional virus which causes scrapie can induce some morphological changes in mice very similar to those of Alzheimer disease. To date, transmission of SDAT to animals has not been accomplished.

---

1 Discussion of dementia in this paragraph is restricted to SDAT, the *terra incognita* of the complex of dementia disorders.

Neurophysiology
Much basic work has to be done on the mechanisms by which the brain regulates its various functions, for example on the neurotransmitter input to and from the basal forebrain.
Genetics
The existence of families at high risk for senile dementia of the Alzheimer type, possibly due to autosomal dominant expression, is a phenomenon that lends itself to international study.
Molecular Biology
Techniques of molecular biology and genetic engineering would be useful in helping to understand the cause of SDAT. A practical way to accelerate research in this field might be for nuclear material from demented and non-demented neurons to be made available to molecular biologists for investigation. For example, it may be that changes occur with progressive age in the choline acetyltransferase (ChAT) gene that may decrease its expression and result in the lowering of the enzyme activity, a hypothesis that may be explored by isolating and cloning the ChAT gene of normal and Alzheimer patients.
Environmental Toxins
Further research should be carried out on the possibility that SDAT may be caused by environmental agents. The role of metallic agents such as aluminium evokes much interest in view of the experimental models, iatrogenic intoxications and the disputed elevation of aluminium concentrations in SDAT.
Membrane Studies
Neurochemical studies in Alzheimer brain and controls to investigate membrane properties and enzymes is likely to lead to new knowledge which may be therapeutically relevant.
Psychoneuroendocrinology
Recent WHO-supported studies on psychoneuroendocrinology, aging and behaviour indicate that the baseline activity of the growth hormone secreting system seems to be enhanced, a finding which may be relevant to developing tools for the early detection of the disease. The search for peripheral markers of SDAT needs to be urgently extended to other disciplines such as immunology and genetics (for chromosomal studies of non-mitotic cells), since these are a prime requirement for clinicians.
International Collaboration
Some of the research tasks described above are highly specialized and would not necessarily be accelerated by international collaboration, but rather call for more attention from national funding sources. There is, however, an urgent need for cross-fertilization between neurobiology and other disciplines, for example cell biology. Areas that can be singled out for international collaborative effort are cross-national neuropathological studies and the search for animal models.

Treatment and Prevention

Improving Clinical Drug Evaluation
There are many agents which claim to improve mental function. However, there are no therapeutic agents which stem the mental decline or the dementing process.

(In so far as cerebrovascular pathology bears a strong relationship to multi-infarct dementia, all measures which tend to mediate the prevention of cerebrovascular disease might lead to a parallel reduction in the frequency of MID.) One of the impediments to developing safe and efficacious treatment of dementia is the lack of methods and instruments of evaluation that are generally approved and accepted by the scientific community.

Drugs purporting to affect brain function are numerous and include GABA and its derivatives, ergot alkaloids, neuropeptides, neurotransmitter precursors, drugs which claim to protect the brain against hypoxia, substances lowering blood viscosity and substances alleged to stimulate metabolism of the brain.

It is proposed that WHO takes steps to improve the design of clinical drug evaluation studies and to promote more rational prescription of drugs for this widespread condition. This would involve defining the objectives of therapy; identifying valid and reliable methods of assessing drug-induced changes; making recommendations concerning the criteria for acceptance of nootropic drugs for marketing; and better training in the use of psychogeriatric drugs, especially in the developing world.

Other Therapeutic Interventions

Disappointments on the efficacy of pharmacological intervention extend also to other interventions, such as memory training. However, the efficacy of concomitant interventions by both drugs and behavioural measures may be synergistic and there is a need for rigorously conducted studies of such combined treatment. Intervention studies to improve short memory are urgently needed.

Symptomatic Treatment

Dementia is distressing both for the patient and the relatives and special emphasis needs to be given to improving the management of a condition in which there is progressive deterioration in behaviour in the affected individual. For instance, there has been no attention to systematic behavioural interventions for the treatment of anxiety, for limiting repetitive compulsive behaviours or for managing the manifestations of paranoia. Only a few behavioural techniques are described in the literature for such diverse situations as shaping appropriate eating behaviour, or quelling chronic screaming, controlling incontinence or preventing wandering. Moreover most studies have been carried out in institutionalized settings and few have been directed to supporting and maintaining the individual's autonomy within a community setting. No attention is given to the impact of the environment itself in maintaining positive behaviour on the part of the demented patient by providing an appropriate structure and environmental stimuli.

Prevention for the Carers

Finally, more attention needs to be given to the stress-response syndromes which are increasingly being documented in relatives charged with caring over a very prolonged period of time for severely demented patients. This constitutes an area of research of prime importance and needs the greatest encouragement.

Health and Social Services

Reorientation to Prevention

A large body of evidence has accumulated which indicates that current standards of quality of treatment and care of the mentally impaired elderly, both in long-stay hospital wards and in non-clinical residential accommodation, are all too often inadequate and at times scandalously poor. Moreover, admission to these institutions is regarded in the overwhelming majority of cases as a final disposal with no possibility of further active therapy or rehabilitation.

However, countries are increasingly adapting their mental health care systems to give them a preventive orientation, with the following goals:

1. Preserving good physical and mental health of those who are well
2. Keeping the mildly ill from becoming more severely ill
3. Preventing the severely ill from developing secondary handicaps

To support such preventive-oriented services, studies are imperative of the specific problems of families caring for elderly demented persons at home, and of the forms of help and support that could be expected to afford them greatest relief and assistance. In this connexion the promotion, development and study of self-help groups of relatives, such as the Alzheimer Disease and Related Disorders Societies of several countries, are of increasing significance in a situation in which demands for residential facilities are becoming insupportable. A further area of health services research, directed at improving care, is the development of criteria for monitoring the quality of care and life satisfaction in institutions.

Improving Training

The unsatisfactory standard of diagnosis, treatment and care of the elderly mentally infirm is a reflection on the neglect of geriatric and psychogeriatric training in medical education. It is therefore recommended that the considerable body of knowledge on practical treatment of the mental disorders in the elderly in a variety of settings be critically examined by WHO and be made available as widely as possible in a form that is understandable to primary health care providers. In this respect it is disappointing to note that no effort has been made to enlist family observers to share with health professionals the day-to-day experience of coping with dementing illness.

Social Networks

Sociological investigations are required to determine the character of social links and networks that enable most old people with dementia to remain in their local community, in close proximity to relatives and friends. Such enquiries should include attempts to identify and determine factors that erode indigenous forms of familial and community support that have evolved and survived over past generations. In this context it is important to distinguish the factors that arise as a consequence of fundamental sociocultural changes (for example, aging carers or the increasing proportion of small families) and those linked more directly with modifiable aspects of the social structure (for example, inadequate housing).

Research Issues for Planning

One research issue arising from the different experience of countries in caring for the mentally infirm elderly is the need to prepare, on an international basis, a list of facilities in which dementia patients are cared for and a description of their staffing levels and problems, difficulties and successes. Another issue is whether elderly persons with dementia should be integrated with other psychiatrically ill people or elderly people requiring all sorts of support care. This is an area where there has been little evaluative research to guide decision makers. A further area in which policy makers and planners require guidance is in regard to the economics of health care delivery for those suffering from senile dementia. The paucity of health economic research is incongruous with the size of the health expenditure on the condition of dementia.

Integrated Collaborative Research Programme

The group concluded that WHO should establish an international collaborative research programme in the following five areas:

1. Clinical diagnosis and classification
2. Epidemiology
3. Aetiology, with particular reference to neurobiology
4. Treatment and prevention
5. Health services

WHO initiatives should be concentrated on two overall objectives namely: to promote the training of young scientists and to support the dissemination of information in the above five areas. The basic elements of the integrated collaborative research programme would be, first to convene a group that would be responsible for (a) the development of common nomenclature and (b) the development of criteria for diagnosis and for staging of the disease. This would be undertaken in collaboration with WHO's preparation for the Tenth Revision of the International Classification of Diseases. A second element would be to establish a task force of investigators who are currently engaged or about to embark upon epidemiological studies of senile dementia so that their methodology may be co-ordinated and their experience on instruments of assessment exchanged.

One or more centres should be designated by WHO for the collection and dissemination of information in regard to the five areas of dementia referred to above. A further function of the international collaborative programme would be to encourage existing brain banks to provide material from well researched demented patients to laboratories where such material is not available, for instance to cell biology laboratories. WHO should also take initiatives to encourage the development of experimental models of dementia in laboratory animals.

If extrabudgetary funds become available, the Organization should consider providing support, after peer review appraisal, for cross-cultural epidemiological studies, for studies of support systems, for studies of cost-effectiveness, for international neuropathological investigations and for strengthening research in the nascent aging countries. The mechanisms by which this international research programme would be implemented would be mainly through an extension of the current WHO network of collaborating centres, which might be serviced by a "dementia task force" within the WHO Secretariat.

Summary

The Report of a WHO Scientific Group on Senile Dementia (WHO Technical Report Series No. 730) makes proposals for an international programme of collaborative research in the following interlinked fields:

- Clinical diagnosis and classification
- Epidemiology
- Aetiology, with particular reference to neurobiology
- Treatment and prevention
- Health service delivery

The report presents the scientific community with the challenge of an intractable problem that inflicts great suffering and currently attracts insufficient research interest.

A special targeted effort, supported by WHO, is deemed necessary in order to ensure long-term research commitments of a multidisciplinary nature.

References

The College Committee on Geriatries (1981) Organic mental impairment in the elderly: Implications for research, education and the provision of services. Coll Physicians Lond 15(3):141–167 (Adapted)

WHO (1984) Report of the scientific group on epidemiology of aging. (WHO Technical Report Series No 706)

WHO (1986) Report of the scientific group on senile dementia: Dementia in later life: research and action. (WHO Technical Report Series No. 730)

5 Assessment, Prevention, and Control of Mental Disorders in the Elderly: Biological, Psychological, and Environmental Influences: Prospects for Early Recognition and Intervention

5.1 Measurement of Psychopathology and Impairment in the Elderly

H. Bickel

Introduction

The large majority of mentally ill old people receive no psychiatric treatment, are not in institutional care, and have no contacts with the social welfare services. At the level of primary medical care, many psychogeriatric disorders are either not recognized or not treated systematically. This failure to recognize or to treat the condition may result in much unnecessary suffering for the patients and their families and has long-term prognostic consequences.

It is therefore important to consider what steps could be taken to promote the earlier diagnosis, treatment, and medical care of old age mental disorders. Secondary preventive action, aimed at earlier recognition, diagnosis, and treatment, appears to offer the greatest hope of progress in this field of care (Bergmann 1982). Essential conditions for such action are access to high risk groups among the elderly and the use of case-finding methods. Techniques for screening and assessment must be available, which can be applied in community settings.

First-Stage Screening and Detection Methods

Screening has been defined as:

> the presumptive identification of unrecognized disease or defect by the application of tests, examinations or other procedures which can be applied rapidly. Screening tests sort out apparently well persons who probably have a disease from those who probably do not. A screening test is not intended to be diagnostic. Persons with positive or suspicious findings must be referred to their physicians for diagnosis and necessary treatment (US Commission on Chronic Illness 1957).

In recent years, the possibility of psychiatric screening as a preventive measure has begun to attract attention (Eastwood 1971) and has been recommended for high-risk groups, such as the elderly, above all for frequently occurring disorders with typical symptom patterns (Goldberg 1974). Short psychiatric scales have found application mainly in two-stage methods of case identification (Duncan-Jones and Henderson 1978), or as an economic alternative to detailed interview procedures for assessing psychiatric morbidity in various populations (Goldberg 1981). There are also many reports on the use of such scales in clinical investigations. Hardly anything, however, is known about the value of these methods in primary health care, in relation to case finding, early intervention, or the consequent benefits to the affected persons (Cooper and Bickel 1984). At this stage, conclusions can be drawn only as to the types of method which would lend themselves to use in this context.

Since there are as yet no reliable biological markers for most forms of mental disorder, the choice of available instruments is in practice limited to self-reports or complaint inventories, ratings of symptoms and abnormal behavior observed by an interviewer or reported by key informants, and simple psychological tests, especially of cognitive functioning.

Standardized procedures of this kind are used in the clinical setting to give a more accurate description of psychopathology for differential diagnosis and for assessment of changes associated with treatment. Since they are here applied in cases of already identified illness, their value for early recognition does not come in question. The conditions necessary for case finding in the community serve to limit the number of potentially useful methods.

In screening for global cognitive impairments, which may indicate possible dementing processes, the use of complex psychometric tests or test batteries is inappropriate. They are too time consuming, call for special skills and training, and cannot be conducted with many old people because of poor comprehension, motor or sensory impairments, or low motivation (Kuriansky et al. 1976; Kahn and Miller 1978).

In this context, short, standardized clinical tests with fixed cut-off scores have proved useful. The various tests do not differ greatly from one another in their essential content. Nearly all include questions on orientation for time, place, and person, together with simple tests of memory and general knowledge. The shortest have only ten items and can be administered orally. Among the best known such procedures are the Mental Status Questionnaire (Kahn et al. 1960) and the Short Portable Mental Status Questionnaire (Pfeiffer 1975). The somewhat longer procedures with up to 30 items also test, in varying measure, comprehension of speech, verbal abstraction, and simple arithmetical or psychomotor performance (Folstein et al. 1975; Jacobs et al. 1977; Pattie and Gilleard 1979). The superiority of these longer procedures over the shortest ones has not yet been convincingly demonstrated.

Tests of this kind are simple, require no intensive training, and appear to be acceptable to most old people (Qureshi and Hodkinson 1974; DePaulo et al. 1980), more especially since many of the questions can be incorporated into a short history taking (Comfort 1978). The interrater reliability is ensured by a high degree of structuring (Kahn et al. 1960; Jacobs et al. 1977). Test – retest reliability over a period of up to 1 month has been shown for several of the tests to be in a satisfactory range of over 0.8 (Folstein et al. 1975; Pfeiffer 1975; Pattie and Gilleard 1979).

Investigations of the validity of the tests have shown a good agreement between a high test score and the diagnosis of an organic psychosyndrome (Wilson and Brass 1973; Pfeiffer 1975; Pattie and Gilleard 1975, 1976; Haglund and Schuckitt 1976; Smyer et al. 1979; Cresswell and Lanyon 1981), so that one may say that the validity of these scales has in general been confirmed for inpatient populations. So far, however, there has been a dearth of cross-validation studies on unselected samples of the elderly population.

In view of the cognitive impairments of dementing old people, the use of self-assessments as an indicator must be judged unreliable (Kahn et al. 1975). Complaints of forgetfulness and loss of concentration appear to be associated more closely with affective than with cognitive disorders. For this reason, cognitive and behavioral performance can be assessed more reliable by dementia rating scales, based on the judgment of an interviewer (Lawson et al. 1977; Reisberg et al. 1982; Hughes et al. 1982). According to Kay (1977), the dementia rating scale developed by the Newcastle group correlated more closely with pathological changes in the cortex than did scores on a cognitive scale. The usefulness of judgmental scales for screening purposes is, however, limited by their dependence on the clinical competence of the rater. Reports by key informants are also of restricted value in community surveys, because of the relatively high proportion of old people for whom no reliable informant is available.

While no information is available about the usefulness of behavior rating scales (Hall 1980; Smith 1979; Honigfeld 1981) in case finding, the fact that these have been developed largely for the assessment of severely disturbed, uncooperative, or uncommunicative hospital patients, and that they are based on the assumption of continuous observation in a closed environment, makes it seem improbable that they will find any large-scale application for purposes of early recognition and diagnosis. Somewhat similar objections apply to the use of clinical procedures for assessment of the frequency, duration, or severity of depressive symptoms (Mayer 1977; Blöschl 1981), since these are also intended for use primarily in the detailed assessment of already diagnosed illnesses. Little information is available about their applicability to old people (McDonald 1980). Intergeneration comparisons have shown age-related differences in symptom profiles, with in particular an increase of somatic symptom scores among the elderly (Zemore and Eames 1979). There are as yet, however, no scales of this kind which have been developed especially for elderly patients (Kochansky 1979; McNair 1979; Cresswell and Lanyon 1981).

Some findings have been reported on the use of short forms of psychogeriatric interviews. Thus, a highly structured short version of the Geriatric Mental Status Schedule has been tested on old people (Bond et al. 1980). The agreement with psychiatric diagnostic classification was found to be high for organic mental disorders, rather lower for affective disorders and neurosis, and very low for schizophrenic and paranoid disorders.

A short form of the Comprehensive Assessment and Referral Evaluation (CARE), so-called CORE-CARE, containing about one-fifth of the items, has also been developed for use in community studies. In addition, there is a so-called SHORT-CARE, focused on the assessment of depression, dementia, and disability. The findings of a cross-national study in New York and London have provided extensive information about the use of a dementia and a depression scale (Gurland et al. 1983).

Instruments of this kind afford a possibility of screening for cognitive and affective disorders in tandem, which seems indicated in view of the considerable overlapping between the symptom profiles of dementing and depressive illnesses (DePaulo et al. 1980).

Nearly all the scales mentioned are highly structured and in so far suitable for computer-based automation (Editorial 1983). To what extent automated methods will be useful for psychogeriatric screening purposes remains an open question. One may, however, assume that microcomputers will find extensive application quite soon in many medical fields (Carr and Ancill 1983). If they come to be used in the primary medical care sector for collecting and storing data on patients, they could also have a place in psychiatric case finding. Initial clinical studies with questionnaire procedures and tests have given some encouraging results (Margo et al. 1983; Ogden et al. 1984). There may also be other possible applications: for example, since Bech (1981) has submitted a depression inventory to Rasch scaling and, furthermore, homogeneous scales can also be extracted from the CARE interview schedule (Gurland et al. 1983) it is conceivable that with the further progress of computerized testing so-called tailored testing will become possible in the foreseeable future; that is to say, that sequential test procedures will be feasible, even at item level (Watts et al. 1982).

Second-Stage Case Identification and Diagnostic Procedures

If screening procedures of this kind do prove useful in psychogeriatric case finding, the question then arises as to what second-stage diagnostic assessment should be undertaken in order to reach decisions concerning treatment and management. Because of the potentially large numbers involved and the understandable reluctance of many old people to undergo special investigation, diagnostic clarification must in most instances be undertaken in a community setting. For this task, the physicians or other health professionals must have techniques available which enable them to carry out systematic examination of suspected cases and to describe and classify any existing psychiatric disorders. Considerable progress in this direction has been achieved with the development of semistructured psychiatric interviews (Wing et al. 1967; Goldberg et al. 1970; Spitzer et al. 1964) and the introduction of more precise diagnostic criteria and more refined diagnostic classifications (Feighner et al. 1972; Spitzer et al. 1978), and possibly also by the trends toward computerized diagnosis (Wing et al. 1974; Spitzer and Endicott 1968). In the meantime, there are already a number of standardized psychogeriatric interviews which are based on clinical diagnostic concepts but make also use of scores derived from rating scales or test methods.

The Geriatric Mental Status Schedule (Copeland et al. 1976), for example, grew out of the Combined Mental Status Schedule, a procedure for younger age groups, which in turn developed from English and American diagnostic procedures (Wing et al. 1967; Spitzer et al. 1964) in the setting of the US/UK Diagnostic Project, supplemented by items more or less specific to psychogeriatric diagnosis. The Comprehensive Assessment and Referral Evaluation (CARE) (Gurland et al. 1977) is a comprehensive, semistructured interview for assessing the health and social problems of old people in the community. The psychiatric section contains the most important and best discriminating items for the description of more than 20 psychopathological dimensions, as well as additional items which are intended to detect "minor forms of psychopathology" that occur frequently in the elderly population, and others which are thought to be useful in discriminating between Alzheimer-type and multi-infarct dementia.

By integrating self-ratings, interviewer ratings, test items, and reports from informants, these interviews seek to achieve an exhaustive coverage of the main psychopathological phenomena. Investigations in New York, London, and Canberra have confirmed the satisfactory level of reliability achieved by these methods (Copeland et al. 1976; Gurland et al. 1983; Henderson et al. 1983).

A basic problem arises, however, with respect to the validity of the reported symptoms and their relation to the diagnostic categories. It is often difficult, if not impossible, to decide if a particular symptom has psychopathological significance or if it should not be attributed to some other cause, such as a physical illness. Moreover, the clinical significance of many complaints such as sleep disorder, loss of drive, or loss of concentration, which are common among the elderly, is often unclear, because boundaries between morbidity and normal aging cannot be firmly defined.

The lack of detailed diagnostic criteria is especially significant in early case detection, since without a clear case definition there can be no reliable case identification. The classification systems in general use are strongly oriented toward the needs of clinical psychiatry. In the community, however, mild or borderline forms of mental disturbance are commonly found, for which the available diagnostic criteria are too vague to be made operational in standardized instruments. It is precisely these mild and borderline disorders, such as the so-called mild dementia (Henderson and Huppert 1984), which are especially important for secondary prevention and which in consequence are now attracting increasing attention.

These deficiencies have unfortunately led in the case of the CARE interview to the introduction of idiosyncratic criteria for dementia and depression (Gurland et al. 1980, 1983). It is to be hoped that closer agreement on the diagnostic criteria for psychogeriatric illnesses will soon be achieved. If not, there is a danger that much of the work invested in research will be wasted because of inadequate comparability of the findings from different studies.

Consistency in diagnostic criteria represents, however, only one of the necessary conditions for a successful approach to secondary prevention. For, as Copeland (1981) has emphasized, the concept of a psychiatric "case" is in the last analysis itself a chimera. There are as many case definitions as there are research or preventive aims, and it is only in the light of these aims that the suitability of the case definition can be judged. Applied to questions of early detection and prevention, this principle means that the value of psychiatric diagnosis and classification at community level must be seen in relation to the implications for treatment or more generally for health care. Along these lines it might be possible to develop a catalogue of indications which would give guidance to health [illegible]ling treatment and referral decisions in the individual case. [illegible] and interview procedures represent important [illegible]ent to consider the practical framework in which [illegible]se.

Assessment of Associated Impairments and Disabilities

A preventive approach at community level cannot be confined to psychiatric treatment, independently from other forms of intervention. For this reason, a multidimensional concept is indicated in assessment as well as in care programs (Plutchik 1979; Gallagher et al. 1980). This point is already evident in the introduction of the multiaxial classification system DSM-III, though this system cannot yet be applied in practice because of a lack of suitable operational criteria and, moreover, it seems doubtful if all the proposed axes are appropriate for use with the elderly.

The assessment of psychological symptoms alone provides only limited information with regard to prognosis, need for care, and possibilities for intervention. For the chronic progressive or recurring disorders, which often interfere with activities of daily living and may result in dependency on others, a clinical diagnostic model is insufficient: it must be extended to include the consequences of illness. Here the introduction of the International Classification of Impairments, Disabilities and Handicaps (WHO 1980) may make an important contribution to the development of new concepts. In this scheme, an impairment is defined as any loss or abnormality of psychological, physiological, or anatomical structure or function; a disability is any restriction or lack of ability (resulting from an impairment) to perform an activity in the normal manner; and an handicap is a disadvantage for an individual (resulting from an impairment or disability) which limits or prevents the fulfilment of a normal social role. It is along these three axes, according to the ICIDH system, that the concomitants and consequences of illnesses are to be described. Thus a comprehensive system of reference is created in which the clinical phenomena can be seen in a fuller perspective.

The methods of measurement so far available relate to the axes of impairment and disability (Jefferys et al. 1969; Garrad and Bennett 1971; Lawton 1972; Williams et al. 1976). They do not in fact make the classification system as a whole operational, but their content corresponds closely to some of the categories. In particular, there are many procedures for measuring locomotor disabilities and capacity for personal care, mostly under the rubric "Activities of Daily Living." Some of these have been developed in a clinical setting and depend upon judgments made by nursing staff (Plutchik et al. 1970; Gurel et al. 1972; Pattie and Gilleard 1979). In others, the affected person is questioned about his everyday activities (Lawton and Brody 1969) or is asked to carry out some activities in a performance test (Kuriansky and Gurland 1976). Measurements of this kind have also been incorporated into some psychiatric interview procedures (Gurland et al. 1977; Lawton et al. 1982). Finally, inventories such as the Sickness Impact Profile (University of Washington 1978) and the Vulnerable Elders Index (Branch 1980) have been used in population-based studies for the assessment of illness-associated dysfunctions and need for care.

The availability of these methods should not disguise the fact that disability is essentially a complex construct whose measurement gives rise to a whole series of unresolved methodological and practical problems (Bebbington 1977; Williams 1979; Dunt et al. 1980). Nevertheless, they fulfil some of the conditions necessary for testing the association of psychiatric diagnostic categories with impairment and disability. It can be anticipated that such research will provide clues to prognostic factors and to suitable methods of intervention, as well as making possible a realistic evaluation of preventive programs.

Conclusions

The extensive armory of psychiatric assessment methods contains a number of simple procedures which have yielded satisfactory results in case discrimination, at least in relation to the most frequent forms of old age mental disorder, namely cognitive impairments and depressive states. What value these have for early detection in everyday practical application, how and where they can be successfully introduced, and whether or not they will find public acceptance remains very largely unknown and a matter for speculation. A good deal of evaluative research will be required to test the usefulness of screening methods in real life conditions.

Since it may be said that systematic epidemiological research into psychogeriatric illness first becomes possible with the aid of standardized instruments, one may hope that relatively simple procedures will be developed which can make an essential contribution to early diagnosis. For this purpose it will be necessary to develop firm diagnostic criteria which make possible direct comparison of the research findings at international level. From a preventive standpoint, the validity of these criteria will in the long term depend upon their practical relevance for the selection and the efficacy of methods of treatment and intervention.

Finally, it must be questioned whether a preventive approach to the problem of psychiatric disorder in old age can hope to succeed in isolation from other aspects of health care. Rather there seems to be an urgent need for a coordinated approach to research and to health care, in which the onset, cause, and outcome of psychiatric disorders are seen in relation to physical health and social conditions and attention is focused on those factors which seem to offer the most promising targets for intervention and improvement. The techniques of multilevel assessment developed in recent years thus appear to provide the most suitable working tools for further progress in this field.

References

Bebbington AC (1977) Scaling indices of disablement. Br J Prev Soc Med 31:122–126

Bech P (1981) Rating scales for affective disorders: Their validity and consistency. Acta Psychiatr Scand [Suppl 295]

Bergmann K (1982) A community psychiatric approach to the care of the elderly. Are there opportunities for prevention? In: Magnussen G, Nielsen J, Buch J (eds) Epidemiology and prevention of mental illness in old age. EGV, Hellerup, Denmark

Blöschl L (1981) Psychodiagnostik depressiver Zustände. Z Diff Diagn Psychol 2:7–30

Bond J, Brooks P, Carstairs V, Giles L (1980) The reliability of a Survey Psychiatric Assessment Schedule for the Elderly. Br J Psychiatry 137:148–162

Branch LG (1980) Vulnerable elders. Gerontological Monographs No. 6, Gerontological Society, Washington
Carr AC, Ancill RJ (1983) Computers in psychiatry. Acta Psychiatr Scand 67:137–143
Comfort A (1978) Non-threatening mental testing of the elderly. J Am Geriatr Soc 26:261–262
Cooper B, Bickel H (1984) Population screening and the early detection of dementing disorders in old age: a review. Psychol Med 14:81–95
Copeland J (1981) What is a 'case'? A case for what? In: Wing JK, Bebbington P, Robins LN (eds) What is a case? Grant McIntyre, London, pp 9–11
Copeland JRM, Kelleher MJ, Kellett JM, Gourlay AJ, Gurland BJ, Fleiss JL, Sharpe L (1976) A semi-structured clinical interview for the assessment of diagnosis and mental state in the elderly: the Geriatric Mental State Schedule. I. Development and reliability. Psychol Med 6:439–449
Cresswell DL, Lanyon RJ (1981) Validation of a screening battery for psychogeriatric assessment. J Gerontol 36:435–440
De Paulo JR, Folstein MF, Gordon B (1980) Psychiatric screening on a neurological ward. Psychol Med 10:125–132
Duncan-Jones P, Henderson AS (1978) The use of a two-phase design in a population survey. Soc Psychiatry 13:231–237
Dunt DR, Kaufert JM, Corkhill R, Creese AL, Green S, Locker D (1980) A technique for precisely measuring activities of daily living. Community Med 2:120–125
Eastwood MR (1971) Screening for psychiatric disorder. Psychol Med 1:197–208
Editorial (1983) Psychological assessment by computer, Lancet I:1023–1024
Feighner JP, Robins E, Guze SB, Woodruff RA, Winokur G, Munoz R (1972) Diagnostic criteria for use in psychiatric research. Arch Gen Psychiatry 26:57–63
Folstein MF, Folstein SE, McHugh PR (1975) "Mini-Mental State". A practical method for grading the cognitive state of patients for the clinician. J Psychiatr Res 12:189–198
Gallagher D, Thompson LW, Levy SM (1980) Clinical psychological assessment of older adults. In: Poon LW (ed) Aging in the 1980s. American Psychological Association, Washington
Garrad J, Bennett AE (1971) A validated interview schedule for use in population surveys of chronic disease and disability. Br J Prev Soc Med 25:97–104
Goldberg D (1974) Screening for disease. Psychiatric disorders. Lancet II:1245–1248
Goldberg D (1981) Estimating the prevalence of psychiatric disorder from the results of a screening test. In: Wing JK, Bebbington P, Robins LN (eds) What is a case? Grant McIntyre, London, pp 129–136
Goldberg DP, Cooper B, Kedward HB, Eastwood MR, Shepherd M (1970) A standardized psychiatric interview for use in community surveys. Br J Prev Soc Med 24:18–23
Gurel L, Linn MW, Linn BS (1972) Physical and mental impairment-of-function evaluation in the aged: The PAMIE Scale. J Gerontol 27:83–90
Gurland B, Kuriansky J, Sharpe L, Simon R, Stiller P, Birkett P (1977) The Comprehensive Assessment and Referral Evaluation (CARE) – Rationale, development and reliability. Int J Aging Hum Dev 8:9–42
Gurland B, Dean L, Cross P, Golden R (1980) The epidemiology of depression and dementia in the elderly: The use of multiple indicators of these conditions. In: Cole JO, Barrett JE (eds) Psychopathology in the aged. Raven, New York, pp 37–60
Gurland B, Copeland J, Kuriansky J, Kelleher M, Sharpe L, Dean LL (1983) The mind and mood of aging. Mental health problems of the community elderly in New York and London. Croom Helm, London
Haglund RMJ, Schuckitt MA (1976) A clinical comparison of tests of organicity in elderly patients. J Gerontol 31:654–659
Hall JN (1980) Ward rating scales for long-stay patients: a review. Psychol Med 10:277–288
Henderson AS, Huppert FA (1984) Editorial. The problem of mild dementia. Psychol Med 14:5–11

Henderson AS, Duncan-Jones P, Finlay-Jones RA (1983) The reliability of the Geriatric Mental State Examination. Acta Psychiatr Scand 67:281–289
Honigfeld G (1981) The evaluation of ward behavior rating scales for psychogeriatric use. Presented at the XII. International Congress of Gerontology, Hamburg, July 12–17
Hughes CP, Berg L, Danziger WL, Coben LA, Martin RL (1982) A new clinical scale for the staging of dementia. Br J Psychiatry 140:566–572
Jacobs JW, Bernhard MR, Delgado A, Strain JJ (1977) Screening for organic mental syndromes in the medically ill. Ann Intern Med 86:40–46
Jefferys M, Millard JB, Hyman M, Warren MD (1969) A set of tests for measuring motor impairment in prevalence studies. J Chronic Dis 22:303–319
Kahn RL, Miller NE (1978) Assessment of altered brain function in the aged. In: Siegler J, Storandt M, Elias M (eds) Clinical psychology of aging. Plenum, New York, pp 43–69
Kahn RL, Goldfarb AJ, Pollack M, Peck A (1960) Brief objective measures for the determination of mental status in the aged. Am J Psychiatry 117:326–328
Kahn RL, Zarit SH, Hilbert NM, Niederehe GM (1975) Memory complaint and impairment in the aged. Arch Gen Psychiatry 32:1569–1573
Kay DWK (1977) The epidemiology and identification of brain deficit in the elderly. In: Eisdorfer C, Friedel RD (eds) Cognitive and emotional disturbance in the elderly. Year Book Medical Publishers, Chicago, pp 11–26
Kochansky GE (1979) Psychiatric rating scales for assessing psychopathology in the elderly: a critical review. In: Raskin A, Jarvik LF (eds) Psychiatric symptoms and cognitive loss in the elderly. Evaluation and assessment techniques. Hemisphere, Washington
Kuriansky J, Gurland B (1976) The performance test of activities of daily living. Int J Aging Hum Dev 7:343–352
Kuriansky J, Gurland B, Cowan D (1976) The usefulness of a psychological test battery. Int J Aging Hum Dev 7:331–342
Lawson JS, Rodenburg M, Dykes JA (1977) A dementia rating scale for use with psychogeriatric patients. J Gerontol 32:153–159
Lawton MP (1972) Assessing the competence of older people. In: Kent DP, Kastenbaum R, Sherwood S (eds) Research planning and action for the elderly. Behavioral Publ., New York, pp 122–143
Lawton MP, Brody E (1969) Assessment of older people: Self-maintaining and instrumental activities of daily living. Gerontologist 9:179–186
Lawton MP, Moss M, Fulcomer M, Kleban MH (1982) A research and service oriented multilevel assessment instrument. J Gerontol 37:91–99
Margo A, Johnson C, Ancill R, Carr T (1983) Assessment of depression by microcomputer. Acta Psychiatr Scand 67:434–435
Mayer JM (1977) Assessment of depression. Adv Psychol Assessment 4:358–425
McDonald RJ (1980) Measuring emotions in the elderly. Paper presented at the XXIInd International Congress of Psychology in Leipzig, GDR, July 6–12
McNair DM (1979) Self-rating scales for assessing psychopathology in the elderly. In: Raskin A, Jarvik LF (eds) Psychiatric symptoms and cognitive loss in the elderly. Evaluation and assessment techniques. Hemisphere, Washington, pp 157–168
Ogden M, Kellett JM, Merryfield P, Millard PH (1984) Practical aspects of automated testing of the elderly. Bull Br Psychol Soc 37:148–149
Pattie AH, Gilleard CJ (1975) A brief psychogeriatric assessment schedule. Br J Psychiatry 127:489–493
Pattie AH, Gilleard CJ (1976) The Clifton Assessment Schedule – further validation of a psychiatric assessment schedule. Br J Psychiatry 129:68–72
Pattie AH, Gilleard CJ (1979) Manual of the Clifton Assessment Procedures for the Elderly. Hodder & Stoughton, London Sevenoaks
Pfeiffer E (1975) A short portable mental status questionnaire for the assessment of organic brain deficit in elderly patients. J Am Geriatr Soc 23:433–441

Plutchik R (1979) Conceptual and practical issues in the assessment of the elderly. In: Raskin A, Jarvik LF (eds) Psychiatric symptoms and cognitive loss in the elderly. Evaluation and assessment techniques. Hemisphere, Washington, pp 19–38

Plutchik R, Conte H, Lieberman M, Bakur M, Grossman J, Lehrman N (1970) Reliability and validity of a scale for assessing the functioning of geriatric patients. J Am Geriatr Soc 18:491–500

Qureshi KN, Hodkinson HM (1974) Evaluation of a ten-question mental test in the institutionalized elderly. Age Ageing 3:152–157

Reisberg B, Ferris SH, DeLeon MJ, Crook T (1982) The Global Deterioration Scale for assessment of primary degenerative dementia. Am J Psychiatry 139:1136–1139

Smith JM (1979) Nurse and psychiatric aide rating scales for assessing psychopathology in the elderly: a critical review. In: Raskin A, Jarvik LF (eds) Psychiatric symptoms and cognitive loss in the elderly. Evaluation and assessment techniques. Hemisphere, Washington, pp 169–186

Smyer MA, Hofland BF, Jonas EA (1979) Validity study of the Short Portable Mental Status Questionnaire for the Elderly. J Am Geriatr Soc 27:263–269

Spitzer RL, Endicott J (1968) DIAGNO: a computer program for psychiatric diagnosis utilizing the differential diagnostic procedure. Arch Gen Psychiatry 18:746–756

Spitzer RL, Fleiss JL, Burdock EI, Hardesty AS (1964) The Mental Status Schedule: rationale, reliability and validity. Compr Psychiatry 5; 384–395

Spitzer RL, Endicott J, Robins E (1978) Research diagnostic criteria: rationale and reliability. Arch Gen Psychiatry 35:773–782

University of Washington (1978) The Sickness Impact Profile: A brief summary of its purpose, uses, and administration. Department of Health Services, SC-37, Seattle, Washington

US Commission on Chronic Illness (1957) Prevention of chronic illness in the United States, vol 1. Harvard University Press, Cambridge, Mass.

Watts K, Baddeley A, Williams M (1982) Automated tailored testing using Raven's matrices and the Mill Hill vocabulary tests: a comparison with manual administration. Int. J Man-Machine Stud 17:331–344

WHO (1980) International Classification of Impairments, Disabilities, and Handicaps. Geneva

Williams RGA (1979) Theories and measurement in disability. Epidemiol Commun Health 33:32–47

Williams RGA, Johnston M, Willis LA, Bennett AE (1976) Disability: a model and measurement technique. Br J Prev Soc Med 30:71–78

Wilson LA, Brass W (1973) Brief assessment of the mental state in domiciliary practice. The usefulness of the Mental Status Questionnaire. Age Ageing 2:92–101

Wing JK, Birley JLT, Cooper JE, Graham P, Isaacs A (1967) Reliability of a procedure for measuring and classifying present psychiatric state. Br J Psychiatry 113:499–515

Wing JK, Cooper JE, Sartorius N (1974) Measurement and classification of psychiatric symptoms. Cambridge University Press, London

Zemore R, Eames N (1979) Psychic and somatic symptoms of depression among young adults, institutionalized aged and noninstitutionalized aged. J Gerontol 34:716–722

5.2 Possibilities of Preserving Physical and Mental Fitness and Autonomy in Old Age

A. Svanborg, S. Berg, D. Mellström, L. Nilsson, G. Persson

This report is based mainly on results from our owen longitudinal, gerontological, and geriatric study of 70-year-olds in Göteborg (H 70) (Rinder et al. 1975; Svanborg et al. 1982a, b). The sample studied are, as far as we can judge, representative of the total population of 70-year-olds. The original sample studied in 1971/72 comprised 30% of the 70-year-old population. In 1976/77 this cohort was followed up and at the same time a new 70-year-old cohort was sampled in order to make an age cohort comparison. The first cohort was re-examined at the ages of 79, 81, and 82. The second cohort of 70-year-olds was followed up at 75. When reference is made in this paper to, for instance, manifestations of aging versus prevalence of definable disorders, as well as of a state in between with obvious risk factors for pathology, this is based on the present longitudinal perspective of 12 years in one cohort and 5 years in the other. Because of the findings of certain important differences between cohorts that are separated by a period as short as 5 years, a third 70-year-old cohort, born in 1911/12 (IVEG) has also been investigated (Table 1). The preliminary data show that there were also certain marked cohort differences between this cohort and the other two cohorts. We have therefore added an intervention study to this third cohort investigation: we have been provided with resources to improve the medical care and general living conditions in a representative group of 70-year-olds to see whether such a change at this age will influence aging and the state of health in a positive way. The addition of an intervention program in the study of the third cohort will, of course, markedly improve our ability to draw conclusions concerning causative relationships between aging and the state of health on the one hand, and environmental factors on the other.

As far as we can see, changes in the genetic basis of this population cannot explain the rather marked differences both in manifestations of aging and in the

Table 1. Investigation periods in the population studies in Göteborg from 1971/72 to 1984/85

Year of birth	Year of investigation							
	1971/72	1976/77	1980/81	1981/82	1982/83	1983/84	1984/85	
1901/02 (H 70)	70 years	75 years	79 years		81 years	82 years	83 years	→
1906/07 (H 70)		70 years		75 years				?
1911/12 (IVEG)				70 years	70 years	72 years	72 years	

state of health found between these three cohorts which are separated by intervals of only 5 years. In the age cohorts studied the migration rate has been quite low.

The survey includes data such as housing conditions, income, social and physical communications, educational level, previous and any present occupation, and the need for and use of health care facilities.

All subjects undergo an examination at the outpatient department of the hospital, at the most including a general medical and ophthalmological examination, blood and urine tests, ECG, and chest X-ray. The subsamples undergo psychological, psychiatric, dental, somatometric, and audiometric examinations; interviews regarding diet; examination of body composition; detailed studies of lung function, cardiac function, and immunoresponse capacity; as well as extensive neurophysiological examinations, including EEG, echoencephalography, cerebral blood flow, auditory brainstem response, and measurement of balance ability (including stabilometry).

Those readers who would like to see prevalence figures for definable mental abnormalities in the first cohort are referred to results published by the psychiatrists Göran Persson and Lars Nilsson (Persson 1980; Nilsson 1983; Nilsson and Persson 1984) (Table 2).

The main aim of this presentation is to illustrate the cohort differences that are apparently caused mainly by environmental factors, and also to show some

Table 2. Prevalence of psychiatric morbidity in an urban sample examined at 70, 75, and 79 years of age (Nilsson and Persson 1982)

Diagnosis	Age 70 (n=392)		Age 75 (n=303)		Age 79 (n=206)	
	n	%	n	%	n	%
Nonstationary mental disorders						
A. Psychoses						
Schizophrenic, paranoid	2	0.5	5	1.7	5	2.4
Affective	4	1.0	7	2.3	2	1.0
Dementias	5	1.3	7	2.3	14	6.8
Combined	2	0.5	1	0.3	1	0.5
	13	3.3	20	6.6	22	10.7
B. Neuroses						
a) Moderate-severe anxiety, depressive, obsessive-compulsive	26	6.6	14	4.6	8	3.9
Asthenic	9	2.3	12	4.0	19	9.2
Combined	2	0.5	5	1.7	1	0.5
b) Mild	31	7.9	18	5.9	12	5.8
	68	17.3	49	16.2	40	19.4
C. "Active" alcoholics not included above	5	1.3	4	1.3	2	1.0
Total nonstationary mental disorders	86	21.9	73	24.1	64	31.1

Table 3. Intelligence and memory test results among 70-year-old people in Göteborg, Sweden 1971/72 and 1976/77. Cohort comparison (Berg 1980)

	1971/72			1976/77			*t*	*P*<
	x̄	S/D	*n*	x̄	S/D	*n*		
Verbal meaning/SRB 1	17.0	6.4	357	18.5	6.7	387	3.18	0.001
Reasoning/SRB 2	12.6	4.6	359	13.9	4.8	392	6.60	0.001
Spatial ability/SRB 3	12.9	6.3	181	15.5	7.3	398	6.96	0.001
Perceptual speed/Psif	15.4	8.2	184	19.1	7.1	391	5.48	0.001
Digits forward	5.6	1.0	178	5.4	1.2	398	1.93	NS
Digits backward	3.8	0.9	178	4.1	1.2	397	2.96	0.01

indirect evidence that might indicate further differences that may appear in the future. The observed environmental influence, not only upon the state of health but also upon processes usually identified as causing aging, also shows that an improvement in the environment of the elderly might influence not only their state of health in a positive way, but apparently also the rate and manifestations of aging. Thus I will try to illustrate some possibilities of preserving physical and mental fitness, as well as autonomy, in old age. It seems more reasonable in this context to refer to postponing measures rather than prevention.

At the present stage of our longitudinal study, we have observed age cohort differences in longevity, cognitive function (Table 3), dental state, body mass and body mass index, and also the general state of health. The psychological studies were performed by, or under the guidance of, Stig Berg (1980). The following intelligence and memory tests were performed: synonyms of SRB 1 measuring verbal ability; figure grouping or SRB 2 measuring inductive and logical reasoning ability; block design or SRB 3 measuring spatial ability; Psif measuring perceptual speed; digit span tests measuring primary memory; and Thurstone memory tests measuring secondary memory.

Further studies of the cohorts at the ages of 75 and 79 have confirmed our pervious conclusion from studies of 70-year-olds, i.e., that intelligence and memory have not changed significantly at the age of 70 but that the perceptual speed has apparently already started to decline in early adult life. The discrepancy in the rate of change with age between the perceptual speed and the parameters of intelligence and memory is, according to our experience, the main reason for overdiagnosis of dementia/senility in the elderly. This is especially the case when the perceptual speed is further lowered because of sensory deprivation, such as unwanted isolation, bereavement, different forms of somatic injuries and diseases, as well as mental depression. The differences previously observed between the cohorts at 70 are also found to be obvious at 75. There are two reports in the literature claiming that the incidence of senile dementia in the Scandinavian population is decreasing. Although we have found a positive difference in cognitive functions, we have not seen any indication of any decrease in the incidence of senile dementia between the ages of 70 and 75. For this reason, we are planning another age cohort comparison at the age of 79, when the prevalence is higher.

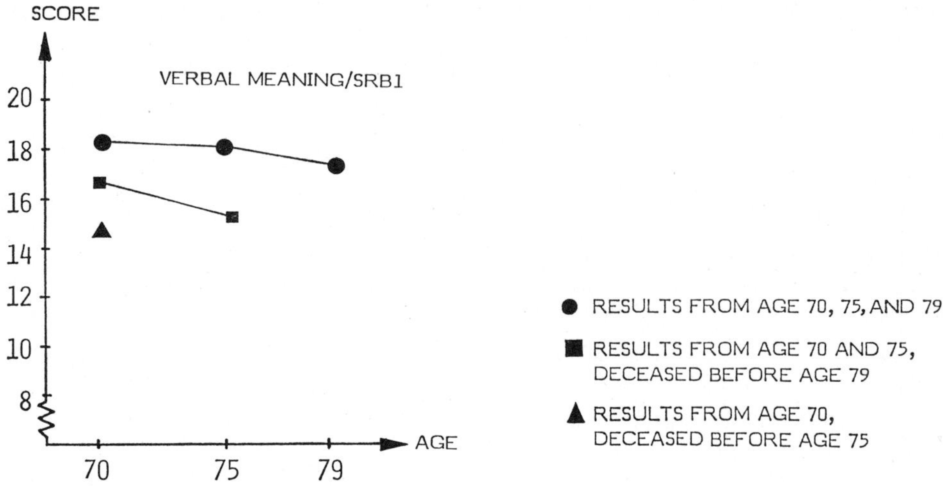

Fig. 1. Results of the cognitive test "Verbal meaning/SRBI" in subjects aged 70, 75, and 79

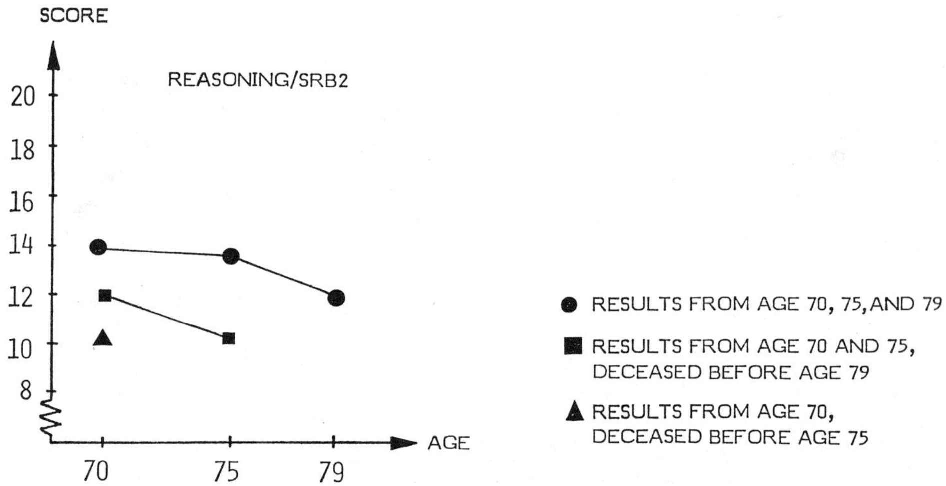

Fig. 2. Results of the cognitive test "Reasoning/SRB2" in subjects aged 70, 75, and 79

Although the prevalence of definable organic brain disorders is low both at 70 and 75 years of age, we can now report a correlation between the results of the cognitive function tests and mortality during the ages 70 – 75 and 75 – 79 (Figs. 1–4). Those who died within the ages 70 – 75 had a significantly lower cognitive ability than those who lived to 75, and those who were still alive at the age of 79 had an even better cognitive ability at the age of 70. Our data indicate that previous conclusions based on cross-sectional comparison, which has demonstrated a rather marked age-related decline in several cognitive functions at these ages, can be mainly applied to the group of elderly who are suffering from either

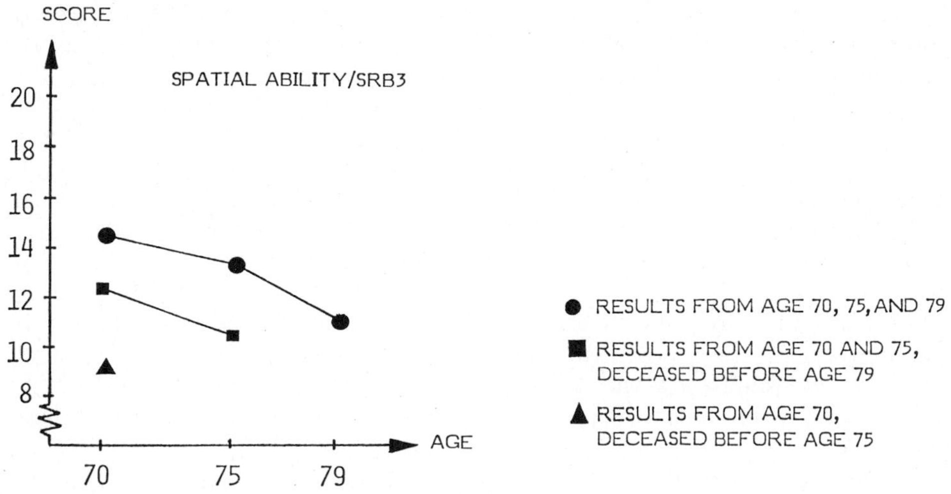

Fig. 3. Results from the cognitive test "Spatial ability/SRB3" in subjects aged 70, 75, and 79

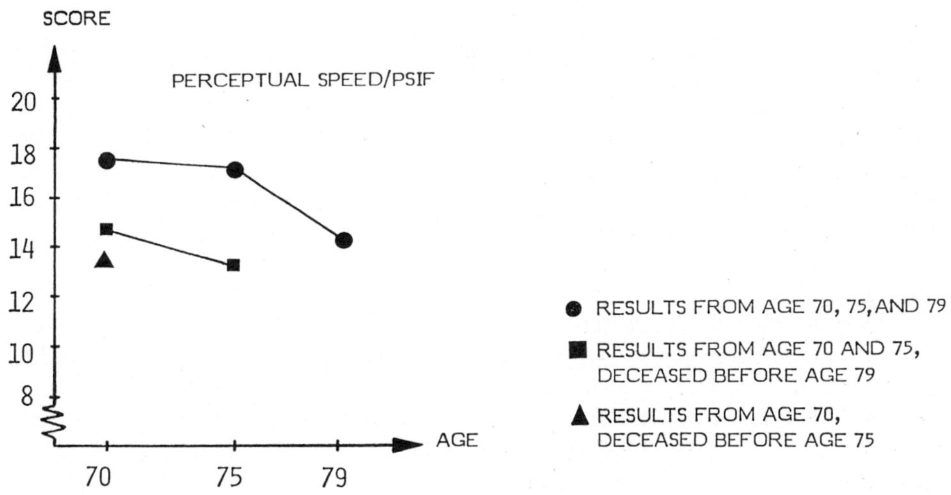

Fig. 4. Results from the cognitive test "Perceptual speed/Psif" in subjects aged 70, 75, and 79

mental or physical disorders (or are already in a phase of accelerated aging). Among those who still lacked signs of definable diseases at age 79, no obvious decline in cognitive function was observed.

We have already published data indicating that people suffering from social isolation have a lower opinion of their state of health and consume more medical and social services as well as drugs (Berg et al. 1981). Now that we have followed them for a longer period, we definitely dare to state that this group is a risk group for overdiagnosis. Apparently, many of them have both mental and physical manifestations that they, and we doctors, are identifying as symptoms of disease.

When we consider that, at least in Sweden, loneliness with such practical consequences is found in about 15% – 20% of the women of around 70, we realize the practical consequences of this type of overdiagnosis and overtreatment. We also realize the opposite, namely, the possibility and challenge that would exist in our societies if another societal organization for the life of the elderly could be established. I would also like to mention the quite dynamic change, not only in the state of health but apparently also in the general physical performance, that can be caused by bereavement at these ages. In this context, we would only like to refer to our previous and published studies showing that in Sweden mortality in the age group 50 – 90 increases by 48% in widowers during the first 3 months of living alone, and by 22% in widows during these first 3 months (Mellström et al. 1982a). In our intervention study, we have focused on this problem both from a biological and from a psychological and sociological point of view. To what extent will it, and would it, be possible to help these people pass this obvious risk period of their lives?

Finally, we would also like to mention some indirect evidence that we have of the future cohort differences. Indirect evidence of future cohort differences has been found in relation to the density of the skeleton, muscle strength and gonadal function (Mellström et al. 1982b; Rundgren et al. 1984). In our study, smokers have an average 30% less skeleton at the ages of 70 and 75 compared with non-smokers. In this context, we are not going to discuss the interesting simultaneous increase in the risk of hip fractures that has been observed by several investigators (for a review, see Zetterberg and Andersson 1982). A discussion of different possible causative factors behind a lower density of the skeleton is beyond the scope of this paper. We will, however, spend a little more time on our observations of changes in the gonadal function among smokers. The best indicators we know of at the present time of the balance between estrogenic and androgenic activity are certain measurements of metabolic effects, and especially the quotient between lecithin and lysolecithin in plasma. According to these measurements, smoking causes a faster rate of decline in the gonadal function (Mellström et al. 1982a). To our knowledge, no study has so far shown that cognitive functions decline more rapidly in smokers, although smokers obviously have a higher risk of developing cardiovascular disease with a negative influence on the nutrition of, for example, brain tissues. Our material has up to now, however, included relatively few cases with defined multi-infarction dementia and we cannot state definitely that multi-infarction dementia is more common among smokers at these ages. In this context, it should, however, be emphasized that we have found *a positive correlation in men between a relative dominance of androgenic activity and better mental health, better energy resources, a greater need to dominate, and a higher degree of sexual activity.* There was *a positive correlation in women between a relative dominance of estrogen activity and better energy resources and lower neuroticism* (Persson et al. 1983). There are, of course, several possible interpretations of this correlation. One is that psychological resistance, personality traits, and the balance between androgenic and estrogenic activity are all related to a common factor concerning vitality. To what extent smoking per se will cause a change in gonadal function, with a secondary influence on personality, remains to be definitely shown.

Finally, we would also like to mention the correlation observed between previous professional work and mortality. These figures are relevant not only to Göteborg but to the whole of Sweden. Although we did find a few differences, both in the rate of aging and the state of health, between workers who had performed heavy physical work all their lives and so-called white-collar workers, they were very minor. But there are still very marked differences in the mortality between different professions in our country, as in some other countries. Farmers and skilled manual workers live longest. Among academically educated people, priests live longest. The shortest life spans are found among sailors, restaurant workers, and journalists. These differences in life expectancy might, of course, illustrate that certain individuals choose certain professions, but in some of these professions sociological and historical analyses do not indicate that the selection process per se should have had a great impact on mortality. Our preliminary conclusions indicate, on the contrary, that also here personal life-style factors, sometimes related to special professional work, have a greater impact on the state of health and mortality than, for example, exposure to the working environment per se. We would, however, like to emphasize that the question of a possible relationship between professional work and the state of health at ages above 70 is an extremely difficult one, and that we, although we now have no less than three cohorts to compare, hesitate to draw any definite conclusions.

To summarize, more and more data indicate that personal life-style and ecological factors have a much greater impact, not only on the state of health but also on the rate and manifestations of aging, than was generally thought. If we turn this causative relationship the other way, obvious conclusions would be that possibilities of preserving physical and mental fitness are greater than believed hitherto.

The intervention study in the third cohort of 70-year-olds started in 1981/82. Before and after the intervention principally the same investigations are performed as in the other "70-year-old studies". The intervention period is 1.5 years. The basic ideas are:

1. Correctly balanced medical care, i.e., to prevent both over- and underdiagnosis. Emergency help and advice in critical situations, such as the loss of a spouse.
2. To improve, when needed and wanted, physical, intellectual, and, if possible, emotional activities. The problem is to find a border zone between load and overload.

A general conclusion from our present experiences is that the elderly in general are more interested in advice and also more willing to try new ideas than is usually believed. It does not seem to be true that "you can't teach an old dog new tricks".

References

Berg S (1980) Psychological functioning in 70- and 75-year old people. A study in an industrialized city. Acta Psychiatr Scand [Suppl] 288, vol 62

Berg S, Mellström D, Persson G, Svanborg A (1981) Loneliness in the Swedish aged. J Gerontol 36:342–349

Mellström D, Nilsson Å, Odén A, Rundgren Å, Svanborg A (1982a) Mortality among the widowed in Sweden. Scand J Soc Med 10:33–41
Mellström D, Rundgren Å, Jagenburg R, Steen B, Svanborg A (1982b) Tobacco smoking, ageing and health among the elderly. A longitudinal population study of 70-year-old men and an age cohort comparison. Age Ageing 11:45–58
Nilsson LV (1983) Prevalence of mental disorders in a 70-year-old urban sample. A cohort comparison. J Clin Exp Gerontol 5:101–120
Nilsson LV, Persson G (1984) Prevalence of mental disorders in an urban sample examined at 70, 75 and 79 years of age. Acta Psychiatr Scand 69:519–527
Persson G (1980) Prevalence of mental disorders in a 70-year-old urban population. Acta Psychiatr Scand 62:119–139
Persson G, Nilsson LV, Svanborg A (1983) Personality and sexuality in relation to an index of gonadal steroid hormone balance in a 70-year-old population. J Psychosom Res 27:469–477
Rinder L, Roupe S, Steen B, Svanborg A (1975) Seventy-year-old people in Gothenburg. A population study in an industrialized Swedish city. I. General presentation of the study. Acta Med Scand 198:397–407
Rundgren Å, Eklund S, Jonson R (1984) Bone mineral content in 70- and 75-year-old men and women. An analysis of some anthropometric background factors. Age Ageing 13:6–13
Svanborg A, Bergström G, Mellström D (1982a) Epidemiological studies on social and medical conditions of the elderly. Report on a survey. EURO Reports and Studies 62. WHO, Copenhagen
Svanborg A, Landahl S, Mellström D (1982b) Basic issues of health care. In: Thomae H, Maddox GL (eds) New perspectives on old age. A message to decision makers. On behalf of the international association of gerontology. Springer, New York, pp 31–52
Zetterberg C, Andersson G (1982) Fractures of the proximal end of the femur in Göteborg, Sweden, 1940–1979. Acta Orthop Scand 53:419–426

5.3 The Role of Medical Treatment in the Prevention and Reduction of Psychiatric Impairment in Old Age

K. Bergmann

It is customary to consider prevention in terms of primary, secondary and tertiary prevention. As the aetiology of the major functional and organic disorders is not understood, medical treatment to prevent or modify these diseases remains a hope for the future. Little of value can therefore be said about primary prevention. However, when considering the subject in a research-orientated setting perhaps some consideration can be given to the necessary preconditions for applying preventative measures. Of necessity, therefore, secondary prevention, the treatment of undetected disease, and tertiary prevention, the better treatment and management of known disease, must remain the main concerns of this paper.

Prevention and reduction of impairment will be examined in relationship to the major diagnostic categories causing serious disability in old age.

Functional Disorders

The two main categories to be considered are depressive disorders and paraphrenia.

Depressive Disorders

The treatment of depression at any time of life leaves much to be desired and so only the special aspects of depressive illness which have a particular bearing on later life will be emphasised. A particular association exists between physical ill health and depression in later life. Thus follow-up studies of samples of middle-aged and elderly patients with affective disorders (Kerr et al. 1969; Kay and Bergmann 1966) reveal a strong association with serious ill health and an increased mortality. The effect of ill health in such cases might be reckoned to be non-specific (Murphy 1982) or the result of generalized pain and discomfort, though some studies (Bergmann 1971; Dovenmuehle and Verwoerdt 1963) identify a special association of affective disorders with cardiovascular disease, cerebrovascular disorders and neoplastic diseases. Endocrine disorders, malnutrition and specific avitaminosis may also be significant. As much physical ill health in old age is occult, a special and more effective assessment of elderly out-patients with depression may both yield undetected disorder and in its treatment improve the prognosis of depression in later life. A more speculative gain might be envisaged if the study of heart disease and neoplastic disorders and their metabolic effects in older people yielded more specific clues on the aetiology of late-life depression.

A more direct approach to the causative factors that especially have a bearing on depression in later life arises from considering aspects of research from a variety of sources.

The Relationship of Dementia and Depression

While there is argument as to whether mental impairment found in severe depression of old age can or should be called a true dementia (Rabins et al. 1984), there is little doubt that in some cases at least the clinical, psychometric and biological findings (Cawley et al. 1973) indicate some grounds for considering the possibility of a biochemical deficit. Furthermore, more recent CAT scan studies (Jacoby and Levy 1980) suggest that the prognosis of elderly depressives may be related to structural changes in the cerebral cortex.

Prognostic Studies

Late-life depression seems in nearly one-third of cases to carry a poor prognosis for recovery (Post 1972; Murphy 1983). Post found that even the advent of oral antidepressant therapy did not confer any advantage on his later follow-up group, who had had the opportunity of this form of treatment.

Studies on Age-Related Changes in Neurotransmitters

A summary of studies on age-related changes in neurotransmitters that aging has substantial effects on catecholamine metabolism: lower levels of noradrenaline, raised levels of monoamine oxidase, and reductions of dopamine and serotonin levels have all been reported.

The Biogenic Amine Hypothesis

The biogenic amine hypothesis is outlined in detail by Zis and Goodwin (1982) and attempts to relate CSF, blood and urinary levels of various catecholamine metabolites to aspects of depressive illness. *Neurobiology of Mood Disorders* (Post and Ballinger 1984) gives detailed critiques of measures of catecholamine activity; in addition, approaches to studies of catecholamine and serotonin receptor responsiveness are described.

In view of the large amount of unremitting invalidism leading not only to increased mortality but also to increased dependency and need for services (Bergmann et al. 1978), the group of patients with chronic persistent depression might provide valuable data on profiles of catecholamine abnormalities and an opportunity to study the use of various types of antidepressants, singly or in combination as long-term substitution therapy. It could also be expected that in elderly patients of this type genetic factors would be less in evidence (Post 1982) and therefore intercurrent biological events relevant to the genesis of the depression would be more readily elucidated.

The position of secondary prevention also needs some discussion. A large number of older people with depressions of some severity remain in their own homes largely untreated and undetected and there is little evidence that the situation has altered substantially since Williamson and his colleagues (1964) reported that more than 70% of depressives are undetected. Though so many elderly people with depression remain unknown to their doctors, it is likely that they suffer from significantly increased morbidity and mortality.

Effective medical treatment of this group requires adequate screening in a primary care setting and health education of primary care practitioners to permit them to exercise the specialized skills required in order to treat elderly people effectively and safely.

Paraphrenia

As genetic factors are not so prominent in this condition as in the schizophrenias of earlier life (Kay 1963), environmental influences would play a greater role, presenting an opportunity for preventative measures. However, the only major factors which might be influenced are those of longstanding deafness and, less commonly, visual impairment; these are commonly found in patients with paraphrenia – more so than in matched controls with affective disorders (Cooper et al. 1976).

It is not beyond the bounds of possibility that better treatment of the conduction deafnesses of middle life might lessen the incidence of late paraphrenia and that better management of deafness in old age, by improved detection of deafness and simple measures to ameliorate hearing, might also have an influence. As regards promoting the viability of paraphrenics in the community and reducing the discomfort of psychotic symptoms, only one factor was of major significance on followup (Post 1980), namely compliance with antipsychotic drugs. Major difficulties arise in initiating and maintaining treatment. Research might be usefully directed at the following areas:

1. The choice of tranquillizer – which is most acceptable, which has the fewest side-effects and what is the optimal dosage range.
2. Which system of care is likely to lead to best compliance – supervision in out-patient clinics, home visits by trained community psychiatric nurses, treatment in the primary care setting or attendance at a day hospital.
3. The need for drug holidays: what is the incidence of various side-effects, especially tardive dyskinesia.
4. What are the indications for the use of long-acting parenteral therapy?

The Problem of the Dementias

The aetiology of the common dementias of old age is unknown and it is doubtful if any therapeutic agent currently available can affect the deficits which characterize them. This does not imply that these conditions are immutably fixed or that there is nor chance of influencing them. A reduction of the incidence of dementia has been demonstrated (Hagnell et al. 1981), which may indicate that temporal changes have occurred affecting the manifestation of the clinical syndrome. The possibility that more effective treatment of hypertension may be a factor cannot be discounted.

Mann and his colleagues (personal communication, 1984) are currently carrying out a prospective investigation of the effects of treatment of hypertension in older people on the subsequent development of dementia in the setting of the methodology of the previous MRC trial of treatment for hypertension.

Other health factors manifesting themselves in earlier life may act as extrinsic causes, though their elucidation rests more in the field of epidemiology than in that of current therapeutic research. The fact that a substantial number of patients who have the clinical syndrome of Alzheimer's disease do not have the corresponding pathological changes (Tomlinson et al. 1970) also encourages the search for extrinsic factors.

The use of psycho-active drugs (nootropics) will not receive consideration here. The current therapeutic problems have been summed up by Kanowski (1983):

1. Their limited efficacy
2. The unreliability of their effects
3. The imperfection of current instruments employed to measure their action

If therapeutic nihilism is not to be the order of the day, implying the abandonment of a medical approach, some principles for assessing the place of medical treatment need to be stated. The natural history of a dementing illness is that of an insidious longstanding condition but the events which lead to referral for medical care are often sudden and may present as acute crises. It seems improbable that the progression of intrinsic brain disease is likely to accelerate to such a degree as to provide a sufficient explanation for such events, especially in the case of Alzheimer's disease. Extracerebral causes of acute crises or decompensations should be evaluated and provide a basis not only for medical but also for social and psychological interventions. In thie paper, however, only the medical aspects of treatment will be considered and briefly enumerated:

1. Major physical ill-health, including illnesses often manifesting a "silent" presentation,
2. Acute cerebral disease: epilepsy, embolism or acute infarction,
3. The presence of symptomatic forms of major psychoses within the dementing illness.

Research issues which require further investigation merit discussion. These would include the prevalence of the above factors in a representative series of patients and evaluation of the efficacy of treatment measures in terms of cognitive improvement, behavioural change and physical capacity. For the symptomatic psychoses careful psychopathological evaluation before and after treatment will be of great importance as a controlled trial under such circumstances might well present clinical and ethical problems. There is scope for a descriptive and "naturalistic" approach without necessarily sacrificing scientific rigour.

The major problems of caring for demented patients are well understood but not well managed. While many aspects of care transcend medication, the role of psychotropic drugs in their management needs further investigation. Among the more intractable features of dementia are:

1. Persistent wandering,
2. Intractable tension and agitation,
3. Unpredictable explosive aggression,
4. Uncontrolled and unacceptable behaviour.

Reliable behavioural measures need to be developed and sensitive indicators of change sought. Systematic investigation of such patients may point the way to more effective and rational ways of employing, in the context of psychological and environmental approaches, psychotropic drugs. It is also important, as Jarvik and her co-workers pointed out for drug trials (1982), to compare the efficacy of psychopharmacological and behavioural approaches.

The knowledge gained in treating known "cases" would permit an approach to secondary prevention. Screening within the community for earlier cases of dementia would then permit the possibility of medical treatments of at least some efficacy, which could then be more readily subjected to controlled trials.

The advances in knowledge which may in the end lead to effective treatments for dementia depend not only on the advances in the fundamental biological sciences but also on (a) the development of sensitive ways of locating early cases and measuring change and (b) the development within the psychiatric services of a preventative approach well in advance of the longawaited scientific breakthrough.

References

Bergmann K (1971) The neuroses of old age. In: Kay DWK, Walk A (eds) Recent developments in psychogeriatrics. Headley Bros., Ashford, pp 39–50

Bergmann K, Foster EM, Justice AW, Mathews V (1978) Management of the demented elderly patient in the community. Br J Psychiatry 132:441–449

Cawley RH, Post F, Whitehead A (1973) Barbiturate tolerance and psychological functioning in depressed elderly patients. Psychol Med 1:39–52

Cooper AF, Garside RF, Kay DWK (1976) A comparison of deaf and non deaf patients with paranoid and affective psychoses. Br J Psychiatry 129:532–538

Dovénmuehle RH, Verwoerdt A (1963) Physical illness and depressive symptomatology. Part 2: Factors of length and severity of illness and frequency of hospitalization. J Gerontol 18:260–266

Finch CE (1977) Neuroendocrine and autonomic aspects of aging. In: Finch CE, Hayflick L (eds) Handbook of the biology of aging. Van Nostrand Reinhold, New York, pp 262–274

Hagnell O, Lanke J, Rorsman B, Öjesjö L (1981) Does the incidence of age psychosis decrease? A prospective, longitudinal study of a complete population investigated during the 25 year period 1947–1972: The Lundby Study. Neuropsychobiology 7(4):201–211

Jacoby R, Levy R (1980) Computed tomography in the elderly. 3. Affective disorders. Br J Psychiatry 136:270–275

Jarvik LF, Miri FT, Stener J, Gerner R (1982) Treating geriatric depression: a 26 week interim analysis. J Am Geriatr Soc 30(II):713–717

Kanowski S (1983) Therapy and preventative aspects of senile dementia. Document presented to the W.H.O. Scientific Group on Senile Dementia

Kay DWK (1963) Late paraphrenia and its bearing on the aetiology of schizophrenia. Acta Psychiatr Scand 39:159–169

Kay DWK, Bergmann K (1966) Physical disability and mental health in old age. J Psychosom Res 10:3–12

Kerr TA, Schapira K, Roth M (1969) The relationship between premature death and affective disorders. Br J Psychiatry 115:1277–1282

Murphy E (1982) Social origins of depression in old age. Br J Psychiatry 141:135–142

Murphy E (1983) The prognosis of depression in old age. Br J Psychiatry 142:111–119

Post F (1972) The management and nature of depressive illness in late life: a follow through study. Br J Psychiatry 121:393–404

Post F (1980) Paranoid, schizoprenia-like and schizophrenic states in the aged. In: Birren JE, Sloane RB (eds) Handbook of mental health and aging. Prentice Hall, Englewood Cliffs, N.J.

Post F (1982) Affective disorders in old age, In: Paykel ES (ed) Handbook of affective disorders. Churchill Livingstone, Edinburgh, pp 393–402

Post RM, Ballinger JC (eds) (1984) Neurobiology of mood disorders. Frontiers of Clinical Science, vol 1. Wilkins and Williams, Baltimore

Rabins PV, Merchant A, Nestadt G (1984) Criteria for diagnosing reversible dementia caused by depression: validation by 2-year follow-up. Br J Psychiatry 144:488–492

Tomlinson BE, Blessed GB, Roth M (1970) Observations on the brains of demented old people. J Neurol Sci 11:205

Williamson J, Stokoe IH, Gray S, Fisher M, Smith A, McGhee A, Stephenson E (1964) Old people at home – their unreported needs. Lancet I:1117–1120

Zis AP, Goodwin FK (1982) The amine hypothesis. In: Paykel ES (ed) Handbook of affective disorders. Churchill Livingstone, Edinburgh, pp 175–190

5.4 Care of Mental Disorders in the Elderly: The Contribution of Social Intervention and Social Programmes

B. Cooper, B. Beck-Dreßler

Nature and Extent of the Problem

Morbidity surveys in a number of countries have consistently shown a high prevalence of mental illness in elderly populations (Kay and Bergmann 1980). In view of present demographic trends, both absolute numbers of cases and prevalence ratios in the over-65 age range must be expected to increase substantially in the coming decades, and this growth will be most pronounced for the severely disabling dementing disorders (Kramer 1980).

Epidemiological research has also repeatedly shown that most mentally impaired old people are to be found living in private households. The numbers in any form of institutional care represent only about a quarter to one-fifth of psychoses, and less than one-tenth of total psychiatric prevalence (Cooper 1984; Kay and Bergmann 1980). Furthermore, mental disorder in the elderly population tends to occur in association with other causes of handicap, and thus to form part of a nexus of ill-health, disablement and dependency in the affected subgroups. In particular, associations have been reported with chronic physical impairment, low socio-economic status, poor housing conditions and – at least in some studies – social isolation and loneliness (Stevenson 1981). Although little information is available about the help received by affected persons, the few studies so far undertaken suggest that social support is generally inadequate (Foster et al. 1976; Levin et al. 1983). There is a growing demand for improvement in both the quantity and the quality of community services for the mentally ill elderly and their families.

In pursuit of this goal, research must be undertaken to define the nature and extent of unmet needs in the elderly population, but also to establish what kinds of service are likely to prove effective, since nothing could be worse than a widespread proliferation of ineffective services. A review of the literature on social care for the elderly (Goldberg and Connelly 1982) reveals that most investigations so far reported have been uncontrolled descriptive studies, while those more ambitious projects which have tried to make use of controlled comparisons have usually failed to reach any firm conclusions because of lack of clear research aims, poor methodology, low response rate or other problems. Any attempt to assess progress in this field must at the present time rely chiefly upon descriptive accounts, rather than on a substantial body of scientific knowledge.

Forms and Aspects of Social Intervention

This short review will be confined to forms of social intervention which are focused on individuals or small groups. We would do well, however, to remember that mental health in the elderly is always subject to the influence of their physical and social environment. National policies in relation to social welfare, retirement and pensions, housing and rents, urban planning and public transport may in the long term prove at least as important in this context as the scale of special-service provision (see the contribution to this volume by D. Mechanic). Moreover, the division between health and social services, though convenient for the present purpose, is in large measure artificial: a point which will be taken up in the concluding section.

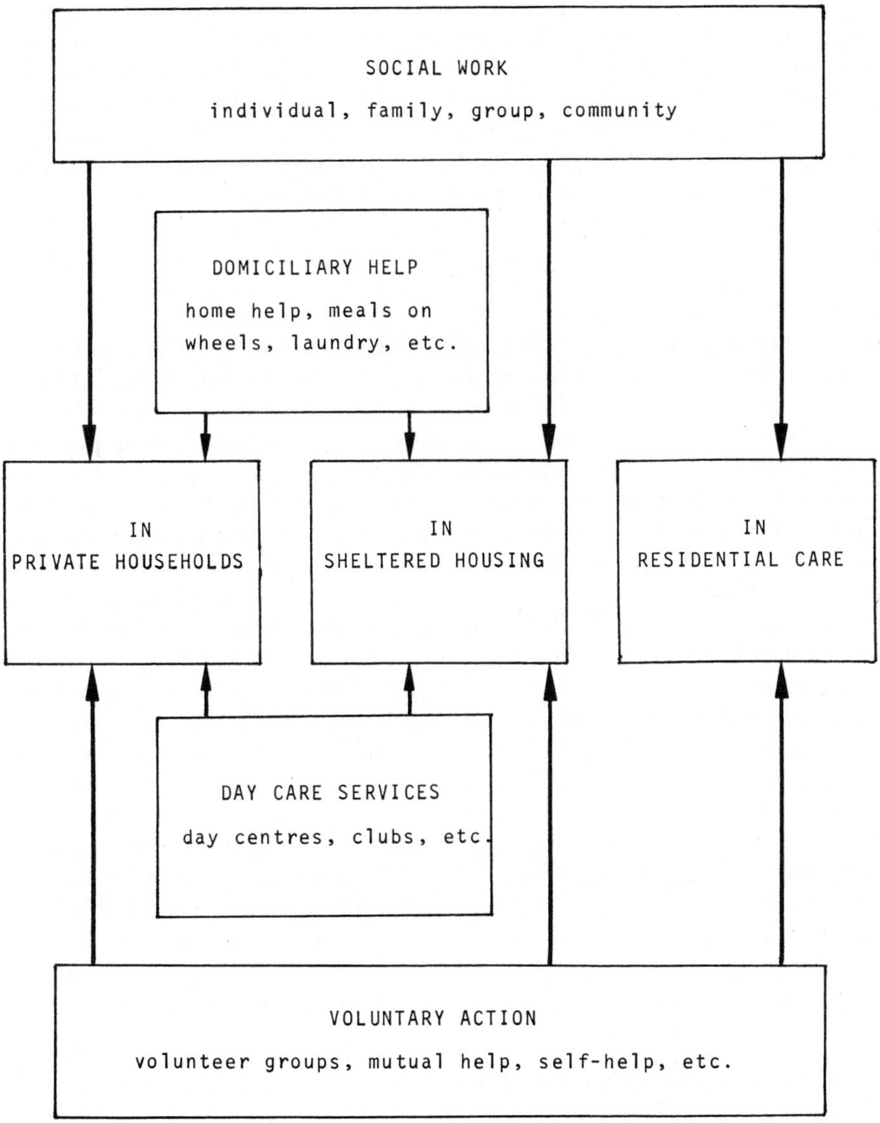

Fig. 1. Main forms and aspects of social care for the elderly

Up to now, very few social agencies have devoted themselves to the problems of mentally impaired old people. In most countries, these matters are dealt with, as part of their wider responsibilities, either by generic social service departments or by social workers in the hospital sector, or by some combination of the two. It is mainly within the area of overlap between these two types of agency that new forms of psychogeriatric care in the community are now beginning to emerge (Hemsi 1982; Lowy 1980).

Developments are occurring simultaneously in several different kinds of social-care provision, which as a rule are not closely co-ordinated with one another. The chief forms of such provision, and their connections to different subsections of the elderly population, are illustrated schematically in Fig. 1. The categories and terminology used here are derived from the comprehensive review of British social services by Goldberg and Connelly (1982). However, analogous service functions are recognized in the U.S.A. (Lowy 1980), the Federal Republic of Germany (Dahlem 1982; Rückert 1979) and other developed industrial countries. Each of the different forms of provision indicated in the figure will be considered briefly in turn.

Social Work[1]

Few people would question that the professional social worker has a key role to play in the care of old people in the community. Indeed, findings of local surveys suggest that the elderly are heavily over-represented in the clientele of social service agencies: in particular, persons aged over 75, those who live alone or with elderly partners and those who experience difficulties with self-care or household tasks as a result of physical or mental infirmity (Dieck 1979; Goldberg and Warbuton 1979). There are, however, no generally accepted guidelines in this field, and many social work departments seem to lack a clear policy in dealing with the elderly. This aspect of social work does not always command interest and enthusiasm, tends to be given low priority, is often relegated to the least trained and experienced staff members and is inadequately represented in training programmes (Radebold 1984; Stevenson 1981). Monitoring studies indicate that most elderly clients are assessed at first contact, given advice or information and, if deemed appropriate, recommended for some form of domiciliary help, after which the case is considered "closed" (Goldberg and Connelly 1982). No doubt the mentally impaired, for whom such an approach would seem unsuitable, figure prominently among the minority of elderly clients who do receive prolonged or intensive support, but if so the numbers involved must be relatively small.

There are now some signs of improvement in this situation. In Britain, the attachment of social workers in certain areas to health centres and general practices represents an important step forward (Clare and Corney 1982). In the Federal Republic of Germany, social "stations" for the elderly have been set up in

1 In this section, the term "social work" is used in the restricted sense of direct professional involvement with individual clients and families in the community. Clearly, social workers may have important tasks in relation to other aspects of social intervention discussed here, just as some traditional social work functions may be shared with other professional or with non-professional groups.

many communities, and a model programme for 18 units of this kind has been undertaken with government support (Brandt 1979). Moreover, these local developments are taking place against a background of change in the functions of social work more generally. Earlier emphasis on open-ended, psychodynamic casework has been giving way, over the past two or three decades, to a more practical, task-oriented approach. The social worker is coming to be seen increasingly as a resource person and a mediator who can also provide skilled personal help in times of crisis. At the same time, a growing awareness of the critical importance of the family as primary care-giver has led to a partial shift in focus from the individual client to the family group: a trend with obvious implications for the care of the elderly (Klusman et al. 1981; Levin et al. 1983). Reviewing these changes, Goldberg and Connelly (1982) conclude that "it is probably the social worker's gatekeeper function, skilled short-term intervention and, above all, her role as mobilizer and co-ordinator of supportive services, that are of crucial importance and need evaluating."

Although there is now an extensive literature on research into the effectiveness of social work (Goldberg and Connelly 1981), few investigations have been focused on the problems of old age, and of these only a handful have made use of a comparative research design. The projects carried out by Blenkner and her associates in New York City (Blenkner et al. 1964) and subsequently in Cleveland (Blenkner et al. 1971) must therefore be regarded as pioneering studies. They illustrate, however, the disadvantages of an approach which fosters the recognition of handicap among the elderly, without a firm policy that support for the handicapped, once identified, should be provided as far as possible in their local communities. The old people in these studies who were allocated to the groups for social worker supervision were later found to have higher rates of institutional admission – and also, incidentally, higher mortality rates – than those placed in matched control groups.

More encouraging are the results of the investigation by Goldberg and her co-workers (1970), in which a sample of 300 old people making contact with social services in one area of London was divided by random allocation into an experimental and a control group. Members of the former group were offered care and support by two experienced psychiatric social workers, whereas those in the latter group had access only to the usual facilities provided by the local social services. A follow-up after 12 months found evidence of greater improvement in the experimental group on a number of indices of health and social functioning, though there was no difference in the frequency of hospital and geriatric-home admission.

Domiciliary Care

Not all forms of social support for the elderly require high levels of training and professional skill. The part played by domiciliary services such as the home help, meals on wheels and mobile laundry agencies may be decisive in enabling many handicapped old people to remain in their own homes. These services should be seen, therefore, as part of the total package of community care of the elderly: a package which also includes general practitioner house calls, home nursing, chiropody and remedial care. Because the personal contacts involved in domiciliary care may be of great significance for the emotional and social well-being of the infirm elderly, there have been proposals that home helps should give first priority to personal care of the client, rather than to cleaning tasks; that they should encourage old people to help themselves as far as possible, and that they should work in closer communication with nurses and social workers (Goldberg and Warbuton 1979).

In those countries with relatively high levels of provision, the multiplicity of different professions and agencies involved in domiciliary care has in recent years received much unfavourable comment (Grunow 1977; Kamerman and Kahn 1976). On the British scene there exists, according to Hopkins (1984), "a hotchpotch of costly and largely autonomous agencies, each with rigid professional demarcations. The co-ordination of these agencies is ineffective and expensive." Demarcation disputes, he adds, must be expected to arise when each member of the so-called team in fact "...has his own captain – often non-playing – off the field." Old people may become alarmed by the tramp of different feet down the garden path. Integrated care, where it exists, has not been generated by the system, but through a deliberate effort to counter the divisive tendencies and conflicts between professional interest groups.

There is evidence that home-help services are often used inefficiently. Goldberg and Connelly (1982) cite a number of local studies which have found no close association between various indicators of need for such services and the pattern of actual provision in elderly populations. This mismatch between need and utilization bears hard on the mentally impaired elderly, because of the difficulty they have in calling attention to their needs and in requesting help. The situation calls, therefore, for a more selective policy of help for those who are severely handicapped, with careful assessment of individual needs, both at the time of first contact and periodically thereafter.

Voluntary Action

In recent years there has been an enormous growth of interest in volunteer, mutual help and self-help movements. The new approaches include sponsorship and promotion of individual voluntary help, organisation of neighbourhood schemes on a part-voluntary, part-paid basis, and self-help initiatives or "pressure groups" formed by relatives and others.

In the Federal Republic of Germany, a stock-taking survey some years ago located nearly 150 self-help groups for old people (Gronemeyer et al. 1979) and the number is growing. A national survey of "good neighbour" schemes in England and Wales, of which there are now several thousand, was carried out by a postal questionnaire enquiry (Abrams et al. 1981). The problems most commonly reported were shortage of helpers and difficulty in recruiting suitable helpers. However, one local scheme (Power and Kelly 1981) was able by means of planned publicity to recruit 63 people, from a total population of 4000, for voluntary work with the aged, and 60 per cent of these were still participating after 18 months. The reservoir of potential helpers may be as high, therefore, as 1% of the general population.

Social workers and other professionals appear to be rather slow in adapting to this development. A British study (Holme and Maizels 1978) found that fewer than 40% of social workers were making use of volunteer help, and then as a rule only for one or two clients each. This reluctance may be largely due to the bureaucratic structure within which the social workers must operate, but no doubt many of them are basically sceptical about the value of voluntary action. Special interest attaches, therefore, to model projects designed to promote better communication and co-ordination between the statutory social agencies and various types of voluntary action. One of the most intriguing schemes, at any rate in its conception, is the Kent Community Project in England (Challis and Davies 1980), in which the participating social workers are each given control of a budget and encouraged to introduce new procedures. To ensure accountability, they are required to record their activities, and the resources they use, on a special case-sheet. The most striking result so far appears to be the recruitment of local people – often neighbours – to perform various helping tasks for small payments. The research team conclude that the social worker's responsibility for a budget encourages a more imaginative use of resources, and a more flexible response to old people's needs, than does the traditional, more bureaucratic approach.

Day Care Services

The aims of day care for the elderly are multiple. Medical aims may include diagnostic assessment, investigation, treatment and rehabilitation of suitable patients, as well as substitution for – or sometimes preparation for – long-term residential care. In addition, however, there are important social functions, including support for bereaved or isolated old people, relief of the strain on caring relatives and alleviation of family crises. The therapeutic and social functions of day care overlap, indeed, to such an extent that it is in practice vital to have close co-operation between day hospitals and day centres, and to ensure a smooth, informal transition from one to the other, as the old person's needs change (Hemsi 1982). Difficulties may arise in achieving this kind of flexibility, because the two types of unit are usually financed and administered by different authorities. It is encouraging that a growing number of partnership schemes have been set up in recent years, and that efforts are being made to evaluate some of these projects (Brandt 1979; Shegog 1981).

Provision of day hospital or equivalent places for the handicapped elderly is still on a very modest scale in most countries. According to a recent survey, for example, there are at most 30 such units in the Federal Republic of Germany (Dahlem 1982). Even if recommended targets of two to three places per 1000 elderly can be reached and if these places are in the event fully utilized, comparison with the epidemiological findings makes it abundantly clear that only a small minority of mentally impaired elderly will be cared for in such units. In order for day care as a whole to make an appreciable impact, large numbers of confused or mentally infirm old people will have to be looked after in centres which do not have medical or psychiatric nursing staff on the premises. Experience in some small projects has shown that this is feasible, and has highlighted the contribution of volunteer helpers who can look after handicapped old people on a one-to-one basis (Goldberg and Connelly 1982). There is a case for extending this type of care by volunteers acting under professional guidance, provided careful supervision and monitoring can be assured.

Few comparative studies of day care have been reported. In one recent British research project (MacDonald et al. 1982), groups of old people in four different types of care setting (day centres, day hospitals, residential homes and long-stay hospital wards) were matched in terms of mental impairment and dependency, and followed up over 9 months. Preliminary findings, using a range of tests, suggest that differences in the type of care do not seem to influence mortality or the severity of mental impairment, but that day care is associated with a lesser degree of dependency. There are, however, obvious difficulties, in this type of non-randomized control study, in excluding confounding variables which may have influenced the original decision concerning the appropriate type of care.

Sheltered Housing and Fostering Schemes

Under modern urban conditions, community housing schemes may fulfil an increasingly urgent need of many old people. Rosenfeld (1978) has described their predicament in graphic terms:

"In the crumbling core of our major cities live many long-time residents – single, insecure, and sometimes sick – fending for themselves in an environment at once familiar but frightening. They huddle in their houses and apartments, fearing the robber and rapist, foraying out for occasional shopping trips, always afraid. Many dream of getting out, of moving to 'someplace nice', but the waiting lists are long for the housing they can afford. Some simply stick it out; others, seeking any route out of constant anxiety, sign into nursing homes. In a more congenial environment, the could manage; bur where they are, it is all too much."

The need is especially apparent among those who are sick or infirm. With or without the benefits of day care, many such persons might be enabled to remain in the general community, if only they could be offered some degree of support and protection in their living situation. This is the aim of sheltered housing projects, and in some places also of fostering or boarding-out schemes for the elderly.

Sheltered housing schemes appear to be highly successful, if one can judge by their growth rate. In England the number of units was estimated at 300 000 in 1975 and at 400 000 5 years later (Goldberg and Connelly 1982). In Federal Germany there are thought to be about 80 000 units (Deutsches Zentrum für Altersfragen 1982, p. 1030), though exact figures are not available. However, the importance of their contribution to mental health care has still to be defined. Critical questions are now arising, as it becomes increasingly apparent that old people, initially accepted as suitable for such accommodation, may be required to leave and to move into institutional care once their health deteriorates. To combat this tendency, there has been a development in some areas of "very sheltered" forms of housing, where severely handicapped old people can remain, and which in effect provide an alternative to geriatric-home care.

Fostering schemes, in marked contrast, appear to be available in only few areas and on a small scale. In such schemes, accommodation is arranged in private households, with persons who are able to offer some degree of help and support, though in practice the amount of care provided may vary a good deal. Facilities of this kind can be useful in giving some respite to family carers, can assist in rehabilitation after hospital discharge, or can give a form of sheltered accommodation over prolonged periods. It is not yet clear which subgroups of the elderly are most likely to benefit from fostering programmes. They may supply a preferable alternative to institutional care for some mentally impaired old people, provided careful selection and supervision of the foster homes is assured.

In Boston, a series of studies were undertaken by Sherwood and her coworkers (1981) to test the effectiveness of community-based alternatives to long-term institutional care. The facilities tested were sheltered congregate housing, foster care homes and public housing with a special alarm system. Preliminary results suggest that institutional admission can be avoided in a proportion of cases; that both congregate housing and foster home care offer feasible alternatives for many elderly persons; that mortality risks are not increased for such persons compared with those in institutional care and, finally, that benefit – cost ratios are relatively high for each type of experimental programme. These are most intriguing findings, whose relevance for services in other countries calls for careful appraisal.

With whatever success community care services for the elderly may be promoted, it is clear from the demographic projections that no fall in the demand for long-stay beds can be anticipated in the next decades: in all probability, the numbers will continue to rise. The implications for mental health care become obvious when one considers that, according to survey findings from a number of industrial countries, over half of all residents in homes for the aged suffer from clinically significant mental disorders. Given the high ratio of geriatric home to psychiatric hospital beds for the elderly, this means that for each mentally impaired old person in psychiatric inpatient care, there are now four to five in geriatric hospitals or homes (Cooper 1984).

The need for active social intervention is underlined by research findings that home residents, like long-stay hospital patients, are often exposed to environmental conditions which aggravate their impairments and compound their handicaps. Townsend (1962) has enumerated six major aspects of social deprivation among the elderly in institutional care; namely (1) loss of occupation and customary activities, (2) loss of independence and self-determination, (3) loss of privacy and personal identity, (4) isolation from family, friends and community, (5) unsatisfactory relationships in the institution and (6) loneliness. What loss of self-determination can mean in practice has been spelt out by Mercer and Kane (1979). For the aged person, they write:

> ...admission to a nursing home is a dramatic departure from life in the community. The range of personal choice is restricted in even the most basic activities – meals, bedtime, rising time, dressing or not dressing, frequency and timing of baths, being with others or being alone, medical examination, use of alcoholic beverages, choice of room-mate, and a host of other details.

The high risk among elderly home residents of becoming socially isolated, as a result of loss of contacts with family and friends, has been documented by a number of empirical studies (Bennett 1980; Cooper et al. 1984).

The relevance for findings such as these of Goffman's (1961) concept of the total institution and its consequences is evident. There is now a growing body of opinion which holds that long-stay homes should not be large, impersonal establishments, but should be planned on a domestic scale – either separately or as semi-autonomous living units within a larger complex – and should be organized to meet the needs of their residents, rather than the convenience of administrators. Increasing attention is being paid to questions of architectural design and construction, to the development of staff training programmes and to the introduction of milieu therapy, reality orientation and other systematic techniques for reducing handicap. While each of these approaches has its importance, there is some evidence that neither a good structural design nor a high ratio of trained staff necessarily leads to good caring practices (Thomas 1981). Equal emphasis must be placed, therefore, on reform and restructuring of the existing care regimes in these establishments.

Those features of the residential environment that are thought to be beneficial represent, in effect, the antithesis of the total institution. They have been enumerated (Goldberg and Connelly 1982) as flexibility of management practice, individual care and encouragement of self-determination among the residents, opportunities for privacy in the home, opportunities for social stimulation and contact with the outside world, social interaction between residents and staff, and a maximum delegation of decision making, combined with a minimum degree of specialization of tasks and roles, among the staff members.

Conclusion

The divisions between geriatric, psychiatric and social forms of care appear largely artificial, when set in relation to the individual needs of old people. The three types of service share in common certain broad aims; namely, to keep the old person active and independent in his own customary environment for as long as possible and, when this can no longer be maintained, to ensure for him an acceptable quality of life in a residential care setting. There is a large degree of consensus among experts as to the kind of service model required to achieve these aims (Shegog 1981). Each area population should have access to a closely co-ordinated group of services, which should include geriatric and psychiatric in-patient units (or joint unit), day hospitals and day centres, homes for the aged, sheltered housing, community-based social workers and domiciliary help. The importance of co-ordination is not confined to the specialist and hospital sectors, but applies equally in the domain of primary care, where general practitioners, community physicians, nurses, social workers and domiciliary agencies must also combine their efforts to meet the needs of individual patients and clients (Williams and Clare 1979). An urgent question for health and social planners, therefore, concerns the manner in which these different professional workers should be deployed so as to achieve a good functional integration. The situation calls for operational and evaluative research, focused on this question. More precisely, it calls for multidisciplinary studies.

The upsurge in recent years of research into various aspects of community care has occurred principally in those countries in which social workers have gained a large measure of professional autonomy; indeed, it can be seen as a by-product of this newly won independence. Most investigations have been planned and undertaken by local social service departments, either alone or in conjunction with university-based social scientists. Whatever the reasons, there has been a dearth of collaborative studies involving geriatricians, psychiatrists or other medical workers. Consequently, even those few studies of the elderly which have made use of a control design and reliable measuring instruments have added little to our knowledge of the special problems and needs associated with mental disorders. Those affected tend to be referred to collectively, in the social work literature, as the "mentally infirm", the "confused", or even simply the "frail" elderly, and to be lumped together in a single category in monaxial social-problem classifications. One result, in an era of rapid progress in neurobiological diagnostic techniques, is a widening of the already formidable gap in communication between neuropsychiatric and social research workers.

The need for improved co-operation and co-ordination between the different disciplines concerned with aging disorders is therefore just as urgent in the field of scientific enquiry as it is in relation to the health and social services. But whereas a better co-ordination between the different services can often be achieved at local level, even within a rigid organizational framework, the available scientific resources are in most countries so few and so scattered that the formation of multidisciplinary working groups at national, or at least at regional, level would seem to be a necessary first step towards the development of an effective programme of applied research.

References

Abrams P, Abrams S, Humphrey R, Snaith R (1981) Action for care: a review of good neighbour schemes. Volunteer Centre, Berkhamsted, England

Bennett R (ed) (1980) Aging, isolation and resocialization. Van Reinhold Nostrand, New York

Blenkner M, Jahn J, Wasser E (1964) Serving the aging: an experiment in social work and public health nursing. Community Service Society, New York

Blenkner M, Bloom M, Nielson M (1971) A research and demonstration project of protective services. Social Casework 52:489–506

Brandt F (1979) Modelle offener Altenhilfe. Schriftenreihe des Bundesministers für Jugend, Familie und Gesundheit, vol 70. Kohlhammer, Stuttgart

Challis D, Davies B (1980) A new approach to community care for the elderly. Br J Soc Work 10:1–18

Clare AW, Corney RH (eds) (1982) Social work and primary health care. Academic Press, London

Cooper B (1984) Home and away: the disposition of mentally ill old people in an urban population. Soc Psychiatry 19:187–196

Cooper B, Mahnkopf B, Bickel H (1984) Psychische Erkrankung und soziale Isolation bei älteren Heimbewohnern: eine Vergleichsstudie. Z Gerontol 17:117–125

Dahlem O (1982) Zu Problemen bei sozialen Diensten für alte Menschen in der BRD. Arch Wiss Praxis Soz Arbeit 13:79–115

Deutsches Zentrum für Altersfragen (1982) Altwerden in der Bundesrepublik Deutschland. Geschichte, Situationen, Perspektiven. vols I–III. D.Z.A., Berlin

Dieck M (1979) Wohnen und Wohnumfeld älterer Menschen in der Bundesrepublik: Bedingungen des Wohnens älterer Menschen in der Bundesrepublik. Quelle and Meyer, Heidelberg

Foster EM, Kay DWK, Bergmann K (1976) The characteristics of old people receiving and needing domiciliary services: the relevance of psychiatric diagnosis. Age and Ageing 5:245–255

Goffman E (1961) Asylums: essays on the social situation of mental patients and other inmates. Doubleday, New York

Goldberg EM, Connelly N (eds) (1981) Evaluative research in social care. Heinemann, London (Policy Studies Institute Series)

Goldberg EM, Connelly N (1982) The effectiveness of social care for the elderly. Heinemann, London (Policy Studies Institute Series)

Goldberg EM, Mortimer A, Williams BT (1970) Helping the aged: a field experiment in social work. Allen & Unwin, London

Goldberg EM, Warbuton RW (1979) Ends and means in social work. The development and outcome of a case review system for social workers. Allen & Unwin, London

Gronemeyer R, Bahr HE et al. (1979) Niemand ist zu alt. Selbsthilfe und Alten-Initiativen. Fischer, Frankfurt

Grunow D (1977) Problemsyndrome älterer Menschen und die Selektivität organisierter Hilfe. Arch Wiss Praxis Soz Arbeit 8:165–195

Hemsi L (1982) Psychogeriatric care in the community. In: Levy R, Post F (eds) The psychiatry of late life. Blackwell, Oxford, pp 252–287

Holme A, Maizels J (1978) Social workers and volunteers. Allen & Unwin, London

Hopkins A (1984) Practical help. Lancet I:1393–1396

Kamerman S, Kahn A (eds) (1976) Social services in the U.S.A. Temple University Press, Philadelphia

Kay DWK, Bergmann K (1980) Epidemiology of mental disorders among the aged in the community. In: Birren JE, Sloane RB (eds) Handbook of mental health and ageing. Prentice Hall, Englewood Cliffs, N.J., pp 34–56

Klusman D, Bruder J, Lauter H, Lüders I (1981) Beziehungen zwischen Patienten und ihren Familienangehörigen bei chronischen Erkrankungen des höheren Lebensalters. (Unpublished research report, University of Hamburg)

Kramer M (1980) The rising pandemic of mental disorders and associated chronic diseases and disabilities. In: Strömgren E, Dupont A, Nielsen JA (eds) Epidemiological research as a basis for organization of extramural psychiatry. Acta Psychiatr Scand 62 [Suppl 285]:382–397

Levin E, Sinclair J, Gorbach P (1983) The supporters of confused elderly persons at home. National Institute for Social Work, London

Lowy L (1980) Mental health services in the community. In: Birren JE, Sloane RB (eds) Handbook of mental health and ageing. Prentice Hall, Englewood Cliffs, N.J., pp 827–853

MacDonald AJD, Mann AH, Jenkins R et al. (1982) An attempt to determine the impact of four types of care upon the elderly in London by the study of matched groups. Psychol Med 12:193–200

Mercer S, Kane RA (1979) Helplessness and hopelessness among the institutionalized aged: an experiment. Health Soc Work 4:91–116

Power M, Kelly S (1981) Evaluating domiciliary volunteer care of the very old: possibilities and problems. In: Goldberg EM, Connelly N (eds) Evaluative research in social care. Heinemann, London, pp 214–234

Radebold H (1984) Altenarbeit. In: Eyferth H (ed) Handbuch zur Sozialarbeit, Sozialpädagogik. Luchterhand, Neuwied, pp 73–83

Rosenfeld AH (1978) New views on older lives. DHEW Publication No. (ADM) 78–687. U.S. Govt. Printing Office, Washington, D.C.

Rückert W (1979) Interventionsmaßnahmen in der BRD: Gegenwärtiger Stand der Altenhilfe. Z Gerontol 12:164–175

Shegog RFA (ed) (1981) The impending crisis of old age. Oxford University Press for Nuffield Provincial Hospitals Trust, Oxford

Sherwood S, Morris JS, Sherwood CC (1981) Cost-effective interventions that prevent or reduce institutionalization. XII. Int. Congress of Gerontology, Hamburg. Abstracts 1:222

Sosna U, Wahl H-W (1983) Soziale Belastung, psychische Erkrankung und körperliche Beeinträchtigung im Alter: Ergebnisse einer Felduntersuchung. Z Gerontol 16:107–114

Stevenson O (1981) The frail elderly – a social worker's perspective. In: Arie T (ed) Health care of the elderly. Croom Helm, London, pp 158–175

Thomas N (1981) Design, management and resident dependency in old people's homes. In: Goldberg EM, Connelly N (eds) Evaluative research in social care. Heinemann, London

Townsend P (1962) The last refuge. Routledge, London

Williams P, Clare AW (eds) (1979) Psychosocial disorders in general practice. Academic Press, London

5.5 Assessment, Prevention and Control of Mental Disorders in the Elderly – Summarising Co-lecture

R. Jones

It is difficult usefully to add to four such highquality papers and impossible to summarise them adequately in a short space. I will attempt only to pick out some key points from each, with some comments of my own, and then add some of our experience in Nottingham to provide further material for discussion.

Dr. Bickel, looking to the prospects for secondary prevention, rightly stresses that comparatively little is known of old age mental disorder in the community. We lack definitive survey instruments to explore more thoroughly. Evidence of an organic psychosyndrome can be detected but we cannot be more specific than this. Mild forms of dementia are not well assessed by current instruments. A similar problem exists with instruments for depression. Whilst some instruments have been extensively used in field studies there remains the problem, both with dementia and depression, of mild forms of disorder and where to draw an appropriate cut-off point between normality and disease. Dementia in particular urgently requires more detailed diagnostic criteria for research – especially with mild degrees as any tools for therapy or secondary prevention must be most likely to be effective in such cases.

Such improved case definition is no less important in depression in old age. High levels of depression have been reported in the elderly community and even higher levels in certain settings, such as an English Social Services Home, as the paper by Dr. Mann and Dr. Graham makes clear. These reports are of great concern but we must be certain we are all talking about the same thing. Clear case definition is obviously crucial to everything else we look at – not least, therapy and outcome.

Turning to Professor Svanborg's paper, the excellence of his longitudinal studies is well known. But his presentation prompts me to some points. Fascinatingly he shows evidence of an important influence of environment, social stimulation and activity on the rate of ageing. We have heard much of the younger onset dementias (type 1) being relatively "endogenous", implying that later onset dementias (type 2) may be more related to environmental factors (Bondareff 1983). There is some evidence that sensory stimulation can be important in actual structural change in the young brain of some organisms. There is evidence of compensatory dendritic branching and growth in the ageing animal brain, and of this growth in humans into old age. Diamond's work suggests the mature rat brain may be induced to such proliferation by an enriched environment (Diamond and Connor 1981). This begins to link together as a coherent story. There is also the report of a fall in the incidence of the dementias in the Lundby study, particularly in the higher age groups (Hagnell et al. 1981). This could be an effect of better environmental conditions on the later cohorts. And we are also reminded of Professor Cooper's work in Mannheim showing a trend towards an increased prevalence of dementia in lower social classes. This again suggests the importance of environmental influences. Professor Svanborg illustrates the value of major longitudinal studies. These and other speculations regarding dementia emphasise the need for a major longitudinal study, specifically on a large group of demented individuals.

Moving to Klaus Bergmann's paper, I would like to insert some points for discussion. His emphasis on the link between depressive disorder – and indeed other old age psychiatric disorder – and physical illness highlights to me the value of joint departments like ours, dealing with all the health of the elderly. Similarly, the work of Elaine Murphy on the social origins of depression, putting together provoking agents and vulnerability factors, identified the threatening life event of serious ill-health as a powerful provoking agent (Murphy 1982). The case for the closest attention to both the psychological and the physical health of the elderly in need is again emphasised.

Concerning deafness and paraphrenia, Herbst, with her study on hearing impairment and the mental state of the elderly at home, highlighted the small proportion of the deaf elderly who actually use hearing aids (Herbst and Humphrey 1980). She noted the likely alienation which could be associated with this and, interestingly, Eastwood recently reported a case of paraphrenic illness apparently controlled by the use of a hearing aid alone (Eastwood et al. 1981).

Summarising a number of avenues to be explored in dementia, Dr. Bergmann alludes also to acute confusional state or delirium. I would like to highlight this area further. The clinical features of this state are in the literature of two thousand years ago. Yet we have made lamentably little progress in therapy and understanding since. We hardly know what the state is in neurophysiological terms but it is a common problem, particularly in the elderly. It is potentially treatable and reversible but often, in fact, leads to death. It seems likely that when it occurs, and certainly when it persists, it is associated with permanent brain defect – but we do not actually know. It seems very likely that different managements or different lines of treatment can achieve much better results than others, but this really has not been looked at properly. There is great scope for improving our knowledge here.

Professor Cooper has contributed a masterly summary but there is only space for me to emphasise a few points. The dominating concern is that whatever we call dementia in the elderly – whether we call it illness or abnormal ageing – the problem will not go away. Under any label there is a massive need in the elderly community for health and social services because of dementia, however we conceptualise it. We are forced to attend to it. Whatever progress we make with neuroradiology or neurotransmitters, we are unlikely to diminish this immediate level of need for some considerable time to come. The name of the game most urgently is proper services – effective services. What is more striking to me in the field of mental health in the elderly is the virtual complete absence of evaluative studies of services. Governments are concerned by the potentially tremendous level of resources required for the elderly and it is pressingly urgent that we establish the most effective, and the most cost-effective, ways of meeting needs and providing services.

The Kent Community Care Project, which is not a psycho-geriatric study, seems to be one of the few evaluative exercises (Challis and Davies 1980). Reportedly, this approach, with social workers all working within allocated shadow budgets to co-ordinate voluntary and statutory support for elderly in the community, has been more cost-effective than traditional ways of working. By definition this has been cheaper than residential care as the "budget" was set well below this level. But some fear the cynical argument that because there has been a reduced mortality with their clientele, decision makers will worry about people being kept alive for longer and costing more over the years in the end. This must make the Kent workers feel they just cannot win.

I am interested by the development of what is called "super-sheltered housing" in Britain. This seems to have potential but, like so much else, needs careful evaluation. But modern technology, particularly microchip technology, now seems to have the capacity to do practically anything we want in terms of monitoring and supervising the disabled elderly. We merely have to invest in the production cost – which brings us back to effectiveness and showing that the cost is worthwhile.

Professor Cooper's final list of research priorities leads back to the need for a co-ordinated multidisciplinary approach and the need to get services working together to meet the multiplicity of needs of the elderly. This, I think, makes it appropriate to say a little about the service model we have developed in Nottingham, which may usefully add more material for our discussion.

The Department of Health Care of the Elderly in Nottingham aims to be readily available, through the general practitioner, to any elderly person in our area. It really does not matter what is wrong, or what the general practitioner thinks is wrong, we encourage him simply to contact us to say there is a health problem and he would like our help. From the point of view of the patient's doctor, the general practitioner, we wish to be seen as a constantly open shop which deals with all the health problems of old people. The core of our Department is a group of old age psychiatrists and old age physicians working together and so we do ask the doctor to say which part of the service he thinks he needs. But we make it clear that he can leave it to us to sort out the most appropriate service. We try to remove, as far as possible, any obstacles inhibiting the doctor from referring. We do not even require a diagnosis – simply an idea of the problem or even just a call for help if that is all that can be given. Referral can be by letter but most are, in fact, by telephone, which we encourage, or even by catching us in the street. The point for general practitioners should be "If you think about referring – do it". More than that, "Whenever you feel there is a problem with an old person, think of us and refer to us". We function as differentiated specialist services – medical and psychiatric – working together, and do not pretend to do each other's work; but we do call on each other and work intimately together with all cases as necessary.

In other words, all the specialist resources of our joint department are available to any patient referred. We cut out accidents of misreferral, games of pass the parcel with the patient; the clinical needs of the patient will be met by our department however the patient comes to us. And further, there will be continuing contact and monitoring as needs change. We will continue to deal with the needs of the patient and his family, or be available to be so involved, as long as those needs exist. It is a touchstone of our approach to give at the outset our reassurance that we will always be available to help.

Being an integrated department also means, I believe, that we bring to bear all aspects of the Health Service more readily for our patients as necessary. Echocardiographic examination becomes available to the psychiatric patient who needs it and the expertise of the clinical psychologist becomes available to the medical patient who needs it. We help to make all the Health Service more available to all our patients. This is so because we combine our expertise – and we even combine yet further with other specialties in our ortho-geriatric unit, for example – and also because we combine our clinical worlds.

Working in this co-operative, integrated way, and very much in a multidisciplinary way, also makes us much more able to work effectively with Social Services. We are probably more flexible and more receptive to their different perspectives because we are already in the business of working with different perspectives. But also, because we deal with all the spectrum of health problems of the elderly, we are a much more useful "business" for them: the shop which deals in everything. They know that there is great benefit from working together with us and, of course, vice versa.

Our service also reaches out into primary care through the medium of our community nurses, who liaise with primary health care team workers and sometimes work fairly directly with general practitioners – though I am sure there is scope for more exploratory work in this area.

This sort of link-up very much illustrates our general approach. Firmly rooted in the local community, we strongly encourage easy early referral and then aim to keep people managing at home as long as decently, humanely possible. The home is where people live and overwhelmingly this is where they wish to stay. To this end we see them at home, assess them at home and aim to help co-ordinate delivery of any necessary support services to the home. This means working together with Social Services, other arms of the Health Service and voluntary agencies. Every patient referred to the psychiatric side of the service is seen at home by a senior psychiatrist and the majority of referrals to the medical side of the department are similarly seen at point of origin.

All our activity is conducted in the full glare of medical student scrutiny. We have medical students with us all through the year. They are constantly watching us grappling with the problems or registering our successes, and constantly, we hope, enthusiastically soaking up all that is good about our approach. Education is very much our business and an integral part of how we work. This is very much so at medical student level, but also for trainee specialists and other specialisms.

This sounds like the description of some perfect ideal which, of course, it is not. But basically our service is straightforward, simple, and very effective – and great fun to work in. So much that is contained in the other papers has surely made it plain that the elderly challenge us with a multiplicity of overlapping problems: physical ill-health, psychological ill-health and social difficulties. This cries out for a co-ordinated, collaborative, integrated response. Unfortunately different services, be they Social Services or Health Services, have not got a terribly good record of co-operating in this manner. At least the record shows there have been problems. An ideal situation would probably be one organisation which met all the needs of the elderly, both for health care and social care. Such a development may come but here, with our department, we are talking about integration of services which are all within the Health Service. All it needs is a little will, and goodwill, for this to be achieved straight away. This style of service, I submit, is an important step forward.

My description of our department has perhaps been rather didactic and certainly enthusiastic, as my purpose has been, of course, to advocate it but also, I would hope, to provoke a desire to study and evaluate this model, and indeed a desire to replicate it.

References

Bondareff W (1983) Age and Alzheimer's Disease. Lancet I:1447

Challis D, Davies B (1980) A new approach to community care for the elderly. Br J Soc Work 10(1):1–18

Diamond MC, Connor JR (1981) A search for the potential of the aging brain. In: Enna SJ et al. (eds) Brain neurotransmitters and age-related disorders. Raven, New York

Eastwood R, Corbin S, Reed M (1981) Hearing impairment and paraphrenia. J Otolaryngol 10:306

Hagnell O, Lanke J, Rorsman B et al. (1981) Does the incidence of age psychosis decrease? Neuropsychobiology 7:201

Herbst KG, Humphrey C (1980) Hearing impairment and mental state in the elderly living at home. Br Med J II:903

Murphy E (1982) Social origins of depression in old age. Br J Psychiatry 141:135

6 Evaluation of Social and Health Service for the (Disabled) Elderly

6.1 The Elderly in the Health Care System: Primary and Specialised Medical Care

C. Godber

Our concepts of the place of the elderly in the health care system tend to be very much influenced by the arrangements which prevail in our own particular countries. These differences owe less to rational planning than to our respective social, political and economic histories and to the varying degree to which the whims and power of the medical profession have been harnessed to the real needs of the population they should be serving. Provision for the elderly has also further varied according to the way the responsibility has been shared between health, social services and private care. The experience which unites most of us has been the inadequate and delayed priority afforded to the elderly in the face of the eminently foreseeable demographic changes.

One country which did positively set out to build up good public services for the elderly when there was still the money to do it was Denmark, and we have much to learn from their experience (Ammundsen et al. 1982; Godber 1982). An important key to their policy was the philosophy that the provision for those with chronic handicap should be regarded primarily as a social service, with specific input from health only when needed. This, coupled with the political pressure for high-quality services for old people, had the advantage that it gave prime emphasis to maintaining the integrity of the individual and his personal environment, especially in the setting of long-stay institutions. In retrospect the high standard of their nursing homes probably led the Danes to invest too heavily in institutional care and there were not really reciprocal economies in the use of hospital beds. They have, though, responded in recent years with some excellent initiatives in community care.

The choice of an Englishman rather than a Dane to give this paper presumably relates to the fact that it is within its Health Service that some of Britain's more creditable developments have taken place. The poor quality of many of our long-stay hospitals and a relatively low health budget have contributed to a strong emphasis on community care. The NHS has always placed heavy reliance on good general practice and has built up the primary care team with its community nursing service through which initiatives in prevention can be developed. In my view one of our major contributions has also been the emergence of the specialties of Geriatric Medicine and Psychiatry, with their different approaches to treatment and rehabilitation of the elderly and their emphasis on multidisciplinary team work and careful rationing of resources. In this paper I will be using this framework to look at what I see as the main growing points in primary and secondary health care for the elderly. I will apologise in advance if my viewpoint sounds rather parochial and if the emphasis is rather heavily on the delivery as opposed to the evaluation of services. As a full-time clinician I am really only competent to point out to others the areas of progress which they might usefully evaluate.

The General Practitioner

Although endorsing the primary care team as the proper centre of gravity of a health service I hasten to admit that its performance in relation to the elderly often leaves much to be desired, in Britain as elsewhere. This subject was recently usefully reviewed by four primary care physicians from Europe and the United States in a report for the Kellogg International Scholarship programme (Almind et al. 1983). They noted the unreliability of the perception of their health needs by many old people and their doctors, and the barriers that inevitably result in a system based on self-referral. It was stressed that these barriers might be reduced by better communication on the part of doctors and their staff, by a readiness to visit old people at home and by ensuring a simple system for 24-hour availability of personal primary medical care. This point echoes the recommendation by a recent WHO Working Group (WHO Regional Office for Europe 1983) for training of primary care workers to act as guides into and through "the system" for their elderly clients.

Better education on the needs and disabilities of the elderly would also improve the performance of GPs on a number of fronts. Their assessment of their older patients should take account of the frequency of multiple pathology, of masked presentation of such common disorders as depression and of the importance of housing conditions and social support networks in determining outcome in both acute and chronic illness. In common with many observers in this field the Kellogg group emphasised the importance of functional (as opposed to a narrow medical) assessment and suggested the development of functional checklists as an aid to those working in primary care. As a corollary to this the GPs should improve team work with other agencies (such as social and paramedical services, voluntary organisations and hospital specialists) to facilitate a joint focusing on the needs of the elderly patient and his carers rather than leave them to bounce from one service to another. As part of his wider role in the primary care team the GP should also participate in health education, support and liaise with neighbourhood groups involved with the elderly, and help to identify those elderly particularly at risk.

Case Finding

This leads to the question of the iceberg of undetected disability highlighted by Williamson et al. (1964) and many others since. As he has pointed out, doctors tend to concentrate on the more striking medical signs and symptoms familiar to them from their hospital training, to the detriment of sometimes more important problems for the patient and his family, such as incontinence, poor mobility, dementia and depression. This can be remedied to some extent by better training of GPs in the problems of old age, by strengthening such services as chiropody and domiciliary physiotherapy and by the influence within the primary care team of nurses with special experience in such fields as psychogeriatrics or incontinence. As with the incorporation of marital and other counsellors in the primary care team, GPs are likely to show a more positive and discerning approach to problems on the fringe of their own competence if they know that those with the appropriate skills or advice are at hand.

The other part of the iceberg comprises the conditions which do not even reach the GP's attention. Experience with screening (in the strict sense of detecting asymptomatic pathology) has shown itself to be largely fruitless in the elderly. As Williamson has emphasised in a recent review of this topic (Williamson 1981), attention needs to be focused on case finding. This is particularly relevant in the mental health field since depression, dementia and paranoid illness are conditions in which self-referral may be inhibited by apathy or lack of insight, and relatives and friends may mistakenly attribute the changes simply to "old age". Depressive illness is also frequently missed because it may manifest itself simply through its exacerbation of symptoms of physical impairment or of difficulty with coping with bereavement, illness or other life events. Work here in Mannheim has shown something of this interaction and of the differing yield of cases by different types of epidemiological approach (Cooper et al. 1982). A number of general practice case-finding studies have been reported (e.g. Tulloch and Moore 1979; Vetter et al. 1984). Postal questionnaires have shown a reasonable yield though there is always the likelihood that depression and dementia will be over-represented among the non-responders. Williamson and others have trained nurses for this type of work (Williamson 1981).

Who Should Do the Case Finding?

In Britain preventive work of this sort has tended to fall on Health Visitors (nurses with extra training geared towards preventive aspects of child care), though in my view the difference in the clientele and their problems makes this inefficient and uneconomical. Our other main species of domiciliary nurse, the District Nurse, is certainly predominantly involved with the elderly but with the emphasis on specific nursing procedures with the severely disabled. I would therefore favour the development of a cadre of nurses with an aptitude for and interest in preventive work specifically with the elderly. They would need appropriate extra training to include a functional approach to assessment, recognition of the marker symptoms of such treatable disorders as depression and the use of simple physical and mental state schedules. They would also need to know the scope of treatment and facilities available to ameliorate the conditions they uncovered and to be able to advise and direct their clients accordingly. Such nurses could also become crucial links between the primary health team and other services involved with the elderly (including social services, housing departments, voluntary groups and relevant hospital specialties).

This sort of arrangement has developed in a few areas in Britain (Norman 1982) but has been inhibited by anxieties over the proliferation of sub-specialties within nursing, some of which stem from vested interests within the specialties that already exist – a reaction with which those specialising in the elderly are only too familiar. As Tulloch and Moore (1979) have stressed, however, there is also the more cogent fear that effective case finding is bound to increase demand, in the short term at least, for a variety of medical, paramedical and social services. As these are likely, however, to result in a reduction of handicap and of the load on carers there should be a lessening of demand in the longer term, especially on the more expensive hospital and residential care. It will of course be by these latter criteria rather than mortality rates that the value of such intervention will need to be measured.

There is no denying, however, that such case finding will incur expense in the early stages at least. In many cases it will also necessitate ongoing surveillance of those so identified. Its cost-effectiveness will depend on the size of the target population. Morbidity rates have been shown to rise steeply from the late 70s and the peak onset for dementia is probably around 80 years of age. From the mental health point of view, therefore, it would be best to aim at the over 80s but also at those over 75 who are living alone, who have recently experienced major illness, bereavement or change of accommodation or who are requesting extra domiciliary social services or residential placements. Such groups are commonly identified as appropriate for listing on at-risk registers.

Secondary Care

The elderly are majority consumers in many areas of specialist and hospital care. This particularly applies in such specialties as orthopaedics, ophthalmology and urology, where technical advances have brought many of the specific disorders of old age within the scope of their treatment. The increasing number of very elderly people and their rather slower recovery and discharge rates have also led to a steady rise in their occupancy of other acute hospital beds.

Many of these patients fit poorly into the acute curative model on which hospitals still tend to base their care; furthermore they may need little of the high technology that makes such beds so expensive. Instead they more often require the careful rehabilitation and planning for discharge which tends to fall outside the interest and skills of the average medical or surgical specialist. This may result in frail old people being discharged precipitately into situations in which they or their carers cannot cope, or alternatively in their being "written off" to long-term institutional care which might have been avoided with better assessment and rehabilitation. These dilemmas are especially likely if there is pressure on a limited pool of hospital beds and may lead to reluctance to admit elderly people in the first place, which may again divert them inappropriately into residential or nursing homes from which they are unlikely to emerge.

Specialised Services for the Elderly

It was this sort of climate that gave rise in Britain to the emergence of the specialty of Geriatric Medicine, and more recently of Geriatric Psychiatry (which for simplicity I will refer to hereafter as Psychogeriatrics). These specialties have had to struggle against the prejudice and inertia of the medical establishment and often a low quality and quantity of the resources available to build up their services. Nevertheless, they have achieved a great deal and, at their best, have undoubtedly produced better and more broadly based services to the very elderly than those achieved by general physicians and psychiatrists alone (Isaacs 1981; Horrocks 1982).

In the process they have added much to the body of knowledge on the disorders of old age and have brought new expertise and optimism to their management. Unfortunately the heavy work-load entailed has often limited those building up such services to descriptive accounts rather than proper evaluation (Arie 1970; Jolley and Arie 1978).

Geriatric Psychiatry (Psychogeriatrics)

In the mental health field the acid test of a specialist service must be its impact on the problems of dementia. Good initial assessment and treatment may of themselves greatly reduce the behavioural problems and complicating factors due to other psychiatric or physical conditions, with resulting benefit to the patient and those caring for him. They will also help in the planning of future care and may avoid or postpone admission to institutions (Krakauer 1978).

A crucial part of the service, however, will be its longer term support of families caring for demented patients, an aspect on which I have elaborated in more detail at a previous WHO meeting (WHO Regional Office for Europe 1983). Essentially this entails surveillance, help in crises and the gradual feeding in of support and relief as the disability advances. In our service the key role is played by psychogeriatric community nurses who also liaise closely with GPs and the nurses of the primary care team. This support is backed up by admission to hospital both on a regular planned basis and to cope with sudden deterioration or crises. Day care is also provided for some patients and my colleague has recently introduced a sitting service using volunteers to supervise patients in their own homes for defined periods to give their carers a break (Rosenvinge 1986). This latter project is being evaluated and seems to be reducing demand on the other parts of the service, incuding the ultimate long-stay admission. Since the psychogeriatric service was started 10 years ago we have monitored the work-load and use of beds. The latter has shifted strongly from custodial towards short-term care; we now have less than half the number of beds occupied by long-stay patients and there is no longer a waiting list for these. This has released beds for short-term use and has also given us the space to provide a comprehensive service for elderly patients with functional illness. Referral rates increased markedly with the introduction of the service and again when a second consultant was appointed and the catchment area extended. In each case the referrals then settled somewhat as if we had worked through a backlog. In 1983, from a population of 50 000 people over the age of 65, we had 730 new cases referred and about 950 admissions. During the year 3.5% of the elderly population were in contact with the service, which contrasts interestingly with the contact rate noted in Cooper's study (Cooper et al. 1982).

The support for demented patients and their families was recently compared with that in a district without a specific psychogeriatric service in a detailed study sponsored by the Department of Health (Ball et al. 1983). The findings were strongly in support of the specialised psychogeriatric service but in both cases emphasised the need for closer collaboration, especially in planning, between different services impinging on the disabled elderly. One's overall impression is that this extension of the psychogeriatric service into community assessment and support, and the guarantee of short-term hospital back-up when needed, has substantially improved the morale of family carers and the tolerance of staff in the residential sector. At the same time it seems to have reduced the pressure on institutional care and inappropriate use of expensive resources in the general hospitals.

What impact, however, can the specialised psychogeriatric service have in the area of treatment and prevention? It is certainly my impression that depressive illness in the elderly has been viewed too pessimistically by the main body of psychiatry. Our experience has been that recognition of the different manifestations that may occur, coupled with an active and eclectic approach to treatment, may produce far better results than the literature would imply (Murphy 1983; Godber 1983). We are currently engaged in a study in which we hope to substantiate these feelings. We have certainly noted a marked increase in the recognition and referral of depression in the elderly by GPs in our district and 55% of our new referrals are of functional illness. This would suggest some impact on Williamson's "hidden iceberg".

It is true that this sort of work is limited to secondary and tertiary prevention but it remains the major priority in this field at present. Copeland (1982) has demonstrated the high prevalence of depression among patients in geriatric and medical units which is a reminder of its cost in terms of failed rehabilitation and delayed recovery. This is just one example of how closer working between Psychogeriatrics and other medical specialties, particularly Geriatric Medicine, may help reduce the cost of general hospital care.

As with its medical counterpart, Geriatric Psychiatry has an important educational and liaison role with the many disciplines which impinge on the elderly. In our unit we have been encouraged by the number of our General Psychiatry trainees who have subsequently decided to specialise in Psychogeriatrics, having learned that it can be a stimulating, rewarding and, above all, useful branch of medicine in which to work. Arie (1983) has stressed the value of the model service for the elderly as a framework for teaching medical students. Coupled with the clear need for more evaluative work on the effects of such services, this argues strongly for the establishment of more such departments in teaching centres.

Conclusion

I must reiterate in my concluding remarks that the clinical and administrative work of managing a busy service limits one's familiarity with the literature and with those researching in this field. The many omissions in this paper merely testify to that. I would stress, however, that we are in this field very much at the pioneering stage. In this we have demonstrated that the scope for supportive management of dementia and treatment of the more reversible psychiatric disorders of old age is much greater than is generally appreciated. The epidemiologists have shown us the size of the problem and the demographers and economists the need to contain it more efficiently. The priority now is to examine the models which appear to be succeeding and to spread the findings to the planners and those in primary medical care who will have to be most involved in putting them into practice.

References

Almind G, Freer CB, Gray JAM, Warshaw G (1983) The contribution of the primary care doctor to the medical care of the elderly in the community. Report from the Kellogg International Scholarship, Programme on Health and Aging. University of Michigan and University of Copenhagen

Ammundsen E et al. (1982) The elderly in Denmark: demographic, economic social and health conditions. Dan Med Bull 29:89–168

Arie T (1970) The first year of the Goodmayes psychiatric service for old people. Lancet II:1179–1182

Arie T (1983) Organisation of services for the elderly, implications for education and patient care. Experience in Nottingham. In: Bergener M (ed) Geropsychiatric diagnostics and treatment. Springer, New York

Ball C, Coleman P, Wright J (1983) The practicalities of achieving collaboration between hospital and community based services for the elderly mentally infirm. Report on a Research Study for DHSS, vol I

Cooper B, Cletthr G, Abt H-G (1982) Psychiatric disorder physical impairments and disability among the elderly in an urban community. In: Magnussen G, Nielsen J, Buch J (eds) Epidemiology and prevention of mental illness in old age. ECV, Denmark

Copeland JRM (19829 Mental illness among the elderly in London. In: Magnussen G, Nielsen J, Buck J (eds) Epidemiology and prevention of mental illness in old age. EGV, Denmark

Godber C (1982) A happier old age in Denmark. Br Med J 284:1729–30

Godber C (1983) Depression in old age. Br Med J 287:758

Horrocks P (1982) The case for geriatric medicine as an age related specialty. Recent advances in geriatric medicine 2. Churchill Livingstone, Edinburgh

Isaacs B (1981) Is geriatrics a speciality? In: Arie T (ed) Health care of the elderly. Croom Helm, London

Jolley DJ, Arie T (1978) Organisation of psychogeriatric services. Br J Psychiatry 132:1–11

Krakauer R (1978) Health screening in residential homes. Lancet II:625–626

Murphy E (1983) The prognosis of depression in old age. Br J Psychiatry 142:111–119

Norman A (1982) Mental illness in old age: meeting the challenge. Centre for Policy on Ageing, London

Rosenvinge H (1986) Sittingservice for the elderly confused: part of an integrated programme of management. Health Trends 17: in press.

Tulloch AJ, Moore V (1979) A randomised controlled trial of geriatric screening and surveillance in general practice. J R Coll Gen Pract 29:733–742

Vetter NJ, Jones DA, Victor CR (1984) Effect of health visitors working with elderly patients in general practice – a randomised controlled trial. Br Med J I:269–272

WHO Regional Office for Europe (1983) Services to prevent disability in the elderly. Report on a WHO Meeting, Copenhagen. (EURO Reports and Studies No 83)

Williamson J (1981) Screening, surveillance and case-finding. In: Arie T (ed) Health care of the elderly. Croom Helm, London

Williamson J, Stokes IH, Gray S, Fisher M, Smith A (1964) Old people at home: their unreported needs, Lancet I:1117–20

6.2 Open and Closed Health Care for the Elderly: Comparison of Family and Home Care

A. Mann, N. Graham

Introduction

The majority of the mentally ill elderly stay within their own homes; only approximately 6% in the United Kingdom are in institutional care. In Western Europe, the numbers of the very old – and therefore the numbers of the mentally ill – among the elderly population will increase disproportionately in the next two decades. Every country provides some form of care for the mentally ill elderly, but because of the population shift there is likely to be increased demand. Therefore, examination of the type and quality of care provided to this group is a matter of urgency.

This paper will examine some necessary components for high-quality care, both at home and in institutions. Research data that are relevant to the current status of the care in each setting will be presented, and some indicators that could be used to show the quality of care will be suggested. Because of the authors' experience, the account will be from the United Kingdom perspective.

Care of the Mentally Ill Elderly in Their Own Homes

The pressure within the United Kingdom has been to maintain the elderly at home as long as possible. This laudable movement depends for its results upon the compliance of the families and/or other supporters and then upon local health and social services. The burden on relatives, who are probably the key to successful home care, is great. The particular effect upon others of maintaining the mentally ill, in this case confused, at home has been shown in a recent research study (Levin et al. 1984). The essential requirements of care for the elderly mentally ill in their own homes will be summarised first:

1. Early identification of mental health problems. The family doctor is the keystone of this activity in the United Kingdom, for every elderly person is registered with such a doctor.
2. Comprehensive assessment of health care problems by the family doctor, with a nurse and/or social worker.
3. Timely referrals to appropriate specialists.
4. Continuing back-up and follow-up by family doctors, physicians, psychiatrists, social workers and community nurses.
5. Active medical and nursing attention by the family doctor and nursing team.
6. Information, advice and counselling on medical problems.
7. Practical and regular help with household and personal care.
8. The provision of breaks, either day care or relief admissions.

9. Financial support.
10. Availability of long-term residential care.

How well these standards are being met and the size of the burden for supporters will now be illustrated by a study in London and its suburbs, directed from the National Institute of Social Work, London. A sampling frame of 900 confused elderly (defined as being over 65 with clear-cut problems in remembering recent events, carrying out everyday tasks, concentration, etc.) living at home and known to community agencies was drawn up. From this frame, a sample of 150 was selected randomly, the sample being stratified into three by size of support system (alone, with one supporter, with two or more spporters). The elderly were interviewed by the research psychiatrists for diagnosis, using the Geriatric Mental State (Copeland et al. 1976) while the supporters were given detailed interviews by social work colleagues. The patient and supporters were re-interviewed a year later.

Of the elderly so identified, 80% were diagnosed as demented, 42% severely so. Sixty per cent had had this condition for less than 5 years, the remainder for more than 5 years. There was a highly significant correlation between the severity of dementia and other reported problems such as falls, incontinence and complaints of pain. It was therefore apparent that a frail, mentally impaired group, who were being maintained at home, had been identified. Interviews with the supporters, approximately half of whom were spouses and half children, showed the following: Most had lived with their elderly relatives for a long time, an average of 36 years. They were close to their elderly relative, wanting to keep him or her at home. Indeed, only 13% initially reported that they would opt for residential care for their relative, if offered. Nevertheless, the age of the supporters averaged 61; two-thirds described themselves as being only in average or poor health, and 50% had some medical disability. Only one-third carried on any kind of significant activity outside the home. Seventy-five per cent reported stress, and one-third – approximately double the expected population rate – indicated probable psychiatric morbidity by questionnaire. Their complaints fell into two broad areas: (a) the elderly person's behaviour and the consequent difficulties in interpersonal relationships, and (b) the effects on their own lives, i.e. a restricted social life and the hard work involved in practical help. Those looking after the most disabled elderly were likely to report the most stress, and to give a positive response to the standard questionnaire indicating psychiatric morbidity. All supporters were grateful for the support services they received. These were: Home Helps providing some assistance with thc routine household work; District Nurses for help with their relative's personal care, such as getting in and out of bed, bathing and dealing with incontinence; Community Psychiatric Nurses for help with persistent and difficult behaviour; day care, allowing the supporter to go out; and relief care, in which case the supporter can go on holiday. Many supporters said that they would like to receive more of these services. There were also considerable deficiencies; for example, 45% of the incontinent were unknown to the visiting nurse, and only 17% of the supporters had been offered any kind of relief.

One year later, 20% of the elderly had died and 30% were in institutional care. Stress reported by the relative at initial assessment predicted that the relative was more likely to be in care 1 year later. An improvement in reported stress was associated with the death or admission of an elderly relative. It was also shown that services are instrumental in maintaining the supporters. Those receiving Home Helps, for example, were least likely to have relatives in care 1 year later, and those with most regular nursing and home help showed the lowest levels of stress.

The results of this study, summarised here, highlight some of the critical features of care in the home. The role of behavioural and interpersonal difficulties – a consequence of the illness of the elderly relative – in producing complaints of stress from the supporter was apparent. The predictive power of such reported stress for the failure of continuing home care has been demonstrated, as have some protective factors for those wishing to operate a satisfactory system of home care. What indicators might there be that a system is running effectively? The following are suggested:

1. There should be no gaps in the system. An ideal community service is one in which no family requiring help for their mentally ill relative is unknown to providers.
2. Behavioural and interpersonal difficulties resulting from the mental illness of the elderly relative should be minimised. Medical nursing or psychological help should be given when appropriate. Failing any improvement, at least some regular contact is invaluable for those living with the disturbed person so that they feel that others know of their difficulties.
3. Stress on the supporter as measured by objective test and by self-report should be low. Personal stress can be relieved by linking each supporter into a system that can respond both by counselling and by relief, by means of the provision of day care or holiday breaks. Supporters, too, should have their "tied" time minimised, allowing them to take up leisure or occupational interests outside the home.
4. For any home care system to be effective, it must operate within economic bounds. Thus duplication and unnecessary provision of services should be avoided.

The above four indicators are all amenable to survey research, preferably conducted by those not directly involved in the provision of care, to minimise bias. Thus the elderly themselves in their homes, their supporters or those providing care could be the subjects. Findings are then fed back to the service planners so that corrective measures can be implemented.

Care for the Elderly and Mentally Ill in Institutions

The extent to which at-home help has developed for the mentally ill elderly varies considerably between the developed countries. Every country, however, has long required some form of institution to house some of this group – those with mental illness of such severity that home support is no longer possible, or those with less severe illness but with no supporter available. It is interesting to compare how different countries have developed such institutions, a recent collaboration between research teams in New York, London and Mannheim having produced some idea of this (Mann et al. 1984). Despite their quite different histories and political and social structures, each of these cities has provided places for between 4% and 5% of their elderly population. However, in New York, two-thirds of these places are in settings that provide skilled nursing to their residents, one-third in a residential setting that provides help with practical daily activities only. In London the proportions are reversed. Mannheim lies between the two, with approximately 50% skilled nursing places and 50% residential places. The study also demonstrated that, in terms of dementia and dependence upon others, the populations housed within these three differing systems of care are probably similar. It seems, therefore, that in one city some people would be treated with a medical regime, whereas in another they might have been placed in a residential setting. Such a finding makes unclear the right way to look after a frail elderly population needing care, many of them with severe mental illness.

As with care in the home, some desirable criteria for a residential care system might be listed. These should be acceptable in most cultures.

1. Admission to residential care occurs after all alternatives have been exhausted, and with the understanding and participation of the elderly person.
2. The health and dependency need are assessed at entry to residential care and are regularly reviewed afterwards; unnecessary medication is avoided, particularly for behavioural difficulties.
3. The subject should not become demoralised or clinically depressed while living in the care system.
4. The institutional system should be a pleasant one, accessible to amenities for residents able to go out and for families to visit.
5. There should be a sense of personal care for each resident, i.e. the institutionalising rituals should be at a minimum.
6. Dependency needs should be met with speed and willingness, and the facilities be flexible enough to contain altering states of dependency (i.e. periods of illness) without the need to transfer the resident.
7. There should be recreation and diversion provided for the resident.
8. Staff should have a high morale, tend to stay in their jobs and be sympathetic to and cognisant of the manifestations of mental and physical illnesses of old age.
9. Finally, and as a general overall criterion, residents, their families and the professional staff should together sense that they are participating in a worthwhile enterprise.

As is suggested by the three-city study, these aims are being approached differently, for no-one is sure of the *right* way of delivering high-quality care. This uncertainty can be illustrated by the issue of the size of the institution. Some propose institutions of at least 100 residents, for it then becomes economical to provide ancillary amenities, such as hairdressing or shops on site for the residents, and to employ full-time professionals, such as physiotherapists and occupational therapists. However, institutions of this size can be impersonal, with many staff on shift-work not familiar to the residents. Thus, small units of six to ten elderly residents are promoted, these being perhaps converted houses with one or two staff to work in each. Here, the non-professional, home-like atmosphere should be pleasanter and a resident with dementia more able to become familiar with surroundings and staff. However, a danger is lack of social stimulus and lack of adequate health care supervision.

How best, therefore, to decide on such issues as size, type of staff or administrative policy for an institution, so that high-quality care is provided? A properly designed research study would require random allocation and follow-up of frail elderly to separate institutions that were identical apart from the particular variables, such as size or staffing ratio, that are to be studied. Such pure research is impossible. A second approach, therefore, is to make a "natural" experiment by comparison of the differing existing systems. As indicated above, New York, Mannheim and London have in fact all made decisions – probably not knowingly or with any coherent plan in mind – on the type of care that they are going to provide for their elderly. Their decisions have differed. In the published comparative study to examine the implication of the differences, a randomly drawn sample of female residents from across the care system in each city was selected, each resident being given a standard interview that elicited evidence of dementia, depression and dependence on others. Staff members were interviewed for details of their training, daily tasks and ambitions. It appeared from the results that the three resident samples contained very similar prevalence rates of dementia and impairment in activities of daily living. However, because of the shape of the London system, with its preponderance of places in a residential setting, many demented and physically dependent people were found in that sector. These residents were similar in profile to those elderly in the nursing sector of that city's care system. In the other two cities, in contrast, there appeared to be a much greater impairment amongst those in the nursing sector compared with those in the residential sector.

Another striking feature of the study was that London residents in both the residential and nursing sectors seemed more depressed than in the other two cities, the contrast being most marked within the residential sector. Depression in this study, because of the nature of the screening questionnaire, implies both the concept of demoralisation and of clinical depression. An interesting finding, too, was that the staff (nurses' aides) interviewed in London reported far less training in aspects of recognition and management of mental illness than their counterparts in the other two cities.

This study was an initial foray using a brief screening instrument, and the findings concerning depression could have many explanations other than the London system being inherently a more disadvantageous one. It must be noted that a comparison of medications prescribed for residents in London and New York indicated that New York residents received many more prescriptions than did those in London. A sharp contrast was found for the demented in care, who were significantly more likely to receive phenothiazines in New York than in London.

It is possible, using data from this study, to draw up a list of indicators that might reflect the quality of care in an institution:

1. The prevalance of demoralisation and depression amongst residents. The presence of these must imply inadequate recognition and management of clinical depression, inadequate physical help and lack of social stimulus.
2. The proportion of residents with uncorrected or unaided disabilities. Here one might note deficiencies in sight, hearing, dentition and chiropody.

3. The proportion of residents with unrecognised dependency needs. This is perhaps controversial; many people suggest that provision of help removes the capacity for independent behaviour. A more cynical view would call this argument a rationale for doing nothing.
4. The presence of staff meetings to discuss and diagnose reasons for undesirable or disruptive behaviour.
5. Evidence of continuity of care. It is important that residents and staff do not become anxious during a phase of illness or recovery that a particular resident may be unable to stay in the institution in which he or she is settled owing to legal requirements or staffing problems.
6. Whether visitors are regularly seen on the premises, report that they enjoy coming, and find it an agreeable place to bring the family.
7. Whether staff stay at their job, report that they are happy, and can be seen to respond professionally and competently to the various demands placed upon them.
8. Evidence of innovation and imagination in the plans of the administrators of the institution.

These suggestions for markers of high-quality care are amenable to research either by interviews with residents and staff or by some form of observational approach.

Comparison of Care in the Home with Institutional Care

In the last 25 years, policy in Britain has been towards community care and away from any kind of institutional care of the elderly, following harrowing accounts of life in long-stay hospitals for elderly physically and mentally ill. The motive is a humane one, but in fact there has been little objective research comparing these two modes of care for quality of life and outcome. Methodological difficulties in mounting follow-up studies of frail elderly are considerable. The major ones are:

1. Entry criteria are complicated: Age, sex and the presence of dementia, dependency or depression all need consideration.
2. Mortality and morbidity both cause a high drop-out for follow-up, the latter causing transfer from the home to institutional care.
3. There are many confounding variables that may affect the follow-up period, such as death of a spouse or change in staff in a residential home. Analysis is therefore complicated.

One study aimed to compare day-care and residential care (MacDonald et al. 1982) in London illustrated all these problems. The results of this large-scale follow-up study were therefore inconclusive. However, this relative failure was compensated by the development and use of a method of direct non-participant observation for use with older people. This method allows an observer to record and quantify activities and personal contacts of elderly subjects in various care settings (Godlove et al. 1980). This method is a way of gauging quality of life in care settings, and is a promising development, as the observation data are quantifiable and thus amenable to analysis.

In Britain, because of the pressure towards community care, there has been a neglect of the potential of residential care. Visits abroad do allow many British workers to see that residential life for the frail and mentally ill need not be as dispiriting as it often appears at home. There is much to learn, while others may benefit from the study of the community and day-care provision that have been pioneered in the United Kingdom. One way forward for all of us in raising the quality of care for the elderly is to keep an open mind, to realise that one's own practice is not necessarily the best or the only one.

References

Copeland JRM, Kelleher MJ, Kellett JM, Gourlay AJ, Gurland B, Sears JL, Sharpe L (1976) A semi-structural clinical interview for the diagnosis of mental state in the elderly. Psychol Med 6:439–450

Godlove C, Richard L, Rodwell G (1980) Time for action (an observation study of elderly people in four different care environments). Social Services Monographs: Research in Practice, University of Sheffield

Levin E, Sinclair I, Gorbach P (1984) The supporters of confused elderly persons at home. National Institute for Social Work Research Unit, Tavistock Road, London

MacDonald AJD, Mann AH, Jenkins R, Richard L, Godlove C, Rodwell A (1982) An attempt to determine the impact of four types of care upon the elderly in London by the study of matched groups. Psychol 12:193–200

Mann AH, Wood K, Cross P, Gurland B, Schieber P, Häfner H (1984) Institutional care of the elderly: a comparison of the cities of New York, London and Mannheim. Soc Psychiatry 19:97–102

6.3 Community Care for Psychiatric Patients

S. Kanowski

"Historically these forms of care preceded institutionalization and continue to provide most services required; community and home care are old ideas that are currently being rediscovered." (Maddox 1980)

Planning of psychogeriatric care systems has to take into consideration the following aspects of mental illness in old age:

– High prevalence of different types of psychic disorder
– Multimorbidity
– Avoidance reactions of older people against psychiatric institutions
– Negative stereotypes held by professional and nonprofessional care-givers against aging as a threatening phase of life
– High risk of psychogeriatric patients being ignored, misdiagnosed, mistreated and placed in an inappropriate treatment setting
– High social vulnerability of older individuals

Each of these problem areas underlines the need for well-developed community-based services. The demand for better organized ambulant care delivery systems is further stressed by epidemiological studies showing that most of the emotionally or mentally ill elderly are living within the community and outside of institutions for long-term care.

Roth (1973), after giving a detailed analysis of the contemporary situation, starts his recommendations for future developments as follows:

"First, facilities for community care for the aged, and the domiciliary services, in particular, require immediate expansion if institutions are not to become gravely over-burdened, and serious encroachment upon the services available to the remainder of the population is to be avoided."

For nearly two decades there has been strong pressure from professionals and the public to reorganize psychiatric services, devoting more efforts to ambulant care programs; hence one might have expected a substantial improvement of ambulant care for older mentally ill individuals. However, Lowy (1980), analyzing the development of mental health services in the community from a sociogerontological viewpoint reaches a rather pessimistic conclusion: "When reviewing history, it seems that the encouragement of community mental health programs may, indeed, have been detrimental to solving the mental health needs of the older population instead of beneficial – as originally envisioned." He refers to the unchanged rate of 2.4 per 100 000 people over 65 being treated by outpatient clinics between 1963 and 1971 and explains the state of the affairs by the reluctance of the community mental health centers to accept older patients and of the older patients to make use of these new services.

Maddox (1980), although in favor of alternatives to strictly medicalized service models, notes in his critical overview of the movement toward the community: "The efficiency and effectiveness of alternatives to the current organization of service continues to be asserted rather than systematically demonstrated." The need for carefully designed research is convincingly demonstrated by Dunlop (1980). He summarizes his commentary as follows: "Benefits assumed by those calling for massive expansion of home health care to include preventive health-supportive services for the dependent aged..... have been the objects of inadequate research and reflection. Advocates are unable to specify exactly what kind of person could benefit or who would seek to use such services."

What emerges from the literature so far appears to be an unsatisfying ambiguity. On the one hand, all authors argue in favor of community-based services for the aged population for several and good reasons; on the other hand, such programs have either not been overwhelmingly successful or have been evaluated rather poorly. I shall now try to discuss some of the problems and barriers that may account for the present state of the art.

Complexity of the Field/Institutional Fragmentation and Competition

More obviously than during earlier periods of life, the development of mental illness in old age is a result of a complex texture of various biological, psychological, and social factors breaking down the individual's coping mechanisms and adaptive capacities. Therefore, there is no single or simple therapeutic approach to cure or improve mental illness in old age. On the contrary, it is imperative to base each individual therapeutic regimen on a comprehensive diagnostic procedure and assessment of the individual's remaining capacities.

Due to specialization of medical and social services, comprehensive diagnostics and therapy involve multiple professional skills which in reality are rarely offered to the population in need in a properly and adequately organized institutional setting. Fragmentation and lack of cooperation and coordination of existing services present an important barrier to the elderly, preventing them from making optimal use of the services offered (WHO 1972).

The dichotomies (a) between social services in general and sociomedical or psychiatric services and (b) between senior citizens' programs and services for the dependent elderly are well-known and extreme examples of barriers, particularly insofar as the Federal Republic of Germany (FRG) is concerned.

These obstacles interfere with impaired awareness of and lack of information on existing services as well as with the limited mobility of dependent older individuals. Instead of providing optimal flexibility to meet the needs of functionally incapacitated older patients, the present services frequently exhibit greater rigidity than their target populations. Medical specialization, for instance, often requires old patients to visit several institutions at different times in order to obtain a thorough and qualified medical diagnosis appropriate to multimorbidity. Even if they overcome these difficulties it is very likely that there will be no doctor who feels responsible for taking the partial diagnoses offered by different specialists and turning them into a comprehensive therapeutic scheme which fits the basic needs of the individual patient and takes into account his ability to understand and perform the therapeutic recommendations. Moreover if there is no engaged member of the family or other related person, nobody takes care to see that the recommended therapeutic interventions are successful.

Two other lines of fragmentation appear between inpatient and outpatient services and between medical hospitals belonging to the public health sector and nursing homes belonging to the social security sector, resulting in a multidimensional system of *disorganisation*: This seems to occur because the interfaces between these facets of the service systems do not exist at all or function by chance (i.e., through channels of personal acquaintance motivated by personal engagement) rather than by rational planning. Both egocentric, competitive struggling of services for patients and overburdened institutions can often be observed within the same community as a paradoxical result of this kind of fragmentation. For example, old peoples' homes and nursing homes shelter an important percentage of severely mentally disturbed old patients (Cooper and Sosna 1983); however, they are seldom reached by or linked with psychiatric services. Particularly in the FRG, the inhabitants are viewed as independently living older community members with regard to medical care, which they are supposed to receive from general practioners or, when in need of psychiatric care, from privately working psychiatrists. This principle fails to work in many respects and prevents the institutions and their patients from receiving the psychiatric help and guidance which both of them so urgently need.

Gaitz and Hocker (1970), Gaitz (1974) and Cohen (1976, 1980) have drawn attention to a detailed analysis of psychosocial barriers and obstacles to the delivery of mental health services to the elderly; this cannot be discussed here, and the interested reader is referred to their publications.

Uncertainty in Defining Target Populations and Appropriate Goals of Care and Treatment

Definition of goals of treatment and care of psychosocial handicaps depends not only on the possibility of perceiving objectively the underlying situation; on the contrary, it is greatly influenced by the following rather unspecific factors: (1) the cultural system of a society (embodying values and beliefs); (2) the available technology; and (3) the social structure of organizations that facilitate or inhibit goal attainment (Perrow, cited after Maddox 1980).

Due to differences in values and beliefs between different sociocultural settings or between subgroups of one sociocultural setting or even between varying institutions in the same country, uncertainty may arise in respect of goal definition. This vagueness in goal definition may be reinforced by divergent standpoints with regard to the adequacy of different therapeutic approaches. Some further factors may contribute to these problems.

In a 1972 report by a WHO working group on psychogeriatrics it was stated that old people were finding their way to psychiatric hospitals, old people's homes, and nursing facilities for reasons other than clear medical ones, and that the populations of these institutions overlapped to a large extent in their medical, psychiatric, and social characteristics. Such a situation can easily lead to inappropriate placement of a person, particularly if one considers the usual difficulties involved in transferring a patient from one institution to another. Of course, the rate of misplacement notified also depends on a proper definition of treatment goals and on the availability of appropriate treatment modalities to secure goal attainment.

Central Principles and Elements of Therapy and Service Delivery in Community Settings

General Principles

There is no doubt that, as in all other fields of psychiatry, it is essential to help psychogeriatric patients to continue their lives in their natural environment as long as this is acceptable for them, their relatives, and the community, to support the social networks they are embedded in, and to give them access to proper medical treatment at a level which is generally considered to be a standard for the population as a whole. Particularly the maintenance of existing supportive networks or the construction of new ones where none exist is of basic importance, since no professional service is capable of giving the same quality and quantity of care as informal natural support systems.

To fulfill these principles some prerequisites have to be met within each community providing psychogeriatric services for the elderly:

- Close cooperation between psychosocial and general social services
- Close cooperation between psychosocial services and all those services provided for the aged population in general
- Provision of channels of information and communication that enable detection of the "invisible" or hidden patient
- Transportation services

Essential Elements of Types of Institution

The most important element for older patients seems to be the general practitioner or family doctor. He is not, of course, an official part of the psychiatric institutional system. However, he should be as closely affiliated with psychiatric services as possible.

In the FRG the basic line of psychiatric defense is constituted by private psychiatrists and public mental health services, the former being the basic distributors of psychiatric diagnostics and therapy, the latter mainly providing counselling, crisis intervention, and control as regards legality.

Private psychiatrists, however, are by no means extensively and effectively involved in the care of psychogeriatric patients, nor are they adequately trained and equipped to care for the needs of the elderly population. For example, private psychiatrists in the FRG have only limited access to social workers and almost no opportunity for integrating occupational therapy or other forms of activation program into individual treatment plans. Cooperation with social workers is poorly developed because private psychiatrists work on the basis of a private enterprise whereas social workers are paid by the state and are thereby functionaries of public institutions. This, of course, does not inspire cooperation! Social therapy, on the other hand, is not incorporated into the refunding list of the public health insurance systems by which more than 95% of the population are insured.

Two developments are clearly needed in order to improve the care of psychogeriatric patients:

1. A mechanism for comprehensive assessment that builds upon existing health programs in the community
2. Provision of treatment programs that meet the needs, fears, and capacities of older patients.

Undoubtedly, in most cities and even in many rural areas, in the FRG there are sufficiently skilled physicians and modern technical equipment to guarantee reliable diagnostic procedures in the face of multimorbidity. However, there is a lack of coordination and geriatric training of professionals in the community health field.

It is obvious that day hospitals which could be attached to general or psychiatric hospitals to take full advantage of the existing technical equipment could perform comprehensive assessment. They could also offer all treatment modalities which seem to be successful in improving mental and emotional disturbances in old age. However, very few of these useful institutions in the field of geriatrics have so far been founded in the FRG.

It would appear most promising for facilities for comprehensive assessment to be run jointly by internists and psychiatrists. This might be pertinent not only in the case of day hospitals but in clinical settings too. Nevertheless, very few such schemes exist, one example being that in Nottingham (Arie 1981). It seems worth testing whether – under the conditions of the FRG – a (psycho)geriatric day hospital could not be run by a joint group of privately working physicians. Unfortunately, the chance of establishing such a model within the national program for improving psychiatric care in the FRG, which has been under way for 5 years, has not been grasped.

Neither has there been any reaction to the recommendation made by the committee of inquiry into psychiatry in the FRG to build up psychogeriatric centers (Bericht 1975). These centers should include three functional units: an assessment unit, a day hospital, and an outpatient clinic. Such a center could be expected to stimulate existing community services and to introduce better cooperation between existing services as well as to deliver care of its own.

Essential Elements of Treatment

Properly adjusted psychopharmacotherapy is the basis for treatment of functional and organic psychoses, even in old age. This requires sound knowledge of the particularities of pharmacology in old age.

Efficient and humane treatment of mental illness in old age, however, must be based on more than drugs: it must also involve various age-adapted forms of psychotherapy and sociotherapeutic approaches. This is indicated by the well-known high social vulnerability of older individuals and the important role social deprivation and isolation play in the context of mental and emotional diseases in old age.

The elements of treatment psychiatric services in the community should offer can therefore be listed as follows:

- General counseling for the aged and their families
- Comprehensive assessment
- Adequate pharmacotherapy
- Individual and group psychotherapy (not confined to a special technique)
- Individual and group programs for activating and stimulating daily and social activities and skills and for improving coping behavior
- Individual counseling and therapeutic groups for relatives or otherwise related persons who take care of patients
- Information for patients and their families on existing basic services for the elderly in the community, and help to arrange all available resources necessary to maintain at least a partially independent life in their homes
- Guidance and help in the case of institutionalization.

Shrinking Financial Resources

In almost all developed countries the financial burden of health services has obviously reached a critical point. Societies feel that further progress cannot be achieved by designating higher amounts of money to the health sector. On the contrary, some countries are trying very hard to reduce their health budgets. As the cost for hospital care accounts for the largest proportion of health expenditure there is a strong demand – at least in our country – for more ambulant care, which is claimed to be less expensive than institutional care.

However, this has not at all been proven. Particularly in psychogeriatrics a few studies carried out in the United States (see Maddox 1980) cast some doubt on the cost-effectiveness of ambulant care, although final conclusions may not be drawn at present. Maddox (1980) refers, for example, to a study done in Ohio in 1977 which yielded three major conclusions:

1. A large number of extremely impaired older persons are maintained in the community.
2. The extremely impaired are maintained at a cost well above the cost of nursing home care.
3. The high cost of noninstitutional care is borne primarily by kin and friends rather than by public agencies.

The latter point deserves special attention as it seems very likely that the cost-saving effect of more ambulant care depends primarily on shifting the financial burden from the public to the individual him/herself or his/her family. Secondly, it could be true that under the present conditions ambulant care is costsaving because less care or care of a lower quality is consumed since better service delivery cannot be obtained.

In any case, the financial burden imposes an important barrier to the elderly in making optimal use of the existing services. Therefore, it is to be feared that further restrictions on the money available for the health services will particularly put the elderly at a disadvantage.

In the FRG, it has emerged that handicaps following upon chronic illness are principally left to the resources of the individual already disabled. Whether this is an adequate policy for a society which purports to compensate for biological and social incapacities seems open to question. Current discussion on whether a new insurance system, *Pflegerisiko-Versicherung,* should be instituted to cover the consequences of chronic illness has to be seen and evaluated against this background. If it were to be introduced in the right way, improved and more frequently used ambulant care might be expected.

Conclusions

1. There is an irritating and surprising discrepancy between the estimated need for psychogeriatric community services and the use which is actually made of them by the elderly. As Cohen (1980) has noted: "Breakthroughs are needed more in the delivery of services to the elderly than in the services themselves. Much knowledge about the treatment of mental disorders in later life is already available. But settings where this knowledge can be applied through viable services are scanty and poorly developed." Therefore, detailed evaluation of the process of service delivery and obstacles which minimize its efficacy is still urgently needed.
2. Improved forms of cooperation which fit into the society's system of values, goals, and beliefs have to be developed and evaluated.
3. Financing of community mental health care has to be critically evaluated and adjusted to the needs of the chronically ill in general and those who are old in particular, based on the humanitarian beliefs accepted by the society as a whole.
4. The various forms of group therapy commonly offered in specialized psychogeriatric settings ought to be evaluated scientifically with view to whether they may be transferred to nonspecialized service programs.

References

Arie T (1981) Considerations for the future of psycho-geriatric services. In: Kinnard J, Brotherston J, Williamson J (eds) The provision of care for the elderly. Churchill Livingstone, Edinburgh, p 169

Bericht über die Lage der Psychiatrie in der Bundesrepublik Deutschland – Zur psychiatrischen und psychotherapeutisch/psychosomatischen Versorgung der Bevölkerung. 7.2 Versorgung psychisch kranker alter Menschen. Drucksache 7/4200, Deutscher Bundestag 1975, pp 246–260

Cohen GD (1976) Mental health services and the elderly: needs and options. Am J Psychiatry 133:65–68

Cohen GD (1980) Prospects for mental health and aging. In: Birren JE, Sloane EB (eds) Handbook of mental health and aging. Prentice-Hall, Englewood Cliffs, p 971

Cooper B, Sosna U (1983) Psychische Erkrankung in der Altenbevölkerung. Nervenarzt 54:239–249

Dunlop BD (1980) Expanded home-based care for the impaired elderly: solution or pipe dream? Am J Public Health 70:514–519

Gaitz CM, Hacker S (1970) Obstacles in coordinating services for the care of the psychiatrically ill aged. J Am Geriat Soc 18:172–182

Gaitz CM (1974) Barriers to the delivery of psychiatric services to the elderly. Gerontologist 14:210–214

Lowy L (1980) Mental health services in the community. In: Birren JE, Sloane EB (eds) Handbook of mental health and aging. Prentice-Hall, Englewood Cliffs, p 827

Maddox GL (1980) The continuum of care: movement toward the community. In: Busse EW, Blazer DG (eds) Handbook of geriatric psychiatry. Van Nostrand Reinhold, New York, p 501

Perrow C (1965) Hospitals: technology, structure, goals. In: March JG (ed) Handbook of organizations. Rand McNally, Chicago

WHO (1972) Psychogeriatrics. Report of WHO scientific group. World Health Organization Technical Report Series no 507

Roth M (1973) The principles of providing a service for psycho-geriatric patients. In: Wing JK, Häfner H (eds) Roots of evaluation. Nuffield Provincial Hospitals Trust by the Oxford University Press, London, p 215

6.4 Self-help: Possibilities and Potentialities in Gerontopsychiatry

H. Radebold, J. Bruder

Today's self-help groups deal with difficulties and deficiencies of a mainly psychosocial character occurring in connection with and as a consequence of physical and psychic diseases. Self-help groups insist that the possibilities available within the framework of social security and treatment should be placed at their disposal (Moeller 1978; Arbeitsgruppe 1982). In the ideal case they work without professional assistance and have as their goal a practical and limited set of problems. They try to avoid a hierarchic structure and control by professional social security organizations.

The self-help movement can now be considered large and is still constantly growing; some years ago one million self-help groups involving at least 15 million people were counted in the United States (Haber 1983).

Self-help means support which is given by laymen. These people do not receive any remuneration and work independently of professional care. One must distinguish between self-help and outside help: in the latter case laymen are active, for example, helpers or collaborators of institutional care (Moeller 1978; Arbeitsgruppe 1982; Lohfert et al. 1983).

It is especially a case of self-help when those who are in a situation involving difficulties or deprivation (either being affected, coaffected, or potentially affected) can aid themselves. Self-help may be undertaken individually by single persons or in a joint effort by a group of people. *Primary self-help* takes place in the traditional social network of the family, the relatives, the neighbors, the parish, and the circle of friends and colleagues. It is, however, always a by-product of the community and not the real aim of an organization. If, on the contrary, a group is formed specifically with the purpose of mutual self-help, we talk of *secondary self-help*. Sometimes such groups are united in self-help organizations.

In respect of the character of support we must distinguish between collective self-help, mutual help, and altruistic self-help (Arbeitsgruppe 1982; Badelt 1980).

Whether the ideal form of self-help referred to above may be applied to and is useful for the elderly and especially for those who are mentally ill remains to be investigated.

Self-help among old people is marginal to the spectrum of the self-help movement as far as the number and innovative potential of such groups is concerned (Arbeitsgruppe 1982; Butler et al. 1979; Gronemeyer and Bahr 1979; Zeman 1983; Donicht-Fluck 1984). It is estimated, for example, that in the Federal Republic of Germany in 1980 0.3% of all people over 60 were members of self-help groups or organizations (Zeman 1983). Very few reports on experiences of and investigations into self-help for physical problems and/or diseases of old age are available, the few that are merely being on groups of relatives, groups for widowed people, and stroke patients (Hiltz 1975; Radebold 1983).

There are also some reports on experiences from state hospitals and homes in which mentally ill elderly were either looked after by younger patients or by old people who were less ill (MacNiel and Verwoerdt 1972).

In view of its aim, self-help would seem a necessary and sensible complement to professional activity, but there is intensive resistance to realizing, utilizing and investigating the possibilities of self-help in gerontopsychiatry. Among the reasons for this resistance are the following:

1. Medical science has not yet developed a holistic conception of diagnosis and therapy which takes into full account psychic and social factors (Gussow and Tracy 1980). Thus self-help among sick persons is looked upon as competition; only with reluctance is it considered useful, and some medical support is given to self-help groups only in respect of certain physical diseases, such as diabetes, cancer, rheumatism, myocardial infarction, stroke, adiposity, epilepsy, multiple sclerosis, and Parkinson's disease (Gussow and Tracy 1980; Schauwecker 1982). As a rule, patients over 60 are not represented in these groups. Lack of interest in geriatrics, an understanding of syndromes as being mainly of organic origin, an orientation in line with the deficit model, and lack of knowledge of therapeutic and rehabilitative measures all have had the result that until now such groups for people over 60 years old have rarely been suggested or initiated with medical support, and that participation of older people has hardly ever been recommended by physicians.
2. Psychiatry has accepted the usefulness of self-help only for certain groups of patients (marginal), such as Alcoholics Anonymous and Neurotics Anonymous and for the above-mentioned groups of chronically sick people in order to avoid psychoreactive depression. If they are more politically orientated, the groups are rejected (Charlier 1979). This negative view of self-help has been adopted by gerontopsychiatry and reinforced by constant experience in clinical life with the symptoms of demented and depressive patients. Although these syndromes represent only a part of gerontopsychiatric morbidity and although only a small percentage of all gerontopsychiatric patients are treated either as outpatients or inpatients in psychiatric institutions (Cooper and Sosna 1983), the question is not raised as to whether the psychiatric viewpoint of the mentally ill elderly regarding their activity, interests, fitness, and ego assertion is only partly applicable.
3. Acceptance of oneself as a mentally ill old person is a prerequisite for initiating or joining self-help groups. It is a well-known fact that especially the affectively sick (but also other older persons) deny the existence of problems and mental disorders on account of the self-concept for which they strive; they are even supported in this attitude by their environment. The prerequisites for joint secondary self-help are experience of stress regarding problems and suffering, conscious perception of the deprivation, motivation to achieve change, and acquisition of competence to aid similarly affected others.
4. Younger mentally ill persons often repeat, in an unconscious transference to older fellow patients, their childhood and adolescent conflicts, rejecting them or, conversely, desiring aid from older people. The needs of the elderly in mixed age groups are not understood.

5. Younger people professionally active in self-help groups look to interested, energetic, socially, and politically active older ones (e.g., after the model of the "Grey Panthers") for help. The "helper mentality" toward older people with physical or mental illness, as well as professional fear of competition, prevents the initiation of self-help.

The present lack of secondary self-help contrasts with apparently extensive primary self-help (from family, neighbors, domestic community, friends, and acquaintances). It is almost unknown which characteristics (age, sex, social stratum, personality structure, etc.) the providers of such help have, and to what extent, through which persons, and in which fields (contact, information, social and material support, care, or advice) help is given.

Besides collective or altruistic self-help, does mutual help exist on a larger scale? What effects has professional aid: is it complementary, initiating, and supporting, is it exchangeable or similar to that offered by the self-help groups, or does it even harm them? (Pilsuk and Minkler 1980; Stein et al. 1982).

The ideal manifestation of secondary self-help, a group centered around a single issue, does not seem practicable for mentally ill old persons. Their situation calls for a holistic approach which includes aid through both young and old laymen and professional experts (at least as regards the initiation of self-help groups and guidance and advice). Peers who, as former patients, find a new purpose in life through helping others are of special importance (Waters et al. 1976).

If such a holistic approach were adopted, the following tasks of tertiary prevention would be possible: guidance of patients and persons close to them during the disease, helping patients to adapt to living with the social and physical consequences of the disease, training of still existing ego functions, and support for conflict-free parts of the personality. Especially the following groups of patients might profit from such self-help: neurotic and reactive depressive patients (some of whom will have suicidal and slight cerebro-organic symptoms), alcohol and drug addicts, and patients suffering from minor maladjustments after long-term organic diseases.

Self-help takes on tasks of primary prevention if the groups offer contacts, leisure activities, new tasks and roles, and mutual support, and if they give special aid in coping with age-related stressful life-events such as retirement from work, loss of partner, and illness (Pilsuk and Minkler 1980; Stein et al. 1982).

It is an open question whether self-help groups may provide direct therapeutic assistance beyond the psychosocial sector, e.g., in respect of persons with reactive depression or drug or alcohol addicts. Successful styles of individual crisis prevention, treatment, and control may assume a model character for the group. To this end, it would to a certain extent seem feasible for elderly people to give advice to others of the same age on their problems. How far individual prejudices and problem-solving strategies may bar therapeutic access to the elderly has not been investigated. Most probably this kind of aid is only possible within the framework of professional care, with support through instruction, guidance, and supervision (Haber 1983; Hiltz 1975; Radebold 1983; Pilsuk and Minkler 1980).

To sum up, it can be said that among the elderly, self-help does not represent an alternative to gerontopsychiatric care and traditional assistance. But it may be *complementary* in the shape of primary or tertiary prevention, since problems and diseases of the elderly *require outside help* with comprehensive professional and material backing.

If self-help among old people is to realize its specific potential, it requires free space for its work without being supervised and swallowed up by professional institutions. The socialization and historical experiences of 70–80 year olds in the Federal Republic of Germany seem to have led to the potential of self-help among the elderly being realized only to a small extent; the "young" aged generation will probably be able to make better use of it in the future.

Necessary Research Goals in the Field of Self-help in Gerontopsychiatry

It is an established fact that in addition to the existing primary self-help – which is known to be very extensive – forms of secondary self-help for mentally ill already exist in various sectors (although the extent is not known). The following investigations appear possible as a first step toward researching the field of self-help among the elderly:

1. Research into the aims, fields of activity, and experiences of the affected persons (both the nonprofessional and professional) in the existing groups.
2. Investigations of the various groups involved in self-help (family, neighbors, younger people, peers, professionals) regarding personality structure, social and structural differences, and the mutual consequences of the assistance.
3. Research into the extent, fields, and consequences of self-help for different diagnostic groups of the mentally ill elderly.
4. Studies of interaction and problem-solving styles, including in relation to competence in self-help.
5. Investigations of interaction among the mentally ill elderly in self-help groups and its effect on the disease process.
6. Implementation of special models on a comprehensive basis (initiation and observation of self-help groups for certain problematic situations and syndromes).
7. Investigations of the environmental conditions of self-help (social, professional, and institutional factors).
8. Research into the necessity of a change in attitudes among professionals in diverse public institutions (including municipal authorities and those dealing with social legislation).
9. Development of instruments to gauge the quantity and quality of assistance provided by self-help groups.

References

Arbeitsgruppe (1982) Fachbericht über Probleme des Alterns: Altwerden in der Bundesrepublik Deutschland. Geschichte-Situationen-Perspektiven. Deutsches Zentrum für Altersfragen, vol 40, I–III. Berlin

Badelt C (1980) Sozioökonomie der Selbstorganisation, Beispiele zur Bürgerselbsthilfe und ihre wirtschaftliche Bedeutung. Campus, Frankfurt

Butler R et al. (1979) Sel-care, self-help and the elderly. Int J Aging Hum Dev 10:95–117
Charlier T (1979) Gemeindepsychiatrie und Selbsthilfegruppen ehemaliger psychiatrischer Patienten. Ein exemplarischer Vergleich zwischen den USA und der BRD. In: Nagel H, Seifert M (eds) Inflation der Therapieformen. Rowohlt, Reinbek
Cooper B, Sosna U (1983) Psychische Erkrankung in der Altenbevölkerung. Nervenarzt 54:239–249
Donicht-Fluck B (1984) Runzlige Radikale – Graue Panther in den USA und in der Bundesrepublik Deutschland. Vincentz, Hannover
Gronemeyer R, Bahr HE (eds) (1979) Niemand ist zu alt. Selbsthilfe und Alteninitiativen. Fischer, Frankfurt
Gussow Z, Tracy GS (1980) Selbsthilfegruppen in der Rehabilitation. In: Trojan A et al. (eds) Gemeindebezogene Gesundheitssicherung. Urban and Schwarzenberg, Munich
Haber D (1983) Promoting mutual help groups among older persons. Gerontologist 23:251–253
Hiltz S (1975) Helping widows: Group discussions as a therapeutic technique. Fam Coordinator 1:331–336
Lohfert C, Lohfert P, Muschter W (1983) Laien- und Selbsthilfe bei psychisch kranken alten Menschen. Evaluationsstudie im Krankheitsbereich "Psychisch kranke alte Menschen". Deutsche Forschungs- und Versuchsanstalt für Luft- und Raumfahrt e.V., Bereich für Projektträgerschaften, Köln
MacNiel J, Verwoerdt A (1972) A group treatment program combined with a work project on the geriatric unit of a State Hospital. J Am Geriatr Soc 20:259–264
Moeller ML (1978) Selbsthilfegruppen. Rowohlt, Reinbek
Pilsuk M, Minkler M (1980) Supportive networks: Life ties for the elderly. J Soc Iss 36:95–116
Radebold H (ed) (1983) Gruppenpsychotherapie im Alter. Vandenhoek and Ruprecht, Göttingen
Schauwecker C (1982) Selbsthilfegruppen in der Rehabilitation. Dtsch Krankenpflege Z 35:739–741
Stein S, Linn M, Stein E (1982) The relationship of self-help networks to physical and psychosocial functioning. J Am Geriatr Soc 30:764–768
Waters E, Fink S, White B (1976) Peer group counseling for older people. Educ Gerontol 1:157–170
Zeman P (1983) Gemeinschaftliche Selbsthilfe im Alter. In: Asam W, Heck M (eds) Soziale Selbsthilfegruppen in der Bundesrepublik Deutschland. Minerva, Munich

6.5 Evaluation of Social and Health Services for the "Disabled" Elderly

E. Strömgren

The field of psychogeriatrics has increased so rapidly that it is no wonder that no final solutions have been found, and there is not even agreement as to which direction future developments should take.

The situation within the field differs greatly within various countries, and it is not always easy to say why that is so. It is therefore of great importance that cross-national studies are being performed. The very illuminating comparative study of conditions in London, Mannheim and New York has already been mentioned. The diversity with regard to solutions is also a reason why international symposia like the present one are useful and necessary.

Many of the differences depend, as Dr. Godber has stressed, more on historical circumstances than on divergence with regard to general viewpoints. Denmark can serve as an example. During the 1920s and 1930s Denmark was a poor country with much unemployment. Old people were the poorest of all, the old-age pensions being very low. For these old people it was very difficult to manage financially, and for many of them the greatest wish was to acquire a room in an old people's home. The mainly socialist governments tried to encourage the establishment of such old people's homes of a reasonable standard, and it became a matter of local pride for a community to have such a home. After World War II this development continued for a while, but in 1957 something happened which changed the situation radically. A new law decreed that old-age pensions and invalid pensions should rise very substantially. This caused, among many other good things, a rush of old people from the institutions, including the old people's homes, out into the community where it was now possible for them to manage reasonably in terms of finance. There was now no unemployment and it was possible for even moderately handicapped persons to join the labor market.

During the same period the aging of the general population sped up, and the proportion of incapacitated old people increased. They now started to replace the healthy or only mildly incapacitated former inhabitants of old people's homes. This had important consequences. Whereas the former inhabitants did not need much attendance and equipment, the new inhabitants were much more demanding. Many of the buildings were inadequate for incapacitated people, and understaffed with regard to this care-demanding clientele. New institutions had to meet much higher standards and the communities became more reluctant to build such expensive institutions. This again reflected on the hospitals. When old patients did not need further hospital treatment, it was difficult to find room for them in nursing homes, and an increasing proportion of hospital beds were occupied by old people.

The rapid increase in the costs of establishing and running institutions is, of course, one of the reasons why the concept of extramural treatment and of community psychiatry has become so popular in practically all circles. But there are indeed many other reasons, of very different kinds. Psychiatrists were among the first to advocate extramural treatment, but not so much for financial reasons. They were first of all impressed by the shortage of beds in the institutions and felt that an efficient outpatient service could make it possible to discharge patients earlier; in addition community mental health services might intervene in such a way that some admissions could be avoided. There could not be any guarantee that this would diminish the need for places in the institutions, but it would in any case have the effect that the beds were occupied by patients who really needed hospital treatment, patients who under present conditions often had been obliged to wait for a long time before they could be adequately treated.

Last but not least, many psychiatrists, especially those who had participated in some kind of field studies, felt that under present conditions a great percentage of those who needed psychiatric treatment never came to the attention of the psychiatric institutional system. If these patients were found and received adequate treatment, the whole mental health situation might be improved radically. The public popularity of the concept of community mental health services has, however, no doubt mainly been based on the hope that it would decrease the need for institutions, i.e., that hospitals could be closed and the staff transferred to extramural psychiatry. Since at least 80% of the cost of running hospitals goes on the staff's wages, administrators and politicians must also have been convinced that running of community mental health services would demand less staff, because only in that case would there be any financial gain in switching efforts from hospitals to the community.

The contrary may be the case. One of the objects of community mental health services should be case finding, the result of such efforts being that many more individuals would come under treatment, some of them being of such a nature that admission to hospital would be necessary for a while. The pressure on the institutions might therefore increase instead of decreasing. The gain would be that much suffering from mental derangement would be relieved; but it would be very likely that the introduction of really adequate community mental health services would demand much more money than is at present spent on the psychiatric system – and that is, of course, not exactly what politicians nowadays are expecting.

One more problem has been stressed very clearly in the introductory lectures; even if community mental health services for the aged are run in such a way that the cost for society does not increase, or is even reduced, the greater part of the costs will have to be met by the supporters of the mentally ill kept at home, not forgetting that the burden on the supporters is not only of a financial nature.

But what do we know about the financial side of transferring mental health services from institutions to the community? It is, of course, very difficult to carry out cost-benefit studies on this problem. In Denmark a community mental health project has been operating since 1957 on the island of Samsø. It is obvious that the population there gets a much better psychiatric service than is available in any other part of the country since many more professional staff are at their disposal. Many patients have been found who were suffering badly from mental disorders but had never received any treatment, so it can safely be stated that the mental health situation of the population has improved. However, admissions to psychiatric hospital have *not* decreased during these 27 years. Many admissions are prevented, but in other cases patients who would never have been admitted under previous conditions have been admitted. The geriatric patients, however, seem to be an exception in the sense that the mental health services can keep them in their homes for a longer time than was previously possible, and this result seems to be achieved with quite moderate means.

One group of disorders has, as could be expected, proved of special importance: the depressions. General Practitioners (GPs) have referred a number of patients who had previously not received adequate treatment. The project started just when tricyclic antidepressants came into use, and it was a very encouraging experience to see the striking effects of these new drugs. But in addition to those patients who had consulted GPs and been referred to the psychiatrists, there was a more problematic group. The GPs knew about certain patients who were known to suffer from some mental disorder but who had never approached their GP. Not without hesitation the psychiatrists decided to pay visits to these patients. It turned out that the psychiatrists were well received. In most cases the patients obviously suffered from endogenous depressions. They were grateful for the visit and were quite willing to receive treatment. The reason why they had not consulted their GP was that they simply did not have the initiative or the courage to do so. In addition they were not always aware of the fact that they were suffering from a disease. Most of these patients responded excellently to antidepressant therapy. There is no doubt that in most populations there are great numbers of these depressed people who never receive any adequate treatment. This is one of the most important targets for case finding within the framework of community mental health services.

Depression is one of the most frequent and important diseases within the psychogeriatric field. The other large group within this field is, of course, dementia. With respect to these states there is only exceptionally a possibility of efficient therapy. Intervention is a question of prevention of decompensation. Since decompensation usually occurs in connection with change in environment, the basic principle should be to keep the patient in the usual environment as long as possible, and in any case there should be continuity in the environment. When it is becoming obvious that a change of environment, transfer to nursing home, etc., is imminent, this change should, if possible, be gradual, the patient taking up contact with the future environment while still living in his or her own home. In many communities the best solution is the establishment of centers for the aged which in addition to nursing sections comprise all kinds of possibilities for outpatient occupational therapy, entertainment, day nursing, ambulatory treatment by geriatric specialists, etc. If such a center can at the same time serve as a kind of community center with library, cinema, etc. which are also visited by the younger generations, the aged may have become acquainted with the center long before they have a real need to seek its help. It is also very important that the nursing sections can receive old people for shorter stays while the supporters are away, or ill, or just need a rest.

So much for the social side of the problem. But what about the medical side? Old patients are often multihandicapped, and some of the handicaps necessitate the help of specialists. It is natural that the GP coordinates the different medical investigations and treatments. Some GPs are interested in this kind of work and are well qualified for it. Others less so. It is therefore also necessary that there are doctors who specialize in geriatrics. They can naturally be attached to centers for the aged, but in addition it seems necessary that regular geriatric departments exist in hospitals. Such departments will then also be the natural centers for research in the field.

In many countries the cooperation between social services and health services is more or less problematic, especially during periods of economic restriction when all administrations try to get rid of as many economic responsibilities as possible. In Denmark there are three administrative units: state, county, and community. Counties have the administrative and economic responsibility for hospitals whereas social services, including nursing homes, are run by the communities, who pay 50% of the costs while the state pays the rest. It is understandable that in periods of economic depression communities are interested that geriatric patients stay in hospital as long as possible because this placement does not cost the community anything. The consequence is that traditionally many geriatric patients who no longer need hospital treatment are obliged to stay there because there is no room for them in nursing homes. Problems of this nature are serious obstacles to the development of adequate services for the aged. Fortunately, in Denmark there is a growing understanding for these problems among politicians, and a feeling for the necessity of a reorganization.

From today's discussions it has become obvious that these administrative and political problems exist in many countries. They may constitute the most important targets for efforts within the field of psychogeriatrics.

7 Mental Health in the Elderly: Recommendations for Research

H. Häfner

Demographic Trends of the Elderly Population

Mental disorders in the elderly constitute one of the most important social and health problems of our generation. One reason for this is to be looked for in the enormous changes in the age structure of the world population, which are reflected in the increasing mean ages of the populations, in the increasing proportions of those aged 65 and over and the disproportionately large increases in the numbers of those aged 80 and above (see Hauser, this volume). In the developing countries this process is still at an early stage, while in the industrialized countries, where it started before the turn of the century, it has now reached an advanced stage. Increased life expectancy, one of the causes of these demographic changes, has resulted in particular from improved hygiene and standards of living and the progress made in field of preventive and curative medicine in combatting acute diseases associated with a high mortality risk. In searching for the causes of and developing effective preventive measures for chronic diseases, however, only moderate progress has been made. The successful combat against life-threatening diseases and the increased further life expectancy, also in higher age groups, have extended the life span of the chronically ill and thus led to a disproportionately large increase in their numbers. In this context the World Health Organization has spoken of a "rising pandemic of chronic ill-health and disability"[1].

For a long time medicine used to focus its main interest on acute diseases and, consequently, on the health problems of childhood, adolescence and adulthood. The fact that illnesses typical of old age hardly attracted the interest of medical professionals and researchers was also due to a wide-spread resignation with regard to the treatability of these conditions. Chronic diseases of old age, especially cerebral atrophies, were largely regarded as inevitable concomitants of the inexorable process of aging of the organism. Only recently have possibilities of differentiation between some chronic illnesses of high frequency in old age and the process of aging as such begun to emerge. But it is yet impossible to say whether aging itself can be influenced to any degree. In the near future, however, if sufficient research efforts are made, it may become possible to prevent or at least slow down chronic diseases of high prevalence that shorten the life span and decisively impair quality of life in old age. Another reason for the increased interest of medicine in the health problems of the elderly is the fact that the aim of medical treatment is no longer limited to the mere restoration of the ability to work, but has also come to include the maintenance and enhancement of quality of life. This aspect is of importance not only for the individual well-being of the elderly, but also in regard to the decreasing opportunities of gainful employment in old age all over the world.

---

1 World Health Organization: Social Dimensions of Mental Health. Geneva, 1981, p. 23

The utilization of health services by the population aged 60 and over by far exceeds the proportion of this age group to the total population. This is due to the high prevalence of chronic disease in old age requiring repeated medical treatment (see Davis, this volume). Another reason is multimorbidity, i.e., the simultaneous presence of several illnesses, e.g., cardio- and cerebrovascular illnesses, cancer, diabetes diseases of the respiratory organs and joints and various mental disorders, in the elderly. Mental disorders in old age are particularly frequent: according to the concurrent results of various epidemiological surveys some 25% of the population over 65 years of age suffer from mental ill-health (see Cooper, this volume).

The most frequent mental disorders in old age are dementia and depression. In both illness groups physical illness and disability constitute both an important risk factor, sometimes even the decisive underlying cause, and important sequelae. For the treatment of depression there is a remarkable and promising arsenal of effective medications and psychotherapeutic approaches available. For the treatment of the most frequent and severest mental disorder in old age, dementia, no such methods are available yet. The frequency of dementia, depending on definitions, is estimated at 3 – 5% of the population over 65. In advanced age it shows a steep increase, amounting to 20 – 30% of those over 85 years of age in the European populations. In contrast, the frequency of functional mental disorders seems to decrease slightly in advanced age, probably due to selective mortality and the difficulties of recognizing functional syndromes if dementia is also present.

In view of the vast demographic changes, the disproportionately high frequency of health problems in the elderly, and the high utilization of health services by this group, research is called upon to direct more attention to the elderly than it has done ever before. Mental disorders not only are very frequent in old age, but the majority also leads to serious impairment, intellectual decline, and as a consequence, to a greater need for care than in earlier stages of life. They also cause considerable loss of quality of life among the patients themselves and their family members and constitute a burden upon society in qualitative and financial terms. It is therefore necessary to pay increased attention to the mental-health problems of the elderly, to search for the causes and the prevention and treatment of mental disorders in old age, and to give them prominence in health research.

Epidemiological Research in Psychogeriatrics

Epidemiological research in psychogeriatrics pursues three objectives: first, to provide a basis for the planning of treatment measures and the implementation of appropriate systems of care by obtaining information on the frequency and distribution of mental disorders in old age; second, to identify the role played by causal factors such as environmental influences, life styles, and genetically determined patterns of responding of the organism in the development of certain mental disorders in old age (knowledge about such causal relationships is a necessary precondition for the development of preventive measures); third, to assess the effects of treatment of the elderly and to conduct cost-analysis on the care systems implemented. Epidemiological research in psychiatry has in recent yers made considerable advances and provided important information on the frequency and distribution of mental disorders in the elderly populations as well as on the interactions between illness frequencies and illness risks on the one hand and the immediate and more comprehensive social environmental on the other (see Henderson, Osuntokun, this volume).

The results so far obtained indicate that life style, nutritional habits and heavy smoking — risk factors that also are of importance for cardiovascular and cerebrovascular diseases in younger age groups — have an impact on certain mental disorders in old age and on time of survival. At the same time, there are indications of protective or compensatory factors' reducing some illness risks (see Lehr, Svanborg et al., this volume). A Swedish study examining three successive birth cohorts at the age of seventy at an interval of five years has revealed an improvement in the overall state of health and the physical and mental capacities in the later birth cohorts. These results point to the possibility of exerting a favourable influence on mental health in old age by improving the environmental or nutritional conditions and changing personal habits (see Svanborg et al., this volume). Therefore, more longitudinal studies inquiring into the medical and the physical status and their changes over time are especially needed, to make it possible to examine the relationships between risk factors and physical and mental illness in old age. It is of primary importance in this context to search for the risk factors and possible causes of senile dementia of the Alzheimer type (SDAT), of cerebrovascular dementia, and of depressive and paranoid illnesses in old age.

Epidemiological research needs transnationally standardized measurement tools, especially for depressive and dementing conditions. The development of such instruments is an urgent task, since it is only through an international exchange and comparisons over populations that psychogeriatric research can yield fruitful results (see Bickel, Cooper & Beck-Dreßler, Henderson, Osuntokun, this volume).

Apart from the need to carry out various epidemiological research projects, a continuous collection of accurately defined data on the physical and mental health status of the elderly in defined populations is necessary. Epidemiological projects yield only discontinuous data, but their informative value and utility for generalizations can be improved decisively by continuously collected, representative data. In addition to national statistics on causes of death, cumulative case registers based on smaller populations are needed. If possible, they should collect both psychiatric and medical data and work on an epidemiological basis.

Well-Being and Mental Health in Old Age

Personality factors such as individual vulnerability for stress, coping resources, and social network, especially the type and quality of support received, are of great importance for individual well-being and mental health (see Veiel, Mechanic, this volume). Almost all studies in this area have been conducted on populations under 60 years of age, although the above factors are presumably operative in old age, too.

The only thing that has so far been proven by studies conducted specifically on the elderly is that loss of partner (death of spouse) and subjectively experienced loneliness – but not necessarily objective isolation – are associated with mental ill-health, particularly with a high frequency of depression. It has yet to be established whether this association is a direct one or whether it can be attributed to common underlying factors, e.g., certain personality traits. What we do know is that insufficient social support reduces the capacity for self-care in advanced age and increases the probability of institutionalization.

Elderly people now not only live longer than previous generations but also have better physical and mental health and retain their capacities longer. Nevertheless, they often become cut off from domains of active functioning in social and working life. Stressful life events, such as loss of social status and living standard and, above all, loss of close relatives, become more frequent in old age, while at the same time the social network and its support potentials tend to diminish[1].

It is a task of multidisciplinary psychiatric and sociological research to find out whether certain characteristics of the social network and certain personality traits have an influence on the individual's ability to cope with the above-mentioned changes and also on physical and mental health risks (see Svanborg et al., this volume) *and to what extent substitutes for social support can reduce risk when losses and deficits in the social network occur* (see Taylor, this volume). *What looks promising in this regard are not only the necessary prospective longitudinal studies but also intervention studies investigating the influence of learning processes on coping behaviour and/or the influence of social-support substitutes on mental health and the capacity of self-care in old age*. Since the same causal factors frequently lead to both mental and physical disorders, it would certainly be fruitful for such studies to measure other types of disorders than just mental or physical disease.

The growing importance of social-network research is also due to the fact that in the future the role of the family as a natural provider of social support in old age will diminish, for demographic and sociocultural reasons. Whether a well-functioning social network can help mentally ill or, particularly, dementing persons to be cared for at home and, thus, to spare them institutionalization is a question of great importance for the elderly themselves, their family members, and the national economy.

This research field, too, lacks generally accepted and sufficiently validated concepts and instruments of measurement. It should therefore be aimed at developing appropriate methods for measuring psychosocial factors that have a bearing upon mental health and quality of life in old age.

Physical Risk Factors of Mental Health in Old Age

With advancing age, *mental disorders caused by cerebral dysfunctions predominate. Knowledge about their causes and risk factors is therefore of decisive importance for research. The first place is occupied by cerebrovascular and cardiovascular diseases and their precursors, particularly diabetes and persistent hypertension* (see Kohlmeyer, this volume). The increased frequency of degenerative processes in the brain in advanced age necessitates some distinction between the process of

1 Häfner H: Psychische Gesundheit im Alter. Gustav-Fischer-Verlag: Stuttgart, 1986.

aging as such and illnesses that might be influenced by preventive or therapeutic measures (see Carlson, this volume). However, aging is indubitably a biologically determined process that inevitably puts an end to human life.

There are enough signs indicating that *aging is a process depending on genetic and environmental factors* as regards its course and manifestation in various organ systems. *Whether it can be delayed by, say, optimal training of physical and mental capacities or by a substitution of the age-related deficit in neurotransmitters or, some day in the future, by genetic engineering is yet impossible to say. Favourable living conditions, the prevention of specific risks and the treatment of illnesses associated with increased risks can probably prevent an early onset of aging and thus prolong the actual time of survival.*

In order to be able to define and measure illness processes, research needs age-group-specific norms for the most important physiological and psychological parameters of the healthy population, from blood pressure to reaction time. In this field, which also has implications for medical practice, there is a considerable research deficit.

In practice, especially for the provision of medical care and social services for the elderly, *the identification of individuals and groups particularly at risk or in need for care* is of special significance. Epidemiological studies have shown that it is for the most part treatable depressions, especially chronic depressive states, that often remain unrecognized and, thus, untreated in the elderly (see Strömgren, this volume). This also applies, though to a lesser extent, to paranoid conditions, which are very frequent in elderly persons living by themselves or suffering from age-related hearing difficulties. Further factors enhancing the risk of mental illness in old age are life events such as death of close relatives, relocation, or hospital admission.

Detection, Prevention, and Treatment of Mental Disorders and Disabilities

The development and validation of screening instruments for the detection of mental disorders in the elderly is an urgent task for research. Such practicable, short procedures have two objectives: first, the identification of such patients in larger collectives as are in need of care and, second, the identification of defined groups of individuals that will receive a more detailed and differentiated examination in research projects (see Bickel, this volume). The aim should be an internationally validated, standardized instrument, to enable comparisons of service data and research findings over countries.

There are already a few standardized measurement methods available that permit a reliable case identification and a quantitative assessment of psychopathological dimensions, such as cognitive and emotional disturbances and behavioural abnormalities, in elderly persons. The areas measured, however, are insufficient, especially in regard to the differential dimensions of the disturbances, and most of *the instruments have not yet been standardized on an international scale.* It is also *necessary to develop instruments enabling an objective, quantitative assessment of disability and the remaining capacities in the elderly. Since the availability of accurate, internationally standardized assessment methods is a prerequisite for successful research in the majority of psychogeriatric fields, the Global Advisory*

Committee for Biomedical Research, a WHO advisory committee on research, has recommended the launching of an initiative with the object of promoting international collaborative research in the development of screening and assessment methods for identifying, assessing, and differentiating mental disorders in the elderly.

In the industrialized countries where the problem has so far been studied, mentally ill elderly people turn for medical treatment mostly to a general practitioner and only in few cases to the specialized mental health services. The general practitioner is indeed an ideal partner, since he can best cope with multimorbidity in the elderly, provided he is familiar with the problems of diagnosis and therapy of psychogeriatric disorders. This, however, is not always so. It is therefore necessary to enhance the psychiatric competence of general practitioners and the medical competence of psychiatrists (see Godber, this volume).

One of the main obstacles to primary prevention of mental disorders in the elderly is the lack of knowledge. The underlying causes of degenerative processes in the brain and of functional mental disorders encountered in old age have not yet been illuminated satisfactorily. Many of the diseases in the elderly may have more than one cause. Some causes and the combination of causes may differ between various populations, for example those living in tropical and temperate zones or those suffering from undernourishment or overnourishment in childhood, etc. Therefore, also national and cross-national studies need to be stimulated.

In medical secondary prevention, however, important approaches have emerged. By an early treatment of diabetes, hypertension, and cardiovascular and cerebrovascular diseases there is a prospect of reducing their mental sequelae. Through a successful treatment of chronic depression or paranoid states, associated with a high risk of chronification, it is possible to reduce the subsequent risk of various physical illnesses and an early need for institutional care (see Bergmann, this volume). Promising results have been obtained not only drug treatment but also by psychotherapeutic interventions.

Psychotherapy

Owing to the development of new and more economical methods of psychotherapy, in the last few decades considerable progress has been made in the treatment of the symptoms of various severe mental disorders and behavioral abnormalities, also such of physical origin. It is highly probable that many of the less severe mental disorders encountered in the elderly can be alleviated or cured by psychotherapeutic methods. In recent times a possibility of achieving lasting successful results in the treatment of chronic depression, which is especially frequent in old age and associated with a high risk of sequelae, has begun to emerge with procedures of cognitive and behaviour therapy (see Diekstra, this volume).

The development and evaluation of psychotherapeutic methods for the treatment of mental disorders, for favourably influencing pathological behavioural patterns in conjunction with chronic, incurable diseases, and for improving the coping resources of the elderly is a research field of high priority. Better psychotherapeutic methods would benefit mentally ill elderly people not only in the clinical context: they would also help to develop appropriate behavioural strategies of coping with the problems of elderly people which could be adopted, for example in homes or day centres. Another urgent task is the training of personnel in the easily applicable methods that research is called upon to develop (see Kanowski, this volume).

Social Intervention for Mental Health in the Elderly

The main social group in which elderly persons are embedded and which shares their fate of old age and, finally, assumes their care in illness and disability is still the family, in spite of sweeping social changes. The care and nursing of the chronically ill and disabled elderly is assumed primarily by their spouses or children. In the coming decades, however, their numbers and availability for this task will decrease in most countries for demographic and sociocultural reasons. It is likely that with the increasing numbers of the elderly and the decreasing numbers of the young, who are the main providers of support and assistance in old age, also the situation of the elderly in society will undergo a substantial change.[1]

The overwhelming majority of the elderly wish to continue to live in their own homes. This is also in line with a sound health and social policy. To support the families in caring for and nursing disabled and chronically ill elderly persons is a task of domiciliary services. Social intervention in a narrower sense is required when the family is no longer in a position to care for the mentally ill elderly person or if family members prepared to assume the task are not available. In such situations mediation of social support and substitute relationships is needed. *Our knowledge about the way these social support systems function is as yet very limited.*

In many countries *the standard of the medicopsychiatric care of the elderly living in social institutions, above all in residential or nursing homes* (see Mechanic, this volume), *and the social aspects of quality of life among hospitalized elderly persons leave much to be desidered. One of the priorities is therefore to develop criteria for the assessment of quality of care in various institutions for the elderly. There is also a lack of good studies on how social intervention programmes affect mental health or help the elderly to retain their capacity for self-care and autonomy as long as possible.*

Promotion of Self-Help, Lay Initiatives, and Domiciliary Care

The promotion of self-initiative in the elderly and of spontaneous organized help in the community has four objectives: (1) the prevention of illness and disability in old age, (2) support in coping with losses of various kinds, (3) support in coping with disabilities and chronic disease to help the elderly to lead an active life and retain their capacity for self-care as long as possible, and (4) the containment of the increasing costs arising from the care of the elderly. *Where possibilities of prevention exist it is necessary to develop and evaluate effective and economical methods of promoting health-conscious, risk-reducing behavior. This applies above all to social and behavioral factors that have an impact on mental health and well-being in the elderly and are accessible to changes during a lifetime.*[2]

---

1 Sartorius N: Opening speech delivered at the Workshop in Epidemiological Studies of Mental Health of the Elderly in Bejing/China on July 15, 1985.

2 World Health Organization: Self/Health/Care and Older People. A Manual for Public Policy and Programme Development. WHO/IPR/ADR 115–02. August, 1984

The USA National Institute on Ageing[1] is of the opinion that it is possible to *slow intellectual decline in the early stages of dementing processes by simple methods of self-training. However, further scientific evidence is needed to prove this assumption.* In order to prevent the budgets of public health care services from soaring further, it is necessary to develop training methods that can be applied by the elderly themselves or practiced in self-help or lay-initiative groups.

The provision of social support in coping with losses of social relationships and of opportunities of participating in social life in old age is an important field of action for lay initiatives and informal self-help groups, particularly where the family as a provider of social support fails or is not available.

A more ambitious objective of self-help organizations is to supplement domiciliary services in their efforts to provide all the additional help that disabled and mentally ill elderly persons require to continue to live in their familiar surroundings as comfortably and as long as possible.

Self-help groups and organizations are spontaneous movements created by private citizens out of altruistic motives, and they should be allowed to develop as spontaneously as they originated (see Radebold, this volume). *The role of research is merely to elaborate a body of teachable knowledge to avoid unnecessary risks and burdens and to improve the efficacy of the strategies used.*

Brain Research – and Dementia Research in Particular – as Integral Parts of Psychogeriatric Research

Dementia, one of the most prevalent mental disorders in old age, is encountered in 3 – 5 % of persons over 65 years of age and in 20 – 30 % of persons over 80 (see Cooper, this volume). In their further course dementing processes lead to severe mental and physical disabilities and thus to need for care associated with high material costs and a heavy psychological burden. The increased proportion of the elderly and the disproportionately large increase in the very old population have caused *dementia* to become, in the form of an insidious epidemic, *one of the most frequent and severest mental disorders in our times*[2].

Where the possibilities of medicine in general fail, the provision of medical care for the elderly suffering from organic brain and related diseases rests primarily with psychiatry. Therefore, psychiatry cannot be exempted from responsibility for research on the causes and origin or on possibilities of prevention and treatment of dementia and related diseases of the brain. Promising research in this field is possible only if in the field of clinically oriented brain research new initiatives are launched or present activities reinforced, possibly in cooperation with the various disciplines engaged in basic research in the neurosciences, at the psychiatric research institutes best suited to this task.

The introduction of the new brain imaging techniques (CT, NMR, PET) has opened up completely new dimensions in dementia research (see Heiss et al., Frackowiak, this volume). These techniques enable a relatively reliable

---

1 World Health Organization: Self/Health/Care and Older People. A Manual for Public Policy and Programme Development. WHO/IPR/ADR 115-02. August, 1984.

2 A.S. Henderson: The Coming Epidemic of Dementia. Australian and New Zealand Journal of Psychiatry (1983) 17:117 – 127.

identification of the different types of brain changes leading to dementia, whereas by means of clinical diagnosis alone it is not possible to distinguish accurately between the various disease processes underlying dementia (see Kohlmeyer, this volume). But we must not forget that even today postmortem examinations of the brain still make indispensable contributions to brain research. *With the new riskless techniques of assigning dementia to certain types of brain changes in vivo the basis has at last been laid for epidemiological, clinical and longitudinal studies on this illness group. At the same time it has become possible to carry out promising studies on risk factors such as genetically determined enzyme defects, various diseases, environmental factors of life styles and to search for the causes as well as possibilities of prevention. Now that a quantitative analysis in space and over time of metabolism processes in the brain has become possible, parallel to an examination of brain functioning in vivo, prospects of achieving decisive progress and new breakthroughs in dementia research have emerged* (see Carlsson, this volume).

According to clinical and neuropathological studies and CT findings, in all populations sufficiently studied so far about 60% of the dementing processes in old age can be classified as "senile dementias of the Alzheimer type" (SDAT). The only exception seems to be the Japanese population[1], a finding in need of replication.

Opinions, however, differ as to *whether the degenerative processes in the brain caused by normal aging and those operative in SDAT are identical, differing only with respect to age at onset, or whether they just resemble each other. Even if they differed only in quantitative terms and with regard to age at onset, there would still remain the important task for research to find out which factors lead to an early onset of the degenerative processes in the brain that finally result in dementia and how they could possibly be influenced.*

Neuropathological and CT studies have shown that *the extent of morphological and histological changes in the brain correlates with the extent of the loss of cognitive and mnemic capacities*. Studies conducted by PET have shown that *there is a clear relationship between regional cerebral blood flow and glucose metabolism on the one hand and the severity of dementia on the other* (see Heiss et al.; Alavi et al., this volume). Of great informative value is the observation that *both cerebral blood flow and oxygen extraction as well glucose and transmitter metabolism in the aging brain possess compensatory mechanisms that apparently fail partly or totally at the onset of dementia* (see Heiss et al., Carlson, Frackowiak, this volume).

The most promising research approach by far to illuminating the brain changes leading to SDAT has been the discovery of a wide-spread deficit in cholinergic activity in the most heavily affected regions of the brain. The acetylcholine deficit seems to result from a specific deficit in the enzyme "choline acetyltransferase", which is needed for the synthesis of the transmitter acetylcholine (ACh).

ACh seems to have an influence on mnemic capacities and vigilance in exogenous psychosis like delirium. In many such cases a rapid improvement in

---

1 Hasegawa K: An epidemiological study on age-related dementia. Japanese Journal of Geriatrics 12 (1975), pp 258–264

brain functioning can be achieved by administering cholinergic substances, e.g., a temporary clearing up of consciousness in exogenous psychosis or a temporary improvement in mnemic and intellectual capacities in mild forms of dementia. These findings have given rise to hopes of achieving not only short-term improvements through a substitution by proper substances after more detailed information on transmitter deficits has been obtained. Research has already produced a fairly differentiated picture of the transmitter metabolism in an aging brain affected by processes of dementia of the Alzheimer type, but it has still a relatively long way go to provide a comprehensive explanation of the relationships and the underlying causes (see Carlsson, Heiss et al., this volume). Nevertheless, it is fairly probable that a decisive breakthrough in explaining the biochemical processes leading to SDAT will be made in the next two decades. Carlsson estimates that in about 10 years it will be possible to draw a kind of neurobiochemical brain map, which gives a topographic description of the relationships between the mental, sensory, and motor functions of the human organism and the regional metabolism processes in the brain.

The detection of similarities between the patterns of disturbances, the neurobiochemical processes and, in particular, the transmitter metabolism in the brain in degenerative processes of a long-term course of the dementia type and those observed in exogenous psychosis of a short-term course is very likely to lead to promising research approaches (see Evans, this volume). The fact that exogenous psychoses mostly take a short-term course provides an opportunity for observing rapidly progressing neurobiochemical derangements, restitution processes, and the efficacy of therapeutic interventions that might also be applicable to the long-term processes underlying SDAT (see Jones, Bergmann, this volume).

The second most frequent condition leading to dementia in later life is arteriosclerosis, with a share of 20%. Analogously to cardiac infarcts resulting from arteriosclerotical changes in the coronary arteries, repeated minor or major infarcts occur in one or both of the cerebral hemispheres, leading, as a secondary effect, to a diminution of the brain volume. These disease processes, too, with all their various subforms can be diagnosed relatively reliably by means of the new brain imaging techniques, in particular the cranial CT and NMR. *The underlying causes of multi-infarct dementia (MID) and the risk factors leading to its genesis probably differ from those of SDAT. So far diabetes mellitus and hypertension have been identified as risk factors* (Evans). *Since, however, hardly any detailed knowledge is available yet, it is necessary to encourage research on the risk factors of cerebrovascular diseases in old age, in particular of MID. Therapy research on MID must take avenues different from those adopted in therapy research on SDAT.* In this field, too, the investigation of oxygen extraction and the hemodynamics in the brain and its functional reserves by means of PET is of great importance. The findings of studies so far conducted have already led to a revision of our views on the frequency of "chronic ischemic syndrome" of "cerebrovascular insufficiency", based on the analysis of cerebral bloodflow and oxygen extraction by traditional methods (see Heiss et al., this volume). *Independently of the above discussed approaches to elucidating the causes of SDAT, it should be examined whether earlier infections caused by certain viruses might lead to an early onset of neuronal degeneration, on the analogy of the slow virus diseases of the central nervous system.* In this context researchers have also referred to retroviruses.

About 20% of dementias either represent kinds of mixed forms, in which both vascular changes and degenerative changes in brain tissue are present, or result from rarer, in many cases treatable causes such as tumors, hemorrhages, etc. The fact that the various forms of dementia can frequently not be distinguished reliably by clinical means illustrates the great diagnostic – and in a small number of cases also the life-saving – value of brain imaging techniques in dementia and other psychoorganic syndromes of old age.

Psychopharmacology and Pharmacotherapy in Old Age

The two main focal points of psychopharmacological research on the elderly and on mental disorders of old age are: (1) age-related problems of drug therapy in psychogeriatric disorders in general, such as multidrug treatment, decreased elimination, etc. (see Loew, this volume), *(2) the search for approaches to the development of a pharmacotherapy for age-specific mental disorders, in particular senile and presenile dementia.*

As to the first objective, clinical and pharmacological studies on a differing sensitivity of elderly people to certain psychotropic drugs are needed. Differences in sensitivity may result from pharmacodynamic and, above all, pharmacokinetic factors and, thus, necessitate changes in dosage.

While in the past the treatment of endogenous psychosis was evaluated by a substantial body of good, controlled studies, hardly any knowledge has yet been accumulated on the medication treatment of exogenous psychosis in old age, such as deliria and confusional states (see Jones, this volume). *The treatment of deliria, as pointed out, can be regarded as a model for the influenceability of progressive functional deficits in the brain by therapeutic measures.* Due to the lack of established research findings the treatment of exogenous psychosis is largely based on medical experience. It is therefore recommended to *promote clinical therapy studies on promising substances that are likely to be developed by biochemical and pharmacological research in the next few years.*

But much more important and innovative is the second focal point, the development and evaluation of pharmacotherapeutic approaches to the treatment of dementing processes in old age in view of the high frequency of these processes and the total lack of effective therapeutic measures. *Priority must be given especially to the efforts of working out causal therapy approaches for the treatment of Alzheimer's disease.* The existent pharmacotherapeutic approaches to the treatment of Alzheimer's disease should be subjected to careful testing and included in well-controlled clinical therapy studies (see Loew, this volume). An important prerequisite for this is the development and validation of measurement instruments for the establishment of differential efficacy.

The substitution-therapy approaches with cholinergic transmitter precursors (choline, lecithin), developed by basic research, have largely proved to be unsuccessful. Some more recent studies, in which the transmitter precursors were combined with acetyl cholinesterase inhibitors or with a nootropic substance represent approaches worth testing. Substitution therapy studies with other transmitter precursors, apart from an experiment with L-dopa, which, however, yielded a negative result, have not yet been conducted. Due to neurochemical changes in other transmitter systems such studies seem worth considering. In the field of nootropic drug research, which has not yet yielded any convincing results, there is now emerging a scond generation of substances that might give rise to promising developments. The recently conducted therapy trials with neuropeptides, the analogues of ACTH and vasopressin, are also very intersting.

The neurobiochemical and pharmacological research on mental disorders in old age is disadvantaged by the fact that hardly any experimental animal models are available in this field. For example, there is no animal model for Alzheimer's disease. This is one reason why psychogeriatric research cannot do without examining the human brain not only at the psychological, but also at the biochemical and the pharmacological level. Consequently, fruitful psychogeriatric research can only be conducted where there is a sufficiently large number of volunteers for such examinations available and/or brains of patients that suffered from such diseases can be investigated post mortem in a sufficient number (see Macfadyen, this volume).

All promising efforts to develop animal models for mental disorders in old age, in particular for Alzheimer's disease, and, thus, to create the basis for rapid progress in basic research on this disease deserve strong encouragement.

Service Research

The aim of psychogeriatric service research is to analyse the effectiveness and costs of the service facilities provided for mentally ill elderly people. It faces the problem that the services available for the mentally ill and disabled elderly show great regional differences, depending on the way the systems have grown.

With regard to the care provided in residential and nursing homes one of the central questions is (see Mann & Graham, this volume) *whether the knowledge about the treatment of mental disorders in old age and the prevention of unfavourable illness courses obtained by research is sufficiently translated into medical and nursing practice.* Closely associated with the latter is the question *what kind of measures for training the personnel working in homes for the elderly and what kind of organizational arrangements are needed so that preventive and therapeutic effects would emanate from the daily life and the care provided in homes for the elderly.* Another important question worth studying is under what conditions and to what extent residential or nursing-home care can be replaced or complemented by the support provided by natural or artificial social networks, in order to improve quality of life among the elderly and their family members.

Conclusions

Mental health in the elderly is about to become one of the main tasks of health research. The reasons for this are to be looked for in the vast changes in the age structure of the world population, which in the developed countries have already caused the proportions of the elderly populations in the total populations to increase considerably. Due to these demographic changes, to the frequency of chronic disease, and to the high frequency of multimorbidity in old age, in developing countries the elderly utilize a growing proportion, in developed countries a very high proportion of the health services. Mental disorders in old age, which account for a considerable proportion of the health problems of elderly people, lead to progressive mental and physical disability, need for institutional care, and, finally, to death more frequently than in younger phases of life. After the great achievements in the medical field in gaining knowledge about and combatting the acute life-threatening diseases of childhood and adulthood, the chronic conditions typical of old age, in particular dementia, now constitute one of the most important unsolved health problems of mankind and, thus, a challenge to medical research.

In the last few years, after a long period of stagnation, considerable efforts have been made and a remarkable body of knowledge has been accumulated in the field of psychogeriatric research. Credit for this goes not only to psychiatric research in the narrower sense, but also to the social sciences, psychology, biochemistry, and neuropathology. Important contributions have also been made possible by the new brain imaging techniques, CT, NMR and PET.

Psychogeriatric research, more than any other domain of psychiatric research, depends on various levels of research, i.e., medical, psychological, morphological, and biochemical methods. Therefore, psychogeriatric research appears most promising where the boundary of psychiatry proper is crossed in well-organized, fruitful cooperation with those disciplines that are needed as partners for the investigation of the various fields. The solution of the important problems of psychogeriatric research, such as the development of standardized transnational measurement instruments enabling comparisons of research results over countries, additionally require a concerted action of international collaboration, as proposed and already initiated by the World Health Organization. If we succeed in convincing the governments and research-promotion institutions of the necessity of a sustained encouragement of psychogeriatric research in the future, spectacular breakthroughs in this important research field will become very likely in the next two decades.